FOOD SERVICE MANUAL FOR HEALTH CARE INSTITUTIONS

Mary J. Mahaffey
Mary E. Mennes
Bonnie B. Miller

64621

AMERICAN HOSPITAL ASSOCIATION
840 North Lake Shore Drive
Chicago, Illinois 60611

Library of Congress Cataloging in Publication Data

Mahaffey, Mary J.
Food service manual for health care institutions.

"AHA catalog no. 1845."
Bibliography: p.
Includes index.
1. Hospitals—Food service. I. Mennes, Mary E.
II. Miller, Bonnie B. III. American Hospital
Association. IV. Title. [DNLM: 1. Food service,
Hospital. WX 168 A512h]
RA975.5.D5M23 1981   642'.5   81-8036
ISBN 0-87258-330-9   AACR2

AHA catalog no. 1845

©1981 by the
American Hospital Association
840 North Lake Shore Drive
Chicago, Illinois 60611

Previous editions
©1954, 1966, 1972
by the American Hospital Association

10M-7/81

CONTENTS

LIST OF FIGURES

(continued on next page)

LIST OF TABLES

(continued on next page)

PREFACE

In 1954, the American Hospital Association published the *Hospital Food Service Manual*, which was the first comprehensive publication on management of food service for hospitals. A complete revision of that book was published in 1966 as the *Food Service Manual for Health Care Institutions* and an updated edition was done in 1972.

This 1981 edition of the *Food Service Manual for Health Care Institutions* has been completely rewritten to reflect the many changes that have occurred in health care and in food service administration. The text includes current information about management skills and functions; new food service systems and equipment; federal, state, and voluntary regulatory agencies requirements; and nutritional care of patients.

This edition of the *Food Service Manual for Health Care Institutions* was written by:

Mary J. Mahaffey, M.S., R.D., lecturer, Department of Food Science, University of Wisconsin, Madison; Mary E. Mennes, M.S., professor, Department of Food Science, and extension food service administration specialist, University of Wisconsin, Madison; and Bonnie B. Miller, R.D., former senior staff specialist, Hospital Food Service Management, American Hospital Association, Chicago.

The authors wish to thank Jennifer K. Karr, M.S., R.D., lecturer, Department of Nutritional Sciences, University of Wisconsin, Madison, for her help in rewriting portions of this book.

Editorial services were provided by Ellen Thanas, assistant editor, and Dorothy Saxner, director, Division of Books and Newsletters, American Hospital Association, Chicago.

Organization and Management

OVERVIEW

In our fast-changing society, hospitals and health care institutions face the challenge of bringing the most recent technology and the highest standards of quality to the communities they serve. Effective management of hospitals and other health care institutions therefore requires creative and aggressive action to find ways of delivering the best possible health care while meeting the human needs and aspirations of health care practitioners. In any given institution, all department managers share responsibility for attaining these dual goals. The food service administrator, as one such manager, contributes the scientific knowledge and leadership skills required to meet the fundamental need for good nutrition.

The food service administrator must be able to cope with expansion of federal and state regulations, and with new health-related programs, all of which will continue to impact on the operation of hospitals and extended care facilities. For example, an increase in outpatient services in an acute care hospital would necessitate additional modified diets for inpatients and readily accessible food service for outpatients.

The overall increase in the cost of health care, rising food and labor costs, and pressures to provide greater job satisfaction to employees intensify the need for managerial leadership by the food service administrator. Although the nutritional objectives of food services have changed little over time, patients' numbers, food habits, and needs have altered. Recent cost studies by the Hospital Administrative Services (see Bibliography) of the American Hospital Association show that in any hospital budget approximately 8 percent, on the average, is allocated to the food service department. In extended care facilities, the percentage is approximately 18 percent. The data show that more than 50 percent of the total cost per meal in hospitals is for food and expendable supplies. Even though food price increases in the future may be more moderate than those in the 1970s, continued wage increases will intensify the need for effective cost containment in food service operations.

MANAGEMENT RESPONSIBILITIES

The director of the food service department must think and act like a manager if the objectives of the department as well as the overall objectives of the organization are to be met. This means accepting and carrying out certain basic responsibilities. In any operation, regardless of type or size, the manager is the person responsible for getting things done—by planning, organizing, directing, and controlling the use of resources. These are the basic management responsibilities.

The resources of the food service department are food and supplies, facilities and equipment, personnel, time, and money. In carrying out management responsibilities, the food service administrator uses these resources to meet the objectives of the department and the institution.

Although the number of managerial levels varies with the size and complexity of the institution, any person with management responsibilities must have the appropriate skills and the necessary technical knowledge to meet the job requirements. Likewise, although the titles and the scope of supervisory responsibilities differ among various health care organizations, the skills and knowledge needed to be effective are common to all.

ESSENTIAL MANAGEMENT SKILLS

The skills required for any level of management responsibility are job knowledge, leadership qualities, communication and decision-making abilities, and the flexibility to initiate and accept change.

JOB KNOWLEDGE

In order to understand the problems of employees and to be able to effectively train and motivate them to accept new methods and equipment, an effective food service manager must be thoroughly familiar with the technical aspects of all jobs in the department. In order to gain and maintain the respect of employees, it is particularly important that a new manager becomes well versed in the methods, materials, and equipment that are used in the department. This does not mean, however, that the manager has to be as skillful in performing the jobs as the experienced employees in the department. The manager who is consistently performing the work of employees is probably failing to perform the real job of management. The successful manager adds management knowledge to technical job knowledge in order to accomplish the work of the department.

LEADERSHIP ABILITY

Leadership is one of the skills that a manager must develop to be effective in getting things done through other people. Although there are many theories and philosophies about leadership and its development, most management experts agree that when an individual has the basic capacity and desire to be a leader, the necessary skills can be learned. The successful leader must understand not only himself or herself, but the other individuals in the work group as well. The ability to see things as others see them will help the leader become more skillful in understanding, and therefore managing, others. Recognizing individual differences and values is basic to effective leadership because motivation of employees stems from setting conditions that will make the most of the skills and knowledge each person brings to the organization.

The manager who has self-confidence in his or her own ability recognizes that members of the work group must be helped to cooperate with each other in reaching the ojectives of the department and, most of all, to understand how the individual efforts of each contribute to these objectives. By setting an example and reasonable standards, the manager helps others to grow in their ability to be productive and satisfied employees.

COMMUNICATION SKILL

Communication is actually the network that keeps the organization running smoothly by transmitting management's goals, policies, and directions to employees, and employees' attitudes, concerns, and problems to management. Harmony, cooperation, and effectiveness within a department or organization are dependent upon communication that creates understanding of the tasks to be accomplished and of why and how they should be done.

Because communication means "creating understanding," a person who wants to communicate effectively must first of all understand clearly what it is that must be communicated. Then, all means of communicating that idea must be used: written communications, verbal communications, and even physical action (body language or nonverbal communication).

Communication is a two-way process. A manager does not communicate merely by putting ideas into words, no matter how carefully the words are chosen. Words first must be received and interpreted by the employee, and then they must be acted upon. The process is affected by noise, distractions, previous personal experiences, and different meanings that the same words have for different people. The communicator must be able to listen and read nonverbal signs that tell whether or not the message has been received and understood. For that reason, oral face-to-face communication is usually the most effective. Feedback from the listener is immediate and, when necessary, messages can be clarified. Feedback can take many forms, such as questions, comments, or facial expressions.

The needs and wants of the listener affect communication. If an employee feels insecure in a job, a manager's critical comment may be interpreted as a threat, even though none is intended. Past experience, education, and background color the way people react to certain kinds of messages. For example, an individual who cannot take criticism or suggestions from above or below, for whatever reason, will not be an effective communicator.

Barriers to effective communication among people exist in most organizations. Unfortunately, some of the barriers may be erected by the manager's own attitude. Some managers believe that in order to show their authority, they must make employees come to them for all information and that employees should be given only a minimum of information. The reasons why a job is performed or why a certain procedure is used are frequently omitted from directions because of the mistaken idea that employees do not need to know the reasons behind the actions but should follow instructions blindly.

A manager who feels superior to those of lower status may withhold information that employees need, may antagonize them by talking down to them, and probably will be insensitive to or make poor use of feedback.

Fear is another barrier to understanding. A fearful manager may inadvertently communicate negative attitudes about administration to the whole staff. An employee who fears or resents persons of higher status may tell supervisors or administrators only what they want to hear. Good news will be communicated, but problems or difficulties will remain hidden.

Surmounting these and other communication barriers requires constant alertness to techniques that create understanding. To be effective, the ability to see things as others see them is needed, and communication must be planned with the listener in mind. Words and actions should be geared to the listener, and questions and comments should be encouraged. Communicating completely means transmitting and receiving not only the message itself, but also the reasons for it and the expected actions or results. As many ways of communicating as possible should be used. Just because a message was sent does not automatically mean that it was actually understood. Rumors thrive in the absence of complete and accurate information and can create problems that are disruptive to everyone involved.

DECISION-MAKING ABILITY

Managers' jobs exist because decisions have to be made. Even though much of the work in a food service operation can be organized into routine procedures, there are still day-to-day situational changes that require decisions. Problems develop and need solutions that affect all of the resources of the food service operation. Choosing a course of action to solve a particular problem is an accurate definition of managerial decision making.

When asked how they make decisions, most managers are likely to reply that they do not really know. Therefore, many managers enter the job with little instruction or consciousness about a task that constitutes a major part of their job. The process for making good decisions can be learned; largely it involves becoming conscious of some of the things that have been done unconsciously all along.

The **first step** in decision making is to recognize the need for a decision and to define the problem. This is a critical step, because many seemingly apparent problems turn out to be merely symptoms of a larger problem. For example, a manager may notice more employee complaints about work conditions than usual, absenteeism up slightly, more accidents in the kitchen, or dependable employees failing to complete jobs on time. Although it is easy to jump to the conclusion that today's employees are simply undependable and careless, such symptoms actually indicate that a crisis may be on its way. An alert manager would explore further to find the causes of these symptoms. The cause might be a rumor about the likelihood of layoffs or no pay increases, or it might be that employees sense that management does not really care how they do their work. Whatever the cause for unusual disruptions or changes in the way the operation is running, it pays to look for the real problem and define it. Time and effort can be wasted in treating the symptoms while the real problem remains undetected. A clearly defined problem simplifies the rest of the decision-making process. It may even turn out that no decision is needed.

With the problem clearly in mind, the decision maker can move on to the **second step** in the process. This involves analyzing the problem or situation by separating it into parts and examining each of these parts separately. Once a problem has been clearly defined, only the pertinent facts need to be accumulated.

The **third step** in decision making is to develop possible solutions. At this point, all possible ways and means to change or improve the situation should be considered. An open mind to all ideas and suggestions for solutions is imperative. The most creative solutions are not usually the first that occur and may well be suggested only after all persons involved in the problem are also involved in searching for a solution. Each possible solution must be evaluated by considering the strong and weak points and identifying the risks involved. Alternatives should be evaluated in terms of which will give the best results in reaching the department's objectives and in using the available resources. Possible solutions then should be tried out, reevaluated, and revised if necessary.

The **trial stage** should be carefully planned, and the persons involved should be prepared for the process. It helps to try to anticipate possible questions, resistance, or difficulties, and to follow up on the implementation of the solution to be sure that the desired results are being achieved. Necessary corrections or changes can then be made.

Decision making is a skill that develops with practice. Successful managers become adept at making decisions and find satisfaction in meeting the challenges of the operation.

POSITIVE ATTITUDE TOWARD CHANGE

Throughout life, human beings experience continual change. Therefore, it is curious that people of all ages have a tendency to resist change. Resistance is something every manager must contend with, both in employees and in himself or herself. Thinking like a manager requires a positive attitude toward change. Change in products, equipment, methods, and clientele is a fact of life and a necessity for survival. The effective manager not only accepts change but wants to be a part of it and seeks ways to improve the operation of the department.

The manager's role in change begins with self-examination of personal attitudes to impending change and sensitivity to the whys and whats of resistance from employees. Reasons people resist change include fear of economic or status loss and fear of the unknown. Much of the concern over these factors is usually imagined by employees and generally occurs because the reasons for change have not been fully explained. Concern results when employees are not encouraged to participate in the decision-making process.

Many changes seem to imply criticism of the status quo. When changes in procedures or products are suggested, employees tend to feel that their past performance is somehow less than satisfactory and that criticism is implied. Unfortunately, previous unsatisfactory experiences with the implementation of new procedures have a tendency to make some employees suspicious and even angry when a new method is suggested. An alert manager will recognize this condition and make every effort to prepare employees well in advance.

Managing changes means managing people's emotions as well. Sensitivity to the emotional connotations of change helps a manager effect changes smoothly. Setting the stage by creating a healthy climate within the food service department is the first step in the right direction. The next step is for management to cultivate an awareness of and interest in the change process among employees. This will make the trial and adoption stages that follow easier to handle by all involved.

Making employees aware of possible changes that will take place can help prevent anxiety and distrust. Showing awareness of employees' feelings and needs is necessary to help them adjust easily. Generating interest and getting help from employees for trying new plans can result in reinforcing their leadership role. Employees must be able to feel that change will be good for them. The trial-stage evaluation by both employees and management is important. Changes that are well planned and executed go in the direction of growth; unplanned, hasty changes may create problems. A manager's effectiveness can be measured in part by the skill used in initiating constructive plans for change.

MANAGEMENT PROCESSES

Most of the food service administrator's time should be spent in performing the critical management tasks of planning, organizing, motivating, directing, and controlling the food service operation.

PLANNING

Planning is basic to all activities in management. It involves looking ahead to determine how the food service department will carry out and follow the policies of the institution to reach its objectives. Planning is a continuous process of reviewing information, considering alternatives, and devising strategies to make the best use of department resources.

Plans are based upon clear-cut objectives. An objective is a concise statement of what is to be accomplished, and it must be measurable if it is to be the basis for an operational plan. The long-range, broader objectives of the health care institution must be broken down into smaller, more specific, and realistic short-range objectives by each department in the institution. For example, a statement of a broad departmental objective could be: "To improve food quality." Within this framework, several more specific operational objectives can be stated, such as: "To use standardized recipes for all food items," "To ensure that foods are served at proper temperatures," and "To set up and use portion control procedures for all menu items."

Some essential departmental objectives may be of a nature that will require several months or even years to attain. These objectives should be broken down into stages that have shorter time periods so that people do not become frustrated by failure to see visible progress. For example, it may require a long time to develop complete purchasing specifications for all food items, but it would be possible to set up specifications for canned vegetables within a few weeks. When that objective is attained, then another target date is set for a second group of food products, and so forth. By using this kind of specific objective, progress can be steadily noted and measured.

Once objectives are stated, the manager develops an outline of activities that must be undertaken to reach the objectives. In planning, the questions of what is to be done, when will it be done, how will it be done, and who will do it must be answered. Although these may seem like simple questions, many managers fail to deal with all of them when they develop plans. When plans cover these key points, the work of the department proceeds smoothly with a minimum of strife and confusion. Plans are the framework for organizing the work of the department and guiding the use of resources.

Food service managers make many kinds of plans. Perhaps the most critical plan is the menu, because it affects the entire operation. Work schedules, personnel requirements, purchasing plans, equipment usage, production/distribution/assembly time, service, and costs are all affected by and based on the menu. The meal pattern, the selections offered at each meal, and the number of meals served all affect the menu plan. Once the menu is planned, the manager can develop the purchasing plans, the staffing, work, and production schedules, and all of the other plans needed for efficient food production and service in the institution.

Finding and spending sufficient time in planning are sometimes difficult unless managers consciously budget personal time use. Keeping a log of the way time is actually used each day is a useful self-analysis tool. Once actual time use is evaluated, managers frequently find they can have increased planning time if they eliminate activities that should be performed by others. Once managers determine how time is being spent, priorities for improved use of time can be set. The essential tasks can be scheduled and low-priority ones delegated to others or omitted.

Good planning can result in higher productivity, more effective cost control, good morale and employee satisfaction, high-quality work, fewer accidents, and improved relations with other staffs and departments.

ORGANIZING

A useful description and definition of the organizing responsibility of management is (see Haimann and Hilgert reference in the Bibliography):

Organizing means to answer the question "How will the work be divided and accomplished?" To answer this question, the manager has to define, group, and assign job duties. He determines and enumerates the various activities which are required; he assigns these activities; and, at the same time, he delegates the necessary authority for carrying out the activities assigned. Organizing also means designing a structural framework within which various duties are performed, and deciding how they should be performed. This means grouping of work and workers by jobs and departments, allocating space, equipment, and other resources, and defining various relationships among them.

The structural framework of a department must fit into the overall framework of the organization. When an executive designs his organization's overall structural framework, he must make sure that authority relationships between various departmental supervisors are appropriately aligned. This requires the executive to delegate authority, which is absolutely essential for a supervisor to possess in order to manage effectively. In performing his own organizing function, the supervisor in turn clarifies problems of authority and responsibility within his department.

The organization chart is a useful tool for the head of the department. An organization chart shows the vertical and horizontal lines of organization and responsibility within the food service department and within the entire institution. The charts illustrated in figures 1, 2, and 3, pages 10, 11, and 12, demonstrate the way in which the organization of the food service department can be varied with the size and need of the institution and availability of trained personnel. Solid lines on the charts indicate direct responsibility for a function and the formal chain of command and communication for each position or work unit. Broken lines indicate advisory and communication responsibility for a function, but not direct authority. Dotted arrows indicate areas where there is need for individuals at comparable levels to maintain a constant informal exchange of information and to fill in for each other when necessary.

An example of an organization chart for a food service department in a large hospital is shown in figure 1, next page. Large hospitals have a food service administrator who may be a registered dietitian or an individual with specialized education and training in food service management. In addition, there are one or more assistant administrators to whom responsibility for various functions is delegated. In this type of organization, the food service administrator is responsible to an assistant hospital administrator for the management of the department and to the chief of the medical staff for the therapeutic functions. There are two assistant directors, one in charge of nutritional care services to patients and the other in charge of administrative and food production functions.

An example of an organization chart for a food service department with a part-time dietitian is shown in figure 2, page 11. The dietitian is directly responsible to the food service administrator for some of the department management functions and to the medical director or advisory physician for therapeutic functions. The dietetic technician or dietetic assistants are responsible to the food service administrator for administrative activities and to the dietitian for the day-to-day operation of the nutritional care activities of the department.

Figure 3, page 12, shows an example of an organization chart for a food service department with a dietary consultant. In this type of organization, a food service administrator, dietetic technician, or dietetic assistant is responsible to the administrator of the institution. The dietary consultant and the director of nursing have advisory responsibility. Under the direction of the administrator, the consultant provides whatever services are requested.

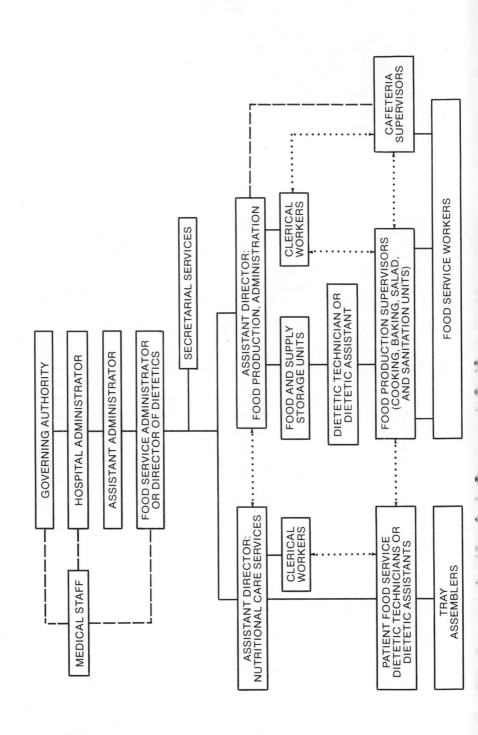

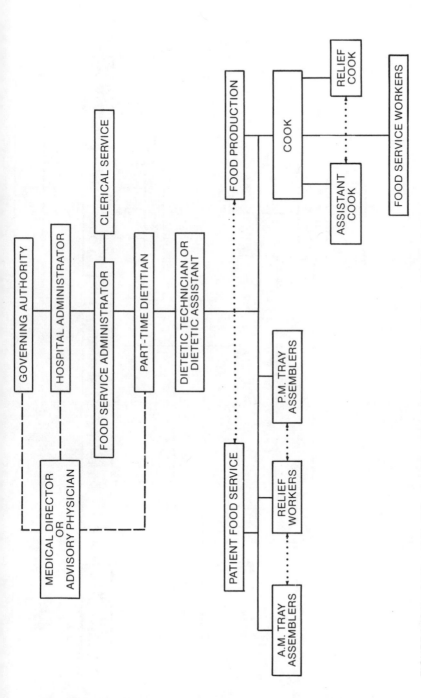

FIGURE 2. Organization of Food Service Department with Part-Time Dietitian. This type of organization is usually found in small hospitals and extended-care institutions (less than 150 beds).

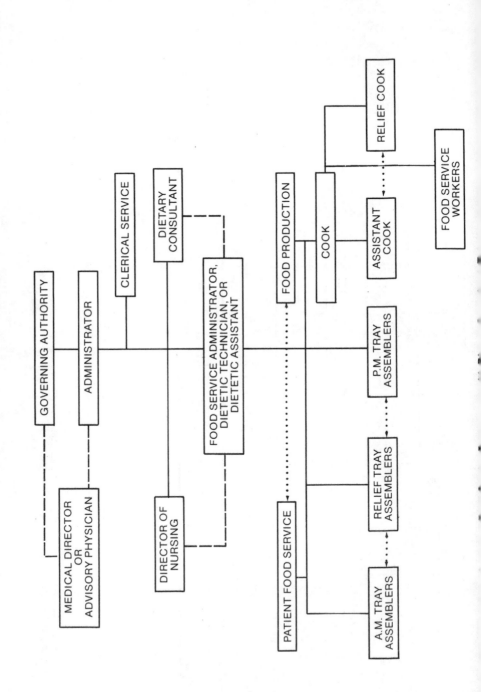

In the absence of a dietitian or dietary consultant, the head nurse frequently advises the food service supervisor with regard to therapeutic aspects of patient care. In these small institutions, the clerical tasks of the food service department may be performed by the administrator's clerical staff. The food service administrator, dietetic technician, or dietetic assistant is responsible for the day-to-day operation of the department.

The Joint Commission on Accreditation of Hospitals (JCAH) specifies that:

> The dietetic department/service shall be directed on a full-time basis by an individual who by education or specialized training and experience is knowledgeable in food service management. The director shall be responsible to the chief executive officer or his designee. The director shall have the authority and responsibility for assuring that established policies are carried out; that overall coordination and integration of the therapeutic and administrative dietetic services are maintained; and that a review and evaluation of the quality, safety, and appropriateness of the dietetic department/service functions is performed.
> Dietetic services shall be provided by a sufficient number of qualified personnel under competent supervision. The nutritional aspects of patient care shall be supervised by a qualified dietitian who is registered by the Commission on Dietetic Registration of the American Dietetic Association, or has the documented equivalent in education, training, and experience, with evidence of relevant continuing education.

Figures 1, 2, and 3 suggest outlines for the division of responsibility by areas of work and personnel that will provide department organization needed to meet JCAH requirements. The charts in the figures also can be adapted and used for planning and evaluating and for in-service education. A complete list of duties and responsibilities of the food service administrator, consultant dietitian, clinical dietitian, and dietetic technician or dietetic assistant follows (see *J. Amer. Diet. Assn.* reference in Bibliography).

The **food service administrator** or **director of dietetics** is a member of the institution's management team and is responsible to a designated administrator. Duties and responsibilities for this position include the following:

1. Develops long-range and short-range goals and objectives for the department.
2. Develops policies and procedures to attain the stated goals and objectives.
3. Prepares and manages the department budget.
4. Controls department resources through appropriate planning, utilization, evaluation, and data analysis.
5. Develops quality standards for nutritional care, food, and service

and evaluates systems to determine department effectiveness.

6. Coordinates clinical and administrative functions to ensure high-quality nutritional care.
7. Administrates personnel policies in accordance with those established for the institution and the department.
8. Develops educational and employee motivational programs.
9. Plans and coordinates all department activities.
10. Plans and implements food service systems, including department layout, patient and nonpatient food delivery systems, and equipment requirements.
11. Maintains effective communication with department personnel, other departments, administration, and the public.
12. Represents various committees of the health care institution, such as the patient reaction/satisfaction committee, nutrition committee, total parenteral nutrition committee, patient education committee, infection control committee, purchasing standardization committee, internal and external disaster committee, safety committee, shared services/purchasing committee, sanitation committee, cost containment committee, and quality assurance committee.
13. Participates in continuing education activities, such as reading current food service and nutrition journals, and participates in local, state, and/or national education programs.
14. Interprets current information for appropriate application to the food service department.
15. Diligently appraises the quality and cost of food service to patients and nonpatients.

The **consultant dietitian, R.D.,** or **part-time dietitian** is responsible for the nutritional care program of the institution and usually evaluates and makes recommendations concerning the administrative functions. The consultant is usually directly responsible to the institution's administrator. Duties and responsibilities of this position include the following:

1. Evaluates and monitors food service systems, making recommendations for a conformance level that will provide nutritionally adequate quality food.
2. Develops budget proposals and recommends procedures for cost controls.
3. Plans, organizes, and conducts orientation and in-service educational programs for food service personnel.
4. Plans layout design and determines equipment requirements for food service facilities.
5. Recommends and monitors standards for sanitation, safety, and security in food service operation.
6. Develops menu patterns.
7. Assesses, develops, implements, and evaluates nutritional case plans

and provides for follow-up, including written reports.

8. Consults and counsels with clients regarding selection and procurement of food to meet optimal nutrition.
9. Develops, maintains, and uses pertinent record systems related to the needs of the organization and to the consultant dietitian.
10. Develops, uses, and evaluates educational materials related to services provided.
11. Consults with the health care team concerning the nutritional care of clients.
12. Provides guidance and evaluation of the job performance of dietetic personnel.
13. Interprets, evaluates, and utilizes pertinent current research relating to nutritional care.
14. Maintains effective verbal and written communications and public relations, inter- and intradepartmentally.

The clinical dietitian, R.D., is a member of the health care team under the food service department director. Duties and responsibilities for this position include the following:

1. Develops and implements a plan of care based on an assessment of nutritional needs and correlated with other health care plans.
2. Counsels individuals and families in nutritional principles, dietary plans, food selection, and economics and adapts plans to the individual's life-style.
3. Utilizes appropriate tools in the provision of nutritional care.
4. Evaluates nutritional care and provides follow-up for continuity of care.
5. Communicates appropriate dietary history and nutritional care data through written record systems.
6. Participates in health care team rounds and serves as the consultant on nutritional care.
7. Utilizes human effort and facilitating resources efficiently and effectively.
8. Evaluates food served for conformance to quality standards and dietary prescriptions.
9. Compiles or develops educational materials and uses them as aids in nutrition education.
10. Compiles and utilizes pertinent operational data to ensure provision of quality nutritional care.
11. Interprets, evaluates, and utilizes pertinent current research related to nutritional care.
12. Provides nutrition education to students and personnel.
13. Plans and organizes resources to achieve effective nutritional care.
14. Plans or participates in the development of proposals for funding.
15. Maintains effective written and verbal communications and public

relations, inter- and intradepartmentally.

16. Administers personnel policies as established by the department and organization.

The **dietetic technician** should have completed an associate degree program that meets the educational standards established by the American Dietetic Association. The dietetic technician may work in the area of administration under the department director or administrative assistants, or may work under the direction of a clinical dietitian providing nutritional care services to patients. In smaller institutions, this position may include both administrative and nutritional care responsibilities.

The **dietetic assistant,** or **food service supervisor,** should have completed a 90-hour program that meets educational criteria established by the American Dietetic Association. The dietetic assistant frequently has the responsibility for the day-to-day management of the administrative and nutritional care functions in a small hospital or nursing home under the guidance of either a part-time or consultant dietitian.

The duties and responsibilities of dietetic technicians and assistants are determined by the size and complexity of the food service department and may include the following:

1. Plans menus based on established guidelines.
2. Standardizes recipes and tests new products for use in facility.
3. Procures and receives supplies and equipment, following established procedures.
4. Supervises food production and service.
5. Monitors food service for conformance with quality standards.
6. Maintains and improves standards of sanitation, safety, and security.
7. Selects, schedules, and conducts orientation and in-service educational programs for personnel.
8. Participates in determining staffing needs, in selecting personnel, and in on-the-job training.
9. Develops job specifications, job descriptions, and work schedules.
10. Plans master schedules for personnel.
11. Maintains a routine personnel evaluation program.
12. Understands and supports personnel policies and union contracts.
13. Assists in the implementation of established cost control procedures.
14. Gathers data according to prescribed methods for use in evaluating food service systems.
15. Makes recommendations that may be incorporated into policies and develops written procedures to conform to established policies.
16. Recommends improvements for the facility and for equipment.
17. Submits recommendations and information for use in budget development.
18. Compiles and uses operational data.
19. Obtains, evaluates, and utilizes dietary history information for

planning nutritional care.
20. Guides individuals and families in food selection, food preparation, and menu planning based on nutritional needs.
21. Calculates nutrient intakes and dietary patterns.
22. Assists in referrals for continuity of patient care.
23. Utilizes appropriate verbal and written communication and public relations, inter- and intradepartmentally.

A starting point for organizing a department is setting up work units. This is done by breaking down the operation of the department into units of related activities. Each resulting work unit is then an area over which someone has supervisory authority. Organizing work units by the similarity of jobs performed produces a natural grouping of employees, equipment, and space. This is called *functional organization*. In an operation large enough to require unit managers or supervisors, functional organization makes each one responsible for the production of similar products, the equipment used to prepare these products, and the employees who are skilled in that kind of work.

Once work units have been set up, the work must be assigned. Part of the manager's job is matching people with work that needs to be done by taking into account skill, work rate, and emotions. The various work units should be staffed with sufficient personnel to ensure proper work performance, yet not in excess of actual need. If employees are familiar with all tasks that must be performed, absenteeism and emergencies should create fewer problems. Although employees need the security of knowing what is expected of them, they derive satisfaction and job enrichment through a broadened range of skills. Although there may be restrictions to this approach in some operations, it is worth considering.

Coordinating various work assignments among work units is the manager's job. Materials, equipment, and personnel must be synchronized to provide proper timing, quantity, and quality of food production. As a department grows, the coordination of daily activities becomes more complicated and more essential. Planned menus, production schedules, and equipment schedules are management tools that facilitate coordination. In the health care institution, careful coordination with the activities of other departments is also required. The manager must keep this in mind, because most employees are preoccupied with their own work and may not recognize the effect that their activities have on other departments or even within the food service department itself.

Coordination requires management to have the power of authority to direct others by orders and actions. Many supervisors refer to this power as *responsibility, duty,* or other terms that avoid flaunting the traditional boss-subordinate relationship. All managers must have authority to direct employees, to make work assignments, and, if necessary, to take disciplinary measures. Successful managers recognize that simply possessing that authoritative right is not sufficient to ensure that work will be properly performed and that employees will follow orders. They also use motivational techniques based on knowledge of human behavior to secure the kind of performance that will result in successful attainment of objectives.

Whenever the responsibility for getting a job done is delegated to someone else, that individual must also be given sufficient authority to carry out the assignment. Delegation is essential in an organization if the work load is to be distributed effectively. This is sometimes a difficult task for some managers, because it does involve some risks. True delegation involves trusting others to perform a job and giving them the power to make the decisions concerning that job. In a sense, it is allowing a subordinate to act in place of the manager. It is an excellent way to help subordinates grow on the job and develop their capabilities. However, in delegating responsibility to others, managers must provide adequate instruction and guidance and refrain from simply getting rid of tasks they did not want to do themselves.

Delegation is a way to gain the time needed to perform the more difficult management tasks, to utilize manpower effectively, to improve employees' satisfaction and self-image, and to increase productivity. Successful delegation requires that a manager not only assign a task but also give the individual responsible for performing that task some freedom to choose the methods that will be used. Policies and established procedures will provide some guidelines, but overly restrictive delegation may frustrate the subordinate. Some mistakes are to be expected, and criticism as well as credit for the outcome of delegated tasks should be shared.

MOTIVATING

Most of the manager's work revolves around the day-to-day supervision of employees. Once the various tasks of the department are grouped and organized, employees need direction, coaching, and stimulation to perform at their maximum potential. At the department level, managers will spend a large proportion of their time in performing this role.

Modern management theories concerning effective ways of securing employee cooperation and performance are based on research in human behavior and motivational drives. People behave in certain ways because of certain needs. Once a need is felt, a person searches for goals that will help satisfy the need. When basic needs for job security, equitable pay, and decent working conditions are met, employees seek fulfillment of other needs. Most people feel that the work they perform is important, that their individual talents are needed and recognized, and that they are contributing something worthwhile to the organization and to society. These needs become the basis for motivating improved job performance.

Because a manager's job is to get the work done through other people, sensitivity to the needs and values of individual employees is the starting point in motivation. Each person has a need for self-respect. Research has pointed out the importance of recognizing this need and the effectiveness of allowing greater employee participation in setting goals and standards as a way of fulfilling this need. Taking the view that employees want to work and gain satisfaction from approval, support, and recognition of their work is in sharp contrast to older beliefs that employee productivity is directly related to orders, threats, and punishment. As a matter of fact, organizations with high levels of productivity usually have high levels of employee morale because of management's ability to create an atmosphere in which people *want* to work.

Although there is no step-by-step recipe for creating a positive work climate, it is evident that the manager's attitude carries a strong influence. An atmosphere in which people want to work at their fullest and best is the product of a manager who understands and respects people. To help managers improve their understanding of people, psychologists stress the necessity of self-understanding. Individuals must examine their own attitudes toward work, criticism, praise, stress, or crisis; must look at their own strengths and weaknesses; and must examine their prejudices and emotions. It is as possible to change or modify weaknesses as it is to build upon strengths. The process of self-examination helps make a manager more sensitive to the emotions and feelings of employees.

Because individuals possess various emotions and feelings, all employees cannot be treated alike. A manager must learn to recognize, respect, and deal with the individuality of each. Empathizing with another's views does not necessarily mean giving in to or agreeing with those views, but, instead, helps to deal with problems by working out effective compromises.

The effective manager pays attention to the employee's need for self-satisfaction gained through performing meaningful work. In part, this is accomplished by delegating reasonable authority and responsibility to individuals. Good performance is recognized with sincere praise, just as poor performance is noted and corrected without threat or recrimination. Providing a chance for employees to improve existing skills and develop new ones, to be involved in decisions that affect them, and to be in full communication are effective motivators.

DIRECTING

Directions and orders should be carefully planned and carefully given to employees. Using a combination of written and verbal directions helps ensure understanding. Orders should be clear, complete, considerate, and reasonable. Above all, they have to be understood the way they were intended. Once it becomes clear that employees understand, the manager should show confidence in their ability by allowing them to proceed without further overseeing. It is important to indicate how the employees are to report back or proceed once an assignment is completed and to follow through to see that the desired results have been accomplished. This approach to direct supervision is sometimes characterized as maintaining an attitude of helpfulness.

Positive discipline, an essential aspect of good supervision necessary for the purpose of teaching members of the work group to follow policies and procedures, is achieved by creating a climate of mutual respect. Discipline is a framework within which people get things done in an orderly way according to established standards, rules, and requirements. Communication, motivation, training, and fairness contribute heavily to building a willing, responsive, and responsible work group. Most employees accept rules as a necessary work condition and expect fair and equitable treatment when rules are violated. Morale suffers when some employees get away with violations while others abide by the rules. For that reason, prompt and fair disciplinary action is a necessary management activity. Situations requiring disciplinary action should be viewed in terms of how much it will teach, not how much it will punish.

The purpose of disciplinary action is to prevent recurrence of unacceptable behavior and improve the employee's self-discipline. All organizations need clearly stated disciplinary procedures that proceed in logical steps. Most labor contracts outline steps that afford protection for both management and employees. Any breakdown in discipline should be dealt with promptly, but not hastily or in anger. Reprimanding an employee should be done privately. Before taking any action, the manager should thoroughly investigate the reason for the infraction and determine whether or not the employee really understands the rules. Rules should be enforced with consistency, with disciplinary action that fits the seriousness of the offense, and with consideration for any special circumstances that may alter or modify the action taken.

CONTROLLING

Controlling includes all management activities that ensure planned objectives are being attained with the most effective use of resources. Checking progress toward objectives, setting standards and measures for the quantity, quality, and cost of activities, and taking corrective action when plans are not being accomplished are major control procedures. Methods to identify and measure accomplishments are necessary.

Some of the basic food service records of quantities of food produced, over or under production, meals served, food and supply costs, inventories, labor hours and costs, and income are basic control documents (see chapter 5). It is necessary to set up and use adequate reporting procedures for gathering data needed to judge performance and productivity. Managers must train themselves to analyze data at regular intervals so that prompt corrective action can be taken to remedy problems indicated in reports.

CHAPTER 2

Personnel Management

MAKING THE ORGANIZATION PLAN WORK

Unifying or coordinating work groups in the food service department is a daily task for management. Supervisory management personnel have the authority and responsibility, as delineated in the organization chart, to make decisions regarding the use of department resources to produce high-quality products. Further, written policies and procedures are important guides for efficient management decision making.

POLICIES AND PROCEDURES

Policies state what to do, whereas procedures outline how to do it. Policies give direction for action, cover all essential activities, and reduce the need for making decisions about these activities every time they occur.

Health care institutions must have written policies covering almost every aspect of patient care and personnel administration. Within an organization, many policies and procedures will be the same for all departments, but some will differ. Each department develops policies that are applicable to both the department functions and responsibilities and compatible with those of the total health care institution.

The food service department needs written policy statements that are based on its objectives. Each policy should include the following: a statement of the policy; the purpose of the policy; concise, clearly stated procedures for carrying it out; and assignment of the responsibility for implementing the procedures. Standard III of the *Accreditation Manual for Hospitals* (see Bibliography) outlines the requirements:

There shall be written policies and procedures concerning the scope and conduct of dietetic services. Administrative policies and procedures concerning food procurement, preparation, and service shall be developed by the director of the dietetic department/service. Nutritional care policies and procedures shall be developed by a qualified dietitian. When appropriate, concurrence or approval should be obtained from the medical staff through its designated mechanism, and from the nursing department/service. The policies and procedures shall be subjected to timely review, revised as necessary, dated to indicate the time of the last review, and enforced. The policies and procedures shall relate to at least the following:

- The responsibilities and authority of the director of the dietetic department/service and of the qualified dietitian, when the director is not a qualified dietitian.
- Food purchasing, storage, inventory, preparation, and service.
- Diet orders. These should be recorded in the patient's medical record by an authorized individual before the diet is served to the patient.
- The proper use of and adherence to standards for nutritional care, as specified in the diet manual/handbook.
- Nutritional assessment and counseling, and diet instruction.
- Menus.
- The role, as appropriate, of the dietetic department/service in the preparation, storage, distribution, and administration of enteric tube feedings and total parenteral nutrition programs.
- Alterations in diets or diet schedules, including provision of food service to persons not receiving the regular meal service.
- Ancillary dietetic services, as appropriate, including food storage and kitchens on patient care units, formula supply, cafeterias, vending operations, and ice making.
- An identification system for patient trays, and methods used to assure that each patient receives the appropriate diet as ordered.
- Personal hygiene and health of dietetic personnel.
- Infection control measures to minimize the possibility of contamination and transfer of infection. This shall include establishment of a monitoring procedure to assure that

dietetic personnel are free from infections and open skin lesions; and establishment of sanitation procedures for the cleaning and maintenance of equipment and work areas, and the washing and storage of utensils and dishes.
- Pertinent safety practices, including the control of electrical, flammable, mechanical, and, as appropriate, radiation hazards.
- Compliance with applicable federal, state, and local laws and regulations . . . .

Diet Manual/Handbook. A qualified dietitian shall develop or adopt a diet manual/handbook in cooperation with representatives of the medical staff and with other appropriate dietetic staff. The standards for nutritional care specified in the diet manual/handbook should be at least in accordance with those of the *Recommended Dietary Allowances* (1974) of the Food and Nutrition Board of the National Research Council of the National Academy of Sciences. The nutritional deficiencies of any diet that is not in compliance with the recommended dietary allowances shall be specified. The diet manual/handbook shall serve as a guide to ordering diets, and the served menus should be consistent with the requirements in the diet manual/handbook. The diet manual/handbook shall be reviewed annually and revised as necessary by a qualified dietitian, dated to identify the review and any revisions made, and approved by the medical staff through its designated mechanism. A copy of the diet manual/handbook shall be located in each patient care unit. All master menus and modified diets shall be approved by a qualified dietitian.

A checklist such as the one shown in figure 4, next page, is helpful in preparing a policy and procedures manual. An example of a policy and procedure statement for a dietary department in a nursing home is illustrated in figure 5, next page.

STAFFING

The task of staffing the department is time-consuming. However, the time is well spent when it provides the key to achieving an effective staff. Building an effective staff involves decisions about the number of employees, skills needed, and the amount of labor time that is necessary to produce the quantity and quality of meals required. Management has the responsibility to keep labor costs at reasonable levels according to the department's budget.

Several factors within the food service department and the institution affect staffing needs and make it difficult to state specific staffing guidelines that will fit every organization. Some of the variables that managers must consider are:
- Type of meal plan (three, four, and five meal-per-day plans have

One subject per policy; one policy per page.
Policy is not a routine, rule, or regulation.
Procedure—include all steps from beginning to end. Further
explain procedure with "Special Note."
Use short sentences. Make concise statements. Use active verbs.
Use same format for each page.
Date each page.
Have a subject outline for the first page of each part of the
manual.
Illustrate when pertinent.
Use a three-ring notebook for the manual.
*Record names and locations of persons to whom manuals have
been issued.*
Revise manual quarterly.
*Make one person responsible for review and issuing of
corrected copies.*

Reprinted, with permission, from *Hospitals*, published by the American Hospital Association, November 1, 1968, Vol. 42, No. 21.

FIGURE 4. Checklist for Preparing a Policies and Procedures Manual.

Department: Dietary—Nursing home   **Date:** _____

Subject: Menu plans for residents   **Policy no.:** _____

Policy: Menus for general and modified diets are reviewed and revised every six months.

Purpose: To provide seasonal variation in menu items offered and to adjust for changes in food supply and prices.

Procedure	Person Responsible	Special Notes
Review present menus	Manager	
Revise general menu	Manager	Discuss with head cook
Revise modified diet menus and analyze nutritional adequacy	Consulting dietitian	
Review all menus to avoid production problems	Manager and consulting dietitian	

FIGURE 5. Example of a Policies and Procedures Statement.

differing labor needs)
- Variety of menu items offered on general and modified diets
- Number and type of modified diets
- Recipe complexity
- Purchase form of foods
- Patient census
- Number of service options (tray service, dining room, employee cafeteria, coffee shop, and so forth)
- Time available for meal preparation and service
- Type of service system (centralized, decentralized)
- Quality of work expected
- Type of equipment available and efficiency of physical layout
- Type of serviceware and warewashing system

The relationship of these factors to labor requirements is discussed in greater detail in chapter 3, Food Production and Service Systems, and chapter 6, Managing a Nutritional System.

The traditional method for assigning work was to have employees perform specific jobs that were their own from start to finish. Using this approach, a cook, for example, would be responsible for prepreparation, preparation, portioning, and service of specific menu items as well as cleanup of equipment and work space used. For more efficient use of highly skilled employees, many operations have switched to a division of work according to the degree of skill needed to perform a job. This assembly line method of assigning work uses fewer skilled employees for repetitive tasks, such as preliminary preparation of recipe ingredients and cleanup activities. Skilled employees are assigned tasks that use their skills to the best advantage. Both approaches have some inherent advantages and disadvantages. The first approach contributes to employee motivation by providing the opportunity for satisfaction in seeing a task through to completion. However, it requires that skilled employees spend a considerable amount of time in performing tasks requiring lesser amounts of talent.

Perhaps the most feasible approach to work assignment lies somewhere between the traditional and the assembly line approaches. Through application of the centralized-ingredient-area concept, many food service departments have been able to achieve greater control over inventory and product quality. The repetitive tasks of measuring, weighing, and prepreparation of ingredients used in all recipes are transferred from the skilled to the less-skilled employees. Cleanup and maintenance responsibilities also are commonly reassigned. To make the jobs of less-skilled employees more interesting, their work assignments may be varied to include different types of activities along with the primary job tasks. For instance, a tray-line employee also could be assigned to patient service for part of the workday, or to the ingredient area or cleanup activities for some of the scheduled hours per week.

Research in business operations has demonstrated the feasibility of enlarging or enriching jobs to provide greater employee satisfaction and productivity. These practices help meet the pressures of rising labor costs. When jobs incorporate a challenge to employees and reasonable freedom to determine how an assigned task is to be carried out, most employees are happier. Management must be aware of what needs to be accomplished, what the most efficient methods to accomplish these needs are, and the necessary skills required. Motivational factors also should be considered. Positions should be designed according to the duties that need to be performed and the abilities of current employees as observed through the process of job analysis.

JOB ANALYSIS

Job analysis is the process of identifying the purpose and nature of job tasks and the skills needed to perform those tasks. In addition, the mental and physical effort required, equipment used, time needed, and working conditions are evaluated. This information is gathered by observation of and discussion with employees performing the tasks. The manager should ask the who, what, why, where, when, and how questions for each job. Questionnaires can be designed to aid in collecting information. These data are then reviewed by the manager, who determines whether or not to change job assignments. Such a change could result in:

- Better balance of work load among the various positions
- Better use of employees' skills
- Improved work quality
- Increased productivity
- Greater employee satisfaction
- Elimination of unnecessary tasks or duplication of efforts
- Reduction of employee complaints by assigning tasks more equitably and logically
- Reasonable performance standards for each job

Job analysis is not a complicated procedure, but may be time consuming. However, careful job analysis can lead to improved efficiency of the food service department by guiding the manager in the development of training programs and by helping increase employee understanding of the responsibilities and standards of the job. It provides the basis for staffing decisions, job descriptions, performance standards, and performance evaluation.

JOB DESCRIPTIONS

A written description of the job responsibilities for each position should be on record. A job description is based on the information gathered in a job analysis. Every job description includes the following kinds of information:

- Job title and classification (if any)
- Summary of the major responsibilities of the job

- Performance requirements: job knowledge, mental and physical demands and abilities, standards for performance
- Qualifications: education, training, experience, any other special qualities needed
- Job relationships: supervision received, employees supervised, career ladder for promotion
- Work environment: statement of working conditions, equipment used, hazards, if applicable

The job description is an important communication and training tool. All employees should have a copy of their job description and copies should be on file in the manager's office and personnel office. As job duties or responsibilities change, job descriptions must be updated.

In many organizations, job descriptions also include an expanded list of performance standards for every job responsibility. The performance standards are used in performance evaluation by the manager and for employee self-evaluation. An example of a job description with expanded performance standards is illustrated in figure 6, next page.

The job specification is a written statement of the minimum standards that must be met by an applicant for a particular job. It includes essentially the same information as the job description, but in considerably less detail, and provides a convenient guide for matching up specific jobs with specific job applicants.

THE EMPLOYMENT PROCESS

Recruitment and employment are important responsibilities shared by the food service manager and the personnel department of the institution. Good employment practices are needed to help reduce turnover. Employee turnover is costly in expenditure of labor dollars during training and in decreased productivity from that employee until job skills are developed.

Good employment practices are subject to several legal requirements that must be met to ensure fairness in providing job opportunities. All managers must be familiar with federal and state laws concerning fair employment practices and worker's unemployment compensation. The ability to work with unions also must be developed in order to avert infringement of the conditions of union contracts. Pertinent laws are discussed later in this chapter.

Job openings should be advertised and posted to recruit interested applicants. Personal recommendations of staff members, schools that train food service workers, government and private employment agencies, newspaper and radio advertisements, and food service industry publications are potential sources of job applicants. Advertisements and notices should briefly describe the duties, responsibilities, and qualifications for the job. This information is derived from the job specification that corresponds to the job description for the position and gives the prospective applicant

Job Description

Job Title __Baker__   Department __Food Service__   Date __July 1981__

Manager __Food production manager__   Job Code __158__

Pay Grade __4__

Job Summary: Will bake pastries, pies, doughnuts, custards, etc., for patients, cafeteria, and catered functions. If need arises, will cook as needed.

Performance Evaluation

End of Probation _____ (Date)

Annual _____

Special _____ Pay Grade _____

Name _____

Date of Hire/Reclassification _____

Evaluation Due Date _____

Responsibilities	Performance Standards	Percent Attained	How Can 100% Be Attained?
Preparation of breakfast breads, doughnuts, etc., for patient tray line and cafeteria in accordance with production sheet and recipes.	Products are measured accurately and/or weighed and mixed according to instructions on boxes or recipes.		
	Dough is kneaded, cut, shaped, and rolled to correct thickness according to directions on recipe; each cut is equally scaled and neatly shaped.		
	The items are baked at the proper temperature and correct length of time, not undercooked (raw) or overcooked (burnt and dry).		
	Special breakfast items are correctly frosted after baking.		
Preparation of puddings (rice, bread, etc.) and cream pies for patient tray line, cafeteria, and special catered affairs.	Pudding mixes are made according to directions on the box, are of the proper consistency, and are set correctly.		

	Pudding mixes for cream pies are made correctly, are set firmly, and will not bleed when pies are cut. Topping is firm and does not exceed ½ inch.
	All other puddings and custards are made according to recipe and the finished product is attractive and well set.
	Over- or underproduction of food items is recorded on daily production sheets.
Preparation of breads for tray line and cafeteria according to production sheet.	Frozen dough is taken out of freezer, portioned, placed on greased pans, and allowed to rise to correct size at room temperature.
	Other breads are prepared according to instructions on box or recipe.
	Breads are baked at proper temperature for correct period of time until golden brown.
Preparation of cakes, cookies, cupcakes, brownies for patient tray line, cafeteria, and special catered functions.	Mixes are correctly prepared according to instructions on box or recipe.
	Batter is not put in oven until oven is checked for proper temperature.
	Products are baked for required length of time. Cakes should be approximately 2-3 inches high and moist.
	All cupcakes are baked in baking cups, are uniform in size, and are moist.
	All icings are made and properly mixed according to recipe and are creamy smooth.
	All cakes, cookies, etc., are acceptable in appearance (not burnt or undercooked).
	Over- or underproduction of food items is recorded on daily production sheets.

Responsibilities	Performance Standards	Percent Attained	How Can 100% Be Attained?
Preparation of pies and cobblers for cafeteria, tray line, and catered affairs.	Frozen crust pies are slotted and brushed with evaporated milk. Pie crust is golden brown before removing from oven.		
	Cobblers are prepared according to instructions on recipes and top crust is brushed with evaporated milk and golden brown when done.		
	All pies and cobblers are cooled before portioning.		
	Pastries are prepared according to recipes and contain the proper amount of filling and/or topping.		
	Frozen pie shells for cream pies are thawed 10 minutes before bottom and sides are pricked, placed on sheet pan, and baked in 400°F. (204°C.) oven for 10 minutes or until light brown.		
	Over- or underproduction of food items is recorded on daily production sheets.		
Maintenance of sanitary work area, equipment, and work techniques and adherence to safety rules, policies, and procedures.	Employees report to work in clean, neat uniforms, wash hands before preparing foods, and wash hands frequently throughout the day.		
	Employees keep work area clean and in sanitary condition at all times.		
	Employees leave work area and equipment clean before going off duty.		
	Employees get needed food supplies from storeroom, freezer, and refrigerator (check recipes and production sheets) and carry carts for returning items to avoid backtracking.		
	Employees carry out instructions of food		

make necessary changes as directed by management, not reverting to old habits.

Employees cooperate with fellow employees and willingly assist where and when needed.

Employees follow policies and procedures of health center and department.

Employees obey safety rules and regulations of department and report any faulty-working equipment or unsafe conditions to production manager.

Education: No special requirements.

Experience: Should possess ability to prepare, cook, and serve in quantity, especially roasts, entrees, vegetables, and sauces. Must have knowledge of materials and methods used in large-scale food production and of use and care of utensils and equipment. Must have ability to follow oral and written instructions and standard recipes. Must be neat and clean in appearance.

Comments on work habits _____

Manager _____ Date _____ Department Head _____ Date _____

For employee: My manager has reviewed my job description and performance evaluation with me. My signature does not necessarily mean that I agree.

Comments: _____

_____ Signature _____ Date _____

FIGURE 6. Combined Job Description and Performance Evaluation Form.

information needed to decide whether he or she is interested in or qualified for the job.

Applications

All persons interested in a job position should fill out a written application form that is available in the personnel office. The application form should request job-related information that will help the manager determine the applicant's qualifications for the job. Information that is in violation of the individual's legal rights as protected by federal laws and regulations on equal employment opportunities must not be requested. Questions about race, ethnic origin, religion, and sex may not be asked. Marital status information also may be considered as a violation of laws forbidding discrimination on the basis of sex, unless asked of both sexes. Some medical information may be requested only on appropriate medical forms.

It also is illegal to discriminate against mentally or physically disadvantaged persons for non-job-related reasons. Questions concerning convictions for violations of the law are not permitted unless the position requires handling of money or other similar tasks. Some of the other areas of questioning that may be construed as discriminatory include information on height and weight, handicaps, credit references, plans to have children, unwed motherhood, and lowest salary acceptable, as this tends to discriminate against women who have traditionally received lower salaries. In many states, photographs may not be requested in order to protect applicants from racial or other prejudicial stereotyping.

After prospective employees have filled out the application form, the manager or personnel officer should screen all forms and check previous employers and listed references before contacting any applicants for an interview. Applicants should be notified of their status as soon as the screening has been completed.

Interviews

It is essential that a person in charge of selecting an applicant for employment do so carefully. Interviews should be scheduled with all persons whose application forms indicate that the minimum skill and experience requirements for the job have been met. In many organizations, the personnel office conducts preliminary employment interviews to select the most promising applicants for the position. The individuals are then referred to the food service manager for further interviews.

Sufficient uninterrupted time for each interview should be set aside and a definite time schedule kept. Interview questions should be planned in advance so that each applicant is treated fairly.

After making introductions, the applicant should be put at ease as quickly as possible by showing sincere interest in that applicant. If the applicant has not already seen the job description for the position, a copy should be provided and the job requirements briefly discussed, allowing time for questions and comments.

The kinds of questions asked can provide an opportunity for the applicant to demonstrate job-related knowledge and experience. Questions that can be answered *yes* or *no* or ones related to race, religion, birthplace, national origin, or other subjects that are not permitted on application forms should not be asked. Follow-up questions to clarify a point should be asked, if the situation calls for it. Many interviewers make the mistake of talking more than the applicant. Although silences may make some persons uncomfortable, it is important to permit enough quiet time for the applicant to think through a response. Nonverbal communications should be noted, but because physical appearance and other personal attributes can bias judgments, a conscious effort should be made to avoid stereotyping or picking early favorites. Sufficient notes or tape-recorded interviews are essential to get more accurate evaluations of applicants. It is a good practice to assign a preliminary rating of each applicant before interviewing the next. In concluding, the interviewer should indicate to all applicants when they can expect to be notified of their status.

Application forms, test scores, interviewer notes, and any other information about applicants should be kept on file for legal purposes as well as to maintain a file of prospects for future job openings. Reasons for not hiring should be clearly stated and kept on record.

The employment interview can be a productive process for management and prospective employees if it is well conducted. When carefully planned questions are asked, unsuitable or unqualified applicants can be screened out. The interview can be the first step in establishing a constructive relationship with new employees and in creating good will with those not employed but who may reapply for a future opening.

Orientation

The first few days on the job are crucial ones for new employees. They must be introduced to the job, other employees, and the organization. An employee's future performance may be highly dependent on the attitudes and impressions formed during the first days of work. Well-organized orientation procedures are needed to help new employees quickly become productive.

In many institutions, the personnel office is responsible for explaining policies, regulations, fringe benefits, and similar subjects. The new employee should be given a brief history of the institution and a guided tour, which both inspires pride and helps in understanding how the food service department is related in function and physical layout to the rest of the facility.

Large facilities may have handbooks for new employees to help acquaint them with the general policies, rules, and regulations; smaller ones may have this information on mimeographed sheets. The important thing is to have written personnel policies in one form or another, so the employee can become fully acquainted with what is expected by and what can be expected of the employer. Policies should cover the following items:

- Job classification, length of probationary period, job security
- Initial or preemployment physical, checkups, reporting of illness and accident
- Benefits for full-time and part-time employees
- Hours of work, days off, overtime, length and hour of meal periods and coffee breaks
- Pay days, pay period, method of receiving pay
- Holidays, vacations
- Personal-care requirements, including cleanliness, hairnet or cap, low rubber heels, uniforms, and so forth
- Opportunity for promotion

When the new employee arrives in the food service department, the manager should set aside time to personally make the introductions to others in the department. Major job duties and general work area and equipment should be explained, locker space located, and the daily routine described. It is helpful to put the new employee at ease and convey a sincere interest in making the orientation and training period a pleasant one. A manager should recognize that new employees are eager to do well in their jobs, anxious to be accepted by others, hopeful that the job will be important, and, above all, nervous. The manager should not try to cover too much information all at one time but rather indicate that more information will be provided throughout the training period.

Training

Employee training is a major responsibility of the food service manager. A continuous, well-organized training program for all levels of personnel leads to results that are evident in increased productivity, quality, safety, and morale. New employees must be trained and old employees need retraining in new methods, use of new equipment, or in the handling of different job duties. Although some training will be conducted in group sessions, much will be handled on an individual basis.

The department head responsible for the performance of unit managers and employees in a hospital setting has more help today as a facilitator of training than in the past. Resources for training have expanded greatly in the past few years. Many hospitals now have staff members who function as training specialists or serve in some capacity as planners of learning experiences. Such persons can assist in overall programming and in designing specific experiences for all levels of departmental employees. But the ultimate functioning of the employee on the job remains the responsibility of the department head.

Employees hired for the food service department have varied educational and social backgrounds and often are unskilled when first employed. Despite these variations in abilities and backgrounds and in basic skills such as reading, it is essential that all food service employees receive certain training in the responsibilities of the food service department as a part of an entire health care institution.

To help make training a systematic and continuous process, the Hospital Research and Education Trust has prepared a program for training the food service employee. This program consists of a student manual, *Being a Food Service Worker*; an instructor's guide, *Training the Food Service Worker*; and visual aids, *Visual Aid Training Supplement to Training the Food Service Worker*. The program was tested by use in hundreds of hospital food service departments. It was designed to provide a guide to the food service manager charged with the responsibility of training and motivating employees. HRET has also published a training book entitled *On-The-Job Training—A Practical Guide for Food Service Supervisors*, which is based on one of the best-known methods of teaching skills to adults—job instruction training (JIT). In the next section of this chapter, a similar approach is described.

Individual training

In order to be an effective trainer, the manager needs to understand the basic principles of the teaching/learning process. The teacher must develop the ability to see each step in training from the learner's point of view. Prior to beginning a training session, each step should be planned carefully and completely.

1. Use the job description to determine what activities need to be taught.
2. Outline a definite step-by-step procedure to follow for each task taught. State the objective for each session and prepare a lesson plan.
3. Set aside a specific time for each training session. Keep it as free as possible from interruptions.
4. Have all materials, tools, equipment, or other teaching materials ready. Have the workplace arranged properly, just as the employee will be expected to keep it.
5. Prepare the employee for learning. Find out what the employee already knows about the job and begin training from that point. Be enthusiastic and encouraging. A frightened or embarrassed person does not learn effectively.
6. Demonstrate the task to be learned. Explain each step completely and clearly, stressing key points. Show the employee any "tricks of the trade" or shortcuts to make the job easier. Ask questions to see if the employee understands.
7. Let the employee perform the job and explain the steps involved while under observation. Ask questions and correct any errors

patiently. Encourage questions from the employee. Repeat this procedure until certain the employee understands the job.

8. Leave the employee alone and check back periodically to see how he/she is progressing. Designate someone to whom the employee can go for assistance if problems arise. Make sure safety procedures are clear. Taper off in supervision as the employee gains proficiency.

9. Recognize the employee's progress and the successful accomplishment of the assigned task. Discuss the schedule for additional training with the employee and set reasonable goals for learning all necessary tasks involved in the job.

Training trainers

In many food service departments, individual training of new employees is delegated to an experienced employee who performs a similar job. When training is delegated, the employee selected should know how to teach as well as how to do the job itself. Working with the employee in planning the step-by-step method described above helps to avoid some of the common training errors made by inexperienced trainers. These errors are: trying to teach too much at one time, telling without showing, lack of patience, failure to get feedback from the trainee, lack of preparation, and failure to emphasize or explain all key points. The manager should follow through to be sure that the training assignment has been carried out effectively.

Group training

An in-service education program is essential for maintaining an efficient and cost-effective department. Continuing education enables employees to grow on the job by learning new techniques or gaining new information that will help them become more productive in performing their job responsibilities. Well-organized group training sessions are an efficient method for carrying out training, and are required for health care institutions in most states.

A good in-service training program is based on needs identified from indicators in the work situation. Once needs of the food service staff are assessed, priority ratings are given to each and a target group is selected for each priority. Some topics, such as safety, may be pertinent for the entire employee group, whereas others may pertain to only a few employees. A well-planned series of in-service meetings requires that the manager establish a schedule several months in advance. The date, time, and subject for each in-service session should be stated on the schedule.

Because varied work shifts are the norm in food service operations, two or more sessions may need to be planned for subjects pertinent to all employees. Employee work schedules and work loads should be considered when setting the time for in-service sessions. If the daily work routine does not allow time for group meetings during the workday, arrangements may be made to hold training sessions at the end of the workday, or overlapping two work shifts. Personnel policies must be checked to determine if pay or overtime pay is required for such sessions.

For each in-service meeting, the topic to be presented should be carefully defined, narrowing the subject matter to an amount that can be covered effectively in the time available. Most in-service sessions conducted during the workday should be reasonable in length (20 to 40 minutes) because employees who have been working several hours may be too fatigued to learn effectively.

A lesson plan for the session should be prepared, stating the points to be covered, how it will be taught, any visuals or equipment that will be needed, and possible discussion questions. Ample time is needed to involve employees in discussion or demonstration during the session. If resource persons from other departments in the organization or from outside sources are going to be used, they should be contacted well in advance; the date and time should be confirmed later; and they should be asked if visual equipment will be needed. Any visual teaching aids used should be previewed in advance. Often a title may sound ideal for the topic under discussion, but the content may not be suitable or may be difficult to relate to a given work situation. A knowledge of how to operate projectors or any other equipment is essential. Finally, charts or posters should be well prepared and easy to see.

The in-service session should start promptly and if it involves employees who may not know each other, they should introduce themselves. A brief statement of the purpose of the meeting helps the members of the group see how it is important to them. The subject matter should be presented carefully and concisely and supplemented with written materials when appropriate. Explaining how to perform a task can be made clearer by involving members of the group in demonstrations or role-playing and by developing questions that will encourage discussion and comment. At the end of the session, the content should be summarized and questions asked to determine whether key points were understood by the group and to see how the information can be applied in the work situation.

Some subjects to be considered in setting up a continuing in-service program for food service staff include:

- Personal hygiene
- Food handling procedures
- Cleaning techniques and procedures
- Equipment operation and maintenance
- Fire safety plans
- Safety rules and procedures
- Energy conservation
- Future operational changes
- Conversion to the metric system
- Basic nutrition

- Modified diets
- Changes in personnel policies
- Reality orientation (pertinent for institutions serving the elderly and mentally handicapped)
- Other subjects particularly related to the patients served by the institution

It may be useful to keep a list of persons in the community and their areas of expertise. Resource persons can be found in state and local public health agencies, schools, universities, and technical colleges, as well as at meetings of professional organizations with speakers who may contribute excellent ideas to the efficient running of a food service department. Persons from other hospitals and nursing homes, as well as in-house staff from other departments, have useful knowledge that should not be overlooked. Resource persons and teaching aids are available from equipment companies and other suppliers. Commercial movies, slides, and filmstrips can be rented or purchased. It is a good idea to check to see if film materials can be previewed before purchase because some of these may be costly or inappropriate.

PERFORMANCE EVALUATION

Because the success of every food service department is based on the performance of employees, managers must be thoroughly familiar with the activities and abilities of each. Systematic evaluation of the individual employee's job performance is essential to measure progress in developing job skills, to identify substandard performance and correct it, and to provide a basis for recognition, promotions, and merit increases. The process of careful, fair, written evaluation can help establish better work relations and communication between the immediate supervisor and the employee.

Performance standards must be developed before a fair evaluation can take place. Performance standards are based on the job responsibilities outlined in the job description. Each performance standard or behavior desired in the job must be clearly and meaningfully stated, with task-related activities cited in measurable and observable terms.

The general factors that should be part of a written performance evaluation form include those related to quality and quantity of work, relationships and attitudes toward other employees, and work habits and dependability. Attitudes, though important in overall job performance, are difficult to rate objectively. Types of behavior toward other employees and acceptance of supervision are helpful in providing some measurable indicators of attitudes. A rating scale for each performance standard should be developed, using descriptive terms to identify the various points on the scale. An excerpt from a performance appraisal form based on performance standards is shown in figure 7, next page.

| Department: _____ | Date: _____ |
| Job Title: _____ | Evaluator: _____ |

Circle the number on the rating scale that most accurately describes this employee's performance.

Performance Standard	Always	Almost Always	Sometimes	Rarely	Never
Products are accurately measured and/or weighed and mixed according to instructions in recipes or on boxes.	4	3	2	1	0
Keeps work area clean and in sanitary condition.	4	3	2	1	0
Cooperates with fellow employees and willingly assists where and when needed.	4	3	2	1	0

FIGURE 7. Excerpt from a Performance Evaluation Form.

If a manager is not careful, several common errors may occur in the evaluation process. The halo effect is the tendency to let very good or very bad performance in one task overshadow or color the evaluation of other tasks. Some managers err in giving overly lenient ratings or in being too severe in ratings. A rating scale with descriptive gradations that avoids the terms *outstanding*, *superior*, *average*, and *poor* helps overcome these errors, as well as the tendency to mark every trait and every employee as average. Appraisals should be conducted as objectively and fairly as possible at regular quarterly, semiannual, or annual periods. For new employees, monthly ratings can be helpful in noting progress in learning needed job skills.

The second stage in the appraisal process is an interview or conference with the employee. Schedule a conference allowing enough time for a private, thorough discussion of the employee's performance. The conference should be conducted in a positive, cooperative manner, beginning with areas in which performance is good and encouraging continuation of that progress. Constructive suggestions for improving performance and mutual agreement on steps and a timetable to follow can be made if necessary. It is important to be open-minded and note opinions and statements made by the employee. The employee should receive a completed copy of the evaluation, signed by the employee and the immediate supervisor. A copy also should be kept in the permanent personnel file for the institution.

In addition to the formal evaluations, informal day-to-day notations of an employee's performance, accomplishments, or problems can be helpful to the manager in arriving at accurate overall judgments of an employee. A sample form is shown in figure 8, below.

| Employee: _____ | Date: _____ |

Job Title: _____

Action by Manager—Check One

Commendation	Correction	Reprimand	Warning	Suspension	Discharge
☐	☐	☐	☐	☐	☐

Reason for Action—Check One

Outstanding Work	Poor Work	Failure To Carry Out Orders	Attitude	Tardiness	Absence
☐	☐	☐	☐	☐	☐

Comments:

_____
Signature of Manager

FIGURE 8. Manager's Counseling Report.

RECORDS

Every organization is required to keep certain kinds of records for all employees, either in the personnel office or in the food service department. A complete personnel record is not only helpful in training and counseling but also necessary in case of disciplinary action or dismissal procedures. Because of the confidential nature of all personnel records, they should be filed in a place that is inaccessible to unauthorized employees. Some of the information that should be kept in each employee's file includes:

- Complete name, home address, telephone number, Social Security number, name of nearest relative
- Job title or classification, rate of pay (hourly, weekly)
- Report of physical examination

- Promotion record (starting date, later changes in job classification, pay increases)
- All records from hiring process (application form, interview notes, education and training record, references)
- Record of training received by employee
- Vacation, holidays, sick leave, and absentee records
- Record of hours worked, overtime
- Safety or accident data (accident reports, workmen's compensation claims)
- Fringe benefits data (health or life insurance plan participation, pension plans, savings plans, and so forth)
- Reports of performance evaluation (interview notes, forms signed by employee, special awards or recognition, written comments on performance made at times other than formal evaluation)
- Record of any disciplinary actions, grievances, complaints.

If the employee leaves, the termination date and acceptability for reemployment also should be recorded.

SCHEDULING

Careful work analysis leads to the development of coherent, logical job positions covering the essential tasks that must be performed in the food service department. However, scheduling the workweek and specific hours each employee is to be on duty is a key step in achieving efficiency in the use of labor dollars while meeting the service objectives of the institution.

The 40-hour workweek is common in almost every institution. In most organizations, there are actually 35 working hours in that total, because each employee usually is given a 15-minute paid break every 4 hours and a 30-minute unpaid meal period. Although the 8-hour per day, 5-day workweek has been the most common schedule, some innovative food service managers have developed effective 10.5-hour per day, 4-day workweek schedules, with notable results in employee productivity and satisfaction.

In one organization, employees are scheduled to work 4 days, have 3 days off, work 5 days, have 3 days off, and then go back to a 4 and 3 routine without working more than 8 days in any 2-week pay period. Overlapping schedules are avoided by retraining employees to perform a broader range of duties. For example, tray-liners may perform production tasks and some porter duties, and porters may perform some food production and tray-line duties. This flexibility in scheduling has resulted in a significant savings in total number of needed labor hours, less absenteeism and turnover, and increased employee morale because of diversified duties (see article by Welsh in Bibliography).

Several types of schedules may be needed to keep both management and personnel informed of the job positions, scheduled hours, and job

task assignments. For any food service department, these must be developed with consideration for:
- Number of meals per day and time period for meal service
- Menu items offered and number of choices
- Forecast of quantities to be produced
- Type of production system used
- Type of assembly, distribution, and service systems
- Labor regulations (government and union contracts)

One type of schedule will indicate each food service employee's position and the total daily hours needed to complete assigned tasks. Developing a line graph such as that shown in figure 9, below, can be helpful in visualizing the scheduling pattern.

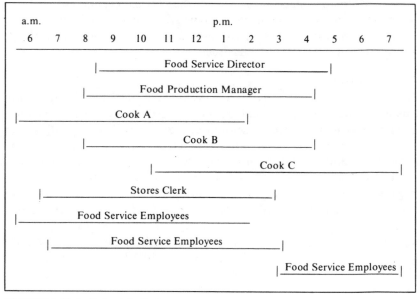

FIGURE 9. Daily Schedule Pattern.

Another type of schedule helpful to the manager and particularly necessary for good employee relations is one indicating days on duty, daily scheduled hours if they vary from one day to the next, days off, vacation days, and so forth. A rotating master schedule, such as that shown in figure 10, next page, should be developed to reduce the amount of time the manager would have to spend in scheduling employees each week. Master schedules are usually developed to tally with the length of the pay period so that each employee gets equal hours of work during the period and so that the number of overtime hours is minimized.

	S	M	T	W	Th	F	S	S	M	T	W	Th	F	S	S	M	T	W	Th	F	S
#1	D/O					D/O					D/O	D/O					D/O	D/O			D/O
#2			D/O				D/O	D/O		D/O		D/O	D/O						D/O	D/O	
#3				D/O	D/O					D/O			D/O	D/O	D/O			D/O	D/O		

FIGURE 10. Rotating Master Schedule. D/O=day off.

Most institutions use part-time help to supplement full-time employees and to extend the service day. With emphasis on cost containment, managers in health care facilities should consider greater use of part-time personnel to reduce labor costs. Highly paid skilled employees should be scheduled to perform tasks requiring their talents only, not routine tasks that can be performed by employees receiving a lower rate of pay. Figure 11, below, is an example of this kind of scheduling.

Week ending: _____

Name—Classification	Sun.	Mon.	Tues.	Wed.	Thurs.	Fri.	Sat.
T. Walker—Cook 1	6-2:30	6-2:30	6-2:30	6-2:30	6-2:30	D/O	D/O
J. Foot—Cook 2	D/O	D/O	8:30-5	8:30-5	8:30-5	6-2:30	6-2:30
I. Shenk—Cook 3	9:30-6	9:30-6	9:30-6	D/O	D/O	9:30-6	9:30-6
M. Smith—Cook 4	8:30-5	8:30-5	D/O	9:30-6	9:30-6	8:30-5	D/O
A. Frank							
B. Tyler							
B. James							

FIGURE 11. Time Schedule.

The manager should examine schedules of specific employees to ensure fairness in daily hours scheduled and days off and to avoid situations in which an employee has the late shift on one day and an early shift the following day. Split shifts are rarely used because most employees prefer a continuous workday. Rotating shifts, in which an employee is scheduled for varying work periods from one week to the next or between pay periods, are frequently used to provide more flexibility for management and employees. Once the master schedule is designed, it can be used without major revision and provides consistency both for staffing procedures and for employees.

Written daily work schedules can be developed to guide each employee's activities during the workday. Such schedules list the duties to be performed during specified time periods and routine cleaning activities for which the employee is responsible. An example of an individual work schedule is shown in figure 12, next page. There are several advantages in providing this type of detailed breakdown of the work responsibilities:

- The employee has written instructions to serve as a guide and does not have to rely on verbal orders
- Deadlines [that assist the employee to set goals for each activity] are established for each job duty

WORK SCHEDULE FOR CAFETERIA COUNTER EMPLOYEE

Name: _____ Hours: 5:30 a.m. to 2:00 p.m.
                                         30 minutes for breakfast
                                         15 minutes for coffee break

Position—Cafeteria Counter Employee—No. 1 Supervised by: _____

Days off: _____ Relieved by: _____

5:30 to 7:15 a.m.	1. Read breakfast menu
	2. Ready equipment for breakfast meal
	   a. Turn on heat in cafeteria counter units for hot foods,
	      grill, dish warmers at 6 a.m.
	   b. Prepare counter units for cold food at 6 a.m.
	   c. Obtain required serving utensils and put in position for use
	   d. Place dishes where needed, those required for hot food in dish
	      warmer
	3. Make coffee (consult supervisor for instructions and amount to be
	   made)
	4. Fill milk dispenser
	5. Obtain food items to be served cold: fruit, fruit juice, dry cereals,
	   butter, cream, etc. Place in proper location on cafeteria counter
	6. Obtain hot food and put in hot section of counter
	7. Check with supervisor for correct portion sizes if this has not been
	   decided previously

6:30 to 8:00 a.m.	1. Open cafeteria doors for breakfast service 2. Replenish cold food items, dishes, and silver 3. Notify cook before hot items are depleted 4. Make additional coffee as needed 5. Keep counters clean; wipe up spilled food
8:00 to 8:30 a.m.	Eat breakfast

8:30 to 10:30 a.m.	1. Break down serving line and return leftover foods to refrigerators
	   and cook's area as directed by supervisor
	2. Clean equipment, serving counters, and tables in dining area
	3. Prepare serving counters for coffee break period
	   a. Get a supply of cups, saucers, and tableware
	   b. Make coffee
	   c. Fill cream dispensers
	   d. Keep counter supplied during coffee break period (9:30-10:30)
	4. Fill salad dressing, relish, and condiment containers for noon meal

10:30 to 11:30 a.m.	1. Confer with supervisor regarding menu items and portion sizes
	   for noon meal
	2. Clean equipment, counters, and tables in dining area
	3. Prepare counters for lunch
	   a. Turn on heat in hot counter and dish warmers at 11 a.m.
	   b. Set up beverage area
	   c. Place serving utensils and dishes in position for use
	4. Make coffee
	5. Set portioned cold foods on cold counter

11:00 to 11:15 a.m.	Coffee break
11:30 a.m. to 1:30 p.m.	1. Open cafeteria doors for noon meal service 2. Replenish cold food items, dishes, and silver as needed 3. Keep counters clean; wipe up spilled food 4. Make additional coffee as needed
1:30 to 2:00 p.m.	1. Turn off heating and cooling elements in serving counters 2. Help break down serving line 3. Return leftover foods to proper places 4. Clean equipment and serving counter as directed by supervisor
2:00 p.m.	Off duty

FIGURE 12. Work Schedule for Cafeteria Counter Employee.

- Work can proceed more smoothly, with less time wasted seeking instructions or directions from the manager
- Tasks are less likely to be forgotten
- The manager can use the individual schedules to check on work-load balance among employees
- Work schedules can be coordinated with the menu cycle and adjusted when the cycle changes

Some organizations set up separate cleaning schedules and rotate these among employees. Rotating unpleasant jobs is usually desirable, but most of the daily and weekly cleaning tasks can be incorporated into individual employee schedules.

LABOR RELATIONS

Although there are many procedures managers can use to organize and direct the efforts of employees, a well-coordinated and cooperative work group depends heavily on the leadership skills of the manager. Successful supervision requires a careful balance between the use of managerial authority and respect for the individual employee. There is no room in today's work situation for a manager who demands performance by exerting the authority of rank with threats or coercion.

Many labor relations problems can be avoided when the manager provides fair and consistent day-to-day supervision. This requires observation of employees as they carry out their assigned duties, as well as the on-paper planning needed to organize the activities of the department. There is no substitute for face-to-face supervisory leadership and guidance.

Order giving is one of the necessary activities of management and demonstrates the manager's skill in motivating employees. Fair treatment and firm direction will inspire employees to willingly carry out the responsibilities of their jobs. Orders should be stated as simply and clearly as possible. Enough information should be provided for the employees to act, without overwhelming them with unnecessary detail. To secure cooperation and not just hostile compliance, orders should be considerate and courteous. Reasonable orders recognize the limitations of time, equipment, or personal abilities.

The employee's feelings should be anticipated if an assignment is going to be particularly difficult or unpleasant, and positive assistance and support should be given. Paying attention to feedback on the orders given, as well as free and direct communication with all employees, is encouraged. Also, an adequate amount of direct supervision will ensure that orders are carried out.

PERSONNEL POLICIES

Even in the most positive work situation, personnel problems can arise.

Clearly stated policies should be available for basic work rules on hours, overtime, pay scales, fringe benefits, training opportunities, promotion policies and possibilities, absenteeism, sick leave, vacation, grievance procedures, and any other pertinent matters affecting personnel. Personnel policies should be published in an easy-to-read, attractive handbook and distributed to all employees. Policies should be periodically discussed with all employees and reviewed by management on a regular basis. Posters, memos, and other appropriate reminders should be used to alert employees to any policy changes and to policies that may not be particularly easy to understand.

Personnel policies should be applied uniformly and consistently for all employees. Making exceptions to the rule, except for extreme cases, may lead to unforeseen legal or morale problems among employees.

DISCIPLINE

Punishment as a form of discipline is inappropriate. Discipline should take a positive approach in order to provide a situation in which employees get things done in an orderly manner according to established and known standards, rules, and requirements. Positive discipline is actually self-discipline: willing obedience to rules. It is based on the belief that normal, mature employees are reasonable, want to do the right thing, carry their share of the work load, and behave themselves. Mature employees will obey rules, meet requirements, and respect regulations if the rules are reasonable.

Self-discipline on the part of employees is related to everything else done by the manager—how work assignments are made, how training is done, effectiveness of communication and motivation, and recognition of good performance. Even a situation requiring disciplinary action should be viewed in terms of how it will teach, not punish.

The purpose of any disciplinary action is to prevent recurrence of unacceptable behavior. Any breakdown in the employee's self-discipline must be dealt with promptly, but not hastily. Before taking any action, the manager must investigate to find out the facts and determine whether the employee actually knew the rules. Reprimands and disciplinary discussions should always take place in private, never in the presence of other employees. A record describing all facts of the occurrence should be kept in the employee's personnel file.

Management has the challenge of disciplining employees fairly when needed. The disciplinary process should begin as soon as possible after a violation occurs. The manager should be certain that all rules, regulations, and requirements are made known to all employees. This underscores the need for clearly stated work rules and policies.

Most operations follow the policy of progressive discipline under which the penalty is increased with each offense, according to previously stated disciplinary procedures that have been made known to all employees. The first step may be only a discussion with the employee. If this does not clear up the problem, an oral warning should be given. Written warnings may be used at this time or saved for a third offense. The written warning should include a statement of the violation and the possible consequences if it is repeated. One copy of the warning should be given to the employee, and another put into the employee's permanent record.

If a written warning does not produce the desired improvement, a disciplinary layoff is used in some situations. When a disciplinary layoff is used, it is coupled with a warning that another violation will be cause for dismissal. Demotion is sometimes used but is not recommended as a disciplinary device. The downgraded employee can become a demoralizing force in the work group. Transfers to other work groups may have similar effects.

Discharge is appropriate only for the most serious offenses and must be well documented by evidence that the employee has been counseled and warned and that each step in the established disciplinary procedures has been followed. Because discharge handicaps the employee in finding other jobs, formal complaints often result in such cases. Consistency in the disciplinary procedure is a requirement. It means that every time an infraction of the rules occurs, the manager must take disciplinary action. Inconsistency can erode employee morale and respect for management and always creates employee insecurity and anxiety. Consistency does not mean rigidity, however. The manager must deal with each case as it comes up and have full information before action. Facts, not gossip or rumor, should be considered and the employee's side of the story should be heard.

Impersonality is another requirement for effective discipline. This requires that all employees who commit the same violation will be penalized, although the precise penalty might vary according to the particular circumstances surrounding the violation. The disciplinary action must seek to correct the unacceptable behavior while avoiding critical attack on the employee as a person. A manager's success at maintaining positive discipline can be measured by how little time is spent in handling grievances and by the employee turnover rate.

GRIEVANCE PROCEDURES

A basic principle of good employee relations is that employees have the right to register complaints and have them fairly considered. A procedure for hearing grievances should be established in every organization, whether or not employees are unionized. Under collective bargaining agreements, grievance procedures are always stated in the contract, with the union steward having the responsibility for helping employees prepare and present grievances to management. However, in any organization, a sound and fair grievance procedure permits employees to express their complaints without fear of recrimination.

Although the specific steps in a grievance procedure vary, most contain the following steps:

1. Conference by employee with the manager, with or without the union steward or other representation. The manager listens and may be able to settle the matter at this step. In any event, the manager must respond with a firm and specific decision to grant or deny the grievance. A written record of action taken should be kept.

2. If the grievance is denied, the employee presents it in writing to the next higher authority in the organization. The manager should have informed his or her superior of the situation so that the grievance will come as no surprise. If the decision at this level still fails to satisfy the employee, the grievance may be taken higher in the organization. In a nonunion operation, this is usually the final step.

3. The last step in a unionized organization is usually arbitration by an outside impartial party. Arbitration occurs when there has been failure to reach an understanding at all levels of management. Both sides agree to abide by the arbitrator's decision. Conciliation, the use of an outsider who tries to help both parties find a common ground for agreement, is another alternative at this stage.

To deal successfully with employee complaints, it helps to listen carefully to facts and be alert to emotions involved. Any complaint is important enough for close attention. Anger or snap judgments should be avoided. Despite the pressure to make a decision, it is best for a manager to wait for a clear and accurate picture of the situation and then give an answer as directly and quickly as possible. The manager should communicate not only the decision, but the reasons for it as well.

A manager's goal should be to handle as many grievances as possible at the first level within the department. This spares the operation the expense of going through the entire grievance procedure and also encourages employees to speak up when they are dissatisfied. The operation of the employee grievance procedure should be reviewed at regular intervals to make certain that it is sufficient and effective.

LEGISLATION AFFECTING PERSONNEL MANAGEMENT

From employment to termination, the management of food service personnel is affected by federal, state, and local laws and regulations. Personnel policies should be in compliance with legal requirements. The food service director should work closely with the institution's personnel and/or legal offices to be sure that pertinent regulations are followed and required records are maintained. Several of the major federal laws that affect personnel procedures are described in this section.

National Labor Relations Act (1935). This act was enacted primarily to prevent unfair management actions against employees who attempted to join a union. Unfair management practices were defined in an attempt to balance the relative power of management and labor. The National Labor Relations Board (NLRB) was created with jurisdiction over any labor dispute affecting interstate commerce. The act was amended in 1947 by the Taft-Hartley Labor-Management Relations Act, which, among other things, defined unfair practices by unions, banned union shops, and established procedures for secret ballot elections in which employees decide whether unions will represent them in collective bargaining.

Social Security Act (1935). This act established a system for payments by employers and employees toward postretirement income. It also established unemployment compensation to protect wage earners and their families against loss of income due to unemployment.

Fair Labor Standards Act (1938). This act, also called the Wage and Hour Law, requires institutions covered by the act to pay employees at least the minimum wage. Any hours worked in excess of 40 hours per week must be paid at the overtime rate. The act provides for annual increases in the federal minimum wage, effective January 1 of each year. Most states also have minimum wage laws that often apply to employees not covered by the federal law.

The Labor-Management Reporting and Disclosure Act (1959). This act was enacted to strengthen internal union democracy while protecting the individual rights of union members and curtailing the economic and political power of unions. Financial reporting requirements for unions were established. The regulations affecting secondary boycotts, informational picketing, and recognitional and jurisdictional strikes also were changed by this act.

The Equal Pay Act (1963). This act, an amendment to the Fair Labor Standards Act, requires employers to pay equal wages to men and women doing equal work on jobs requiring equal skill, effort, and responsibility and being performed under similar working conditions.

Civil Rights Act (Title VII) (1964). Under this act, all discrimination because of race, color, or national origin is banned in places employing 15 or more persons.

Age Discrimination in Employment Act (1967). This law protects job applicants and employees between the ages of 40 and 70 by prohibiting arbitrary age discrimination in hiring, discharge, promotion, compensation, privileges, and other areas of employment because of age. Employment on the basis of ability rather than age is promoted.

Occupational Safety and Health Act (1970). Under this law, employers are required to provide employees a place of employment that is free from hazards causing or likely to cause death or serious physical harm.

Appropriate inspections, record keeping, and reporting are required by the act.

Federal Wage Garnishment Law (Title III, Consumer Credit Protection Act) (1970). An employer is prohibited from discharging any employee on the grounds that their earnings have been subject to garnishment for any one indebtedness. The law also limits the amount of employees' disposable earnings that may be made subject to garnishment for any one indebtedness.

Privacy Act (1974). A prospective employee's privacy is protected from invasions by an employer concerning convictions for offenses against the law, membership in certain organizations when they are irrelevant to employment, and some medical questions that may be asked only on appropriate medical forms.

Workmen's Compensation Insurance is a program administered by the states that covers employers' liability for the costs of any accidental injury incurred by employees on or in connection with the job. The liability insurance premiums are paid by employers.

Rehabilitation Act (1977). Discrimination against the handicapped by recipients of funds from the U.S. Department of Health and Human Services is prohibited by this act.

SAFETY

Maintaining safe working conditions and practices is the responsibility of management in any organization. The federal Occupational Safety and Health Act (OSHA) emphasizes this obligation, placing legal requirements on employers to provide a safe work environment. The primary responsibility for enforcing safety rules and ensuring that employees use safe practices falls upon the department manager. A safety-conscious operation with well-trained personnel also results in a more efficient work force, more peaceful atmosphere, and ultimately better food service.

An effective safety program has several components: safe working conditions, safe equipment, established safety procedures for work activities, fire prevention, and continuous training and self-inspection. General information about OSHA and specific information about food services is contained in *OSHA Reference for Food Service Administrators*, developed by the American Society for Hosptal Food Service Administrators (see Bibliography). Complete records on maintenance, accidents, and safety activities should be maintained. In many organizations, a safety committee made up of employees is appointed or elected. Such a committee can work very effectively with the department manager in carrying out a safety program.

WORKING CONDITIONS

The physical facility must provide several conditions before operating

procedures can be made safe. Some of the necessary conditions include:
- Adequate working space
- Safe clearances for aisles, doors, loading, and traffic areas
- Adequate lighting and ventilation
- Proper electrical installation in accordance with applicable codes
- Sufficient, well-marked exits
- Guarded stairways, platforms, and so forth
- Floor surfaces that are clear, dry, and free from hazards
- Suitable storage facilities for food and nonfood materials

EQUIPMENT

Safe equipment operation includes both equipment construction and use in day-to-day operations:
- Electrical or gas equipment constructed in accordance with the applicable standards and codes: the National Sanitation Foundation codes, Underwriters' Laboratory codes, and National Electrical codes are applicable, as well as any state or local regulations
- Electrical equipment properly grounded and insulated
- Machines with proper guards and enclosures
- Noise levels within those set by OSHA regulations
- Complete, posted operating instructions on or near each piece of equipment
- Locks that open from the inside on walk-in refrigerators and freezers
- Proper insulation or protection from heat-producing equipment, water heaters, condensing units, compressors, and water pipes
- Sharp and properly stored knives

PROCEDURES

To ensure safety at work, the following procedures should be observed:
- Safe clothing and shoes
- Use of ladders for reaching items stored on high shelving
- Use of protective guards and devices on machinery
- Use of proper tools for opening containers and cartons
- Use of leg muscles rather than back muscles to lift heavy objects and use of carts and dollies whenever possible
- Dry hotpads or cloths for handling hot utensils
- Good housekeeping conditions in all work areas, with equipment and materials properly stored and kept clean
- Use of proper operating instructions for all equipment

FIRE PREVENTION

The prevention of fire, as well as the safety of employees during a fire, requires that the following be observed:
- Fire extinguishers should be suitable for the conditions involved,

located in appropriate spots, readily accessible, and kept in operating condition at all times
- All employees should be knowledgeable in the use of fire extinguishers
- Range hoods and other cooking equipment should be kept clean and free from accumulated grease
- Exit doors should be free from obstructions at all times
- All employees should be rehearsed in what to do in case of a fire emergency

TRAINING

The food service director and all work unit managers are key persons in developing a safety-minded work force. Safety training must begin the first day the new employee is on the job and be reinforced by regularly scheduled training sessions. Posters and safety reminders are useful in keeping employees alert to safety procedures. It must be stressed that employees should report any safety hazards immediately to get the problem corrected quickly. The entire department should be periodically inspected for safety compliance in addition to scheduled inspections of equipment by manufacturer's representatives or by the institution's maintenance supervisor. Local fire departments are always helpful in assisting in fire prevention training.

Food
Production
and
Service
Systems

For many years, there were few changes in the way foods were produced and served in health care facilities. However, as food processing technology advanced and costs of food and labor increased, several alternatives in food preparation and service systems evolved. It is not uncommon to find a health care institution using a combination of two or more systems, because modifications in food and equipment continue to develop. Even new facilities may utilize features of more than one production or service system.

Alternative systems are discussed in this chapter. Any health care facility considering a change in system or evaluating the effectiveness of its current system should consider all the factors described here in terms of food quality, microbiological safety, consumer needs, and economics.

FOOD PRODUCTION SYSTEMS

The major food production systems used today are classified as conventional, ready-prepared (cook/chill and cook/freeze), and assembly/serve. The systems differ in the form in which foods are purchased, amount and type of labor required, timing of production relative to service, holding methods prior to service, and equipment requirements. Although each system has certain strong and weak points that have been acknowledged by users and identified in research, all of these production systems have successfully provided food of acceptable quality in operational situations. The key to success lies in managerial control of critical stages in each production system and in thorough employee training.

One of management's greatest responsibilities in a food production system is the prevention of food safety risks. In recent research, the Hazard Analysis Critical Control Point (HACCP) system implemented in the food processing industry was applied to food service systems. Process stages of entree production (control points) wherein microbiological hazards could exist were identified by Bobeng and David (see Bibliography). This system is a preventive approach to quality control that emphasizes microbiological safety.

Figure 13, next page, illustrates the control point during entree processing in four types of food service systems. In the conventional production system, these control points are procurement, preparation, heating, hot holding, portioning/assembly/distribution, and service. Four critical points for these process stages were defined as ingredient control and storage, equipment sanitation, personnel sanitation, and time-temperature relationship. Although careful monitoring of all these critical points during production of menu items is essential to eliminate or reduce microbiological hazards, time-temperature relationship may be considered the most important. Lack of control at any process stage may result in product contamination that cannot be corrected later. During preparation, the time that perishable foods are in a 45 to 140°F. (7 to 60°C.) temperature range must be held at a minimum. During all other stages, foods should be held at temperatures above 140°F., or lower than 45°F. (7°C.).

CONVENTIONAL SYSTEMS

The conventional system has been the traditional method of food production in health care facilities. Modifications have evolved, but in most instances this system is one in which a low percentage of fully prepared food items is used. Most menu items are prepared primarily from basic ingredients on the day they will be served and are held in a hot or cold state until they are served. Production takes place in a kitchen located in the facility or in a central kitchen or commissary that is separate from the service facility.

Although the degree of processing already built into purchased food ingredients varies, the most frequently used prepared items are bakery goods, canned and frozen vegetables and fruits, and ice cream. Few conventional systems purchase primal meat cuts any longer. Portion-cut chilled or frozen meats replace the traditional meat cutting operation. On-premise baking of bread products and dessert items is found in many conventional systems. These are baked using either basic ingredients or a combination of standard production methods along with some mixes or frozen pies,

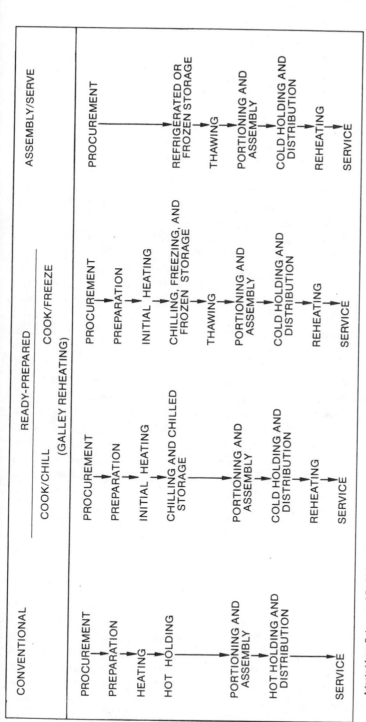

Adapted from Bobeng and David (see Bibliography).

FIGURE 13. Control Points During Stages of Entree Processing in Food Service Systems.

doughs, and other desserts. Vegetables are purchased in many forms: canned, frozen, fresh, prewashed or prepeeled, and dehydrated.

The number of different food items on inventory is relatively high. Availability and cost of labor, equipment, and sources of supply affect the purchasing decisions, but constantly rising labor costs have accelerated the trend toward purchase of more extensively processed foods.

Managers using a conventional system believe they have better control over menus, recipes, and ingredient quality. Menus can reflect changing seasonal supply and market conditions and community ethnic characteristics and can be tailored to the specific standards of the facility. In some cases, however, menu variety may be more limited than in other systems as a result of constraints on production time, skill level of employees, or availability and capacity of equipment used.

A 12- to 15-hour production and service day is common because foods are produced just prior to assembly and service. These peak activity periods occur because of the detrimental effects of hot-food holding on the quality and nutritional value of some foods. However, it is difficult to produce all foods within the ideal time, and the holding that must take place often results in less-than-desired quality.

Both skilled and nonskilled employees are needed in a conventional system. The requirement for skilled employees and more total labor time may lead to a higher labor cost than in some other systems. The availability of skilled employees may be limited because of the community or because of the undesirable schedule of hours people are required to work. Production is scheduled on a 7-day workweek. Labor productivity may not be as high as in other systems because it is difficult to schedule a balanced daily work load that covers service-time peaks, yet minimizes the number of employees during slow periods. Skilled employees are frequently assigned routine cleaning jobs to equalize the work load, even though these tasks could be performed by nonskilled employees.

A wide variety of types and sizes of equipment is needed in a conventional system. Greater total capacity may be needed for certain pieces of equipment because of volume demand and same-day service. Poor utilization of equipment can occur, depending on menu item mix, because both hot-holding and cold-holding equipment is needed. There is some potential for energy savings in using a conventional system because energy for chilling and freezing entrees and other foods is not needed. The ready-prepared and assembly/serve systems require a large amount of electrical energy to chill and freeze foods from the hot stage.

When foods are prepared well in advance of service time, it is difficult to maintain proper temperatures of foods during the hot-holding periods required. Perishability of foods increases with overcooking, and a subsequent loss of palatability and nutrients can occur with late and held trays.

READY-PREPARED SYSTEMS

Ready-prepared systems were developed to overcome some of the labor productivity and cost problems of conventional systems and to decrease food quality deterioration associated with hot holding. Menu items are always prepared and stored in a chilled or frozen state to be ready for assembly and reheating one or more days after production. However, entrees should not be held in the chilled state more than 24 hours. Foods can be purchased at any stage of processing as basic ingredients for recipe preparation, as partially prepared recipe components, or as fully prepared items. After initial preparation, menu items may be individually portioned or stored in bulk. A ready-prepared system requires two stages of heat processing. The first is initial cooking of the food and the second is reheating of the food with a chill (cook/chill) or freeze (cook/freeze) stage in between.

Quality of food can and should be higher in ready-prepared systems because chilled or frozen food is less perishable and retains nutrients longer than food cooked and held in the conventional manner. Menu selections offered to consumers can be greater, particularly when menu items are individually portioned before chilling or freezing. It is possible to offer a hotel or restaurant-style menu because production does not have to occur on the same day as service. Service of items with acceptable sensory attributes also is possible, because initial cooking times for many items in ready-prepared systems are less than in conventional systems. This is because the reheating period continues the cooking. However, an internal oven temperature of at least 140° F. (60° C.) must be reached during the cooking process.

Recipe quantities may need to be increased for large-volume production runs for frozen items. In such cases, traditional steps in preparation are often changed to accommodate the greater volume and save time. For example, canned vegetables are plated without heating and frozen vegetables are only partially cooked.

However, not all foods can be successfully held either in cook/chill or cook/freeze systems without extensive modification of ingredients or recipes. Specialized ingredients, such as thickening agents, are needed for some recipes, and foam or sponge products, gels, coatings, and emulsions pose other problems. When foods are frozen, structural and textural changes occur because of cell damage and protein coagulation. As a result, off-flavors may develop in vegetables and meats.

The extended period between initial preparation of food in cook/chill systems and consumption of the final product provides many opportunities for mishandling of food. Management is responsible for the control of microbiological hazards at critical points in a cook/chill system. This involves monitoring equipment sanitation and time-temperature conditions at all stages from procurement through service. During the production stage, quick-chilling procedures are essential to bring the temperatures of cooked foods to 45°F. (7°C.) or lower within a maximum of 4 hours following initial cooking. Factors that influence the cooling rate of foods include initial internal temperature of the food, batch size and/or depth, dimensions of the food mass, density of the food, and refrigerator temperature and load.

Similar quick-chilling is necessary in a cook/freeze system in order to optimize the sensory quality of the frozen food as well as to have a microbiologically safe product. It is recommended that a temperature of 0°F. (-18°C.) or lower be reached within 1-1/2 hours. Frozen food should be stored at 0°F. or lower and must be properly packaged to avoid dehydration. Entrees should be thawed in a refrigerator and used within 24 hours after thawing. In cook/chill and cook/freeze systems, the temperature of entrees should be maintained at 45°F. (7°C.) or lower during portioning, assembly, and distribution.

As in conventional systems, personnel sanitation is a critical control point at all stages of processing food in ready-prepared systems: initial preparation, portioning, assembly, and service. Personnel may directly or indirectly contribute to microbial contamination through poor personal hygiene.

In either ready-prepared system, whether cook/chill or cook/freeze, production usually can be scheduled into a 40-hour week with regular 8-hour shifts. For this reason, the system may require fewer skilled employees for production tasks demanding their skill levels. In cook/chill systems, plating of food can be spread over a longer period because all items are held cold during plating and tray assembly. This could result in reduction of the number of employees needed and possibly increase employee productivity and satisfaction.

More balanced and efficient use of equipment is possible in ready-prepared systems, because production can be distributed over the entire work shift rather than in the limited time just before service. Total equipment requirements may be less than in a conventional system, but types of equipment and capacities needed will depend on whether it is a cook/chill or cook/freeze system. For example, specialized quick-chill refrigerators are needed for both systems, but blast or cryogenic freezers also are needed for cook/freeze.

Adequate refrigerated space must be available for storing foods and holding foods during the assembly process. The amount of refrigeration space needed for preplated items is greater than for bulk-storage items. Acquisition of all this equipment adds to the capital investment costs. Research also indicates that energy used in either ready-prepared system is higher than that used in a conventional system because of the significant amount of energy needed to chill or freeze, thaw, and reheat foods.

Ready-prepared systems may operate in an on-premise kitchen or may be located in a commissary separate from service areas. Many commissaries use cook/chill or cook/freeze systems, becasue assembly, transport, and delivery of chilled or frozen foods are easier to schedule and control than hot food transport.

ASSEMBLY/SERVE SYSTEMS

The assembly/serve food production system, sometimes called a convenience system, is one in which most or all foods are obtained from a commercial source in a ready-to-serve form. This includes preprepared entree items that come frozen, canned, or dehydrated; ready-to-serve dessert and bakery products that come fresh, frozen, or canned; salads and salad ingredients that come ready to assemble; sauces and soups that come canned, frozen, or dehydrated; fruit juices and beverages that come frozen concentrated, portion packed, canned, or dehydrated; and individual portion packets of condiments such as sugar, jelly, syrup, salad dressing, and cream.

Menu variety can be greater in assembly/serve systems than in most conventional systems, but depends on access to suppliers who can provide a wide range of products. The variety and availability of preplated items has not been as great as that offered in bulk-packaged products. Quality inconsistency among different products and different lots of the same products has been observed. Because of this inconsistency, it is desirable to try several potential vendors before implementing an assembly/serve system. Also, geographic location of the food service and small purchase volumes may intensify problems in obtaining products of the same quality from one purchase period to another.

An assembly/serve system requires a minimum of skilled labor. Labor cost should decrease if the foods used in the system are at a maximum convenience level, but to remain in a reasonable overall cost position, labor savings must compensate for higher food costs.

This system should eliminate the need for most standard production equipment, but in many cases it actually does not. Many institutions are reluctant to abandon the option of on-premise production in case the quality or cost of the convenience system fails to reach expected goals. Thus, a primary economic advantage is lost. Some of the questions related to feasibility of an assembly/serve system are:

- Do the available products meet the nutritional standards established for normal and modified diets?
- Are there sufficient products available to provide variety throughout the menu cycle?
- Do these products meet the quality standards of both the facility and the residents?
- Is the cost per serving within an acceptable range?
- Is there sufficient storage space for disposable ware?
- Will changes in the type and the amount of equipment needed for reheating foods be required?

- Is refrigerator and freezer space adequate?
- How many labor hours can be eliminated with this system?
- How will the method of tray assembly and delivery be affected?
- Will additional packaging materials create trash disposal problems?

In an assembly/serve system, attention must be paid to prevention of microbiological hazards at critical processing stages. Some of the hazards present in other systems are eliminated, because there is little or no on-premise food preparation. Freezer and refrigeration space needs for storing and thawing frozen foods prior to final heating are greater than in conventional systems. Thawing of or tempering frozen products must be carried out under refrigeration, and storage times for purchased chilled foods should be kept to a minimum. Perishable foods must be maintained at 45°F. (7°C.) or lower during portioning, assembly, and distribution. In the reheating stage, foods must attain temperatures of at least 140°F. (60°C.) as rapidly as possible. For maximum safety and palatability, an end-point temperature of 165°F. (74°C.) is recommended for most hot foods. Food temperatures should be routinely checked before service. As in other systems, personnel and equipment sanitation is essential to control microbiological hazards.

SERVICE SYSTEMS

Advances in technology provide many options in patient or resident service systems for hospitals and extended care facilities. Several factors affect the particular choice for each facility: physical layout of the health care institution, patient nutritional and social needs, production system, food and microbiological quality standards set by management, timing of service, skill level of service personnel, and economic factors related to equipment requirements of each alternative system. The various components of each service system should be considered separate from the production system, because many of them can be combined with any or all of the alternative production systems shown in figure 14, next page.

In most health care facilities, the service system includes tray service to patient rooms and a central dining room for visitors, staff, and, in nursing homes, ambulatory residents. The service of food to patient rooms involves tray assembly and distribution to patients, using some means for serving food at the proper temperatures by either temperature maintenance or reheating. The two major categories in patient food service are tray assembly at a central location with varied distribution methods (centralized service) and bulk food distribution to patient floors with plating of food at that point (decentralized service).

CENTRALIZED SYSTEMS

Centralized service systems are prevalent in most facilities today because they permit better control of food quality, portions, temperatures, and

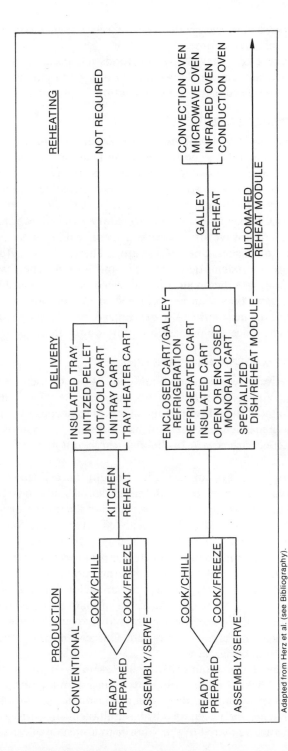

FIGURE 14. Alternative Systems for Food Service to Patients.

Adapted from Herz et al. (see Bibliography).

diet modifications; reduce overproduction and waste; require less equipment; and greatly diminish labor time.

In a centralized tray service system, foods are plated and trays are made up in a central location. Trays are transported to patient floors for service and then returned to the central location for warewashing.

DECENTRALIZED SYSTEMS

In decentralized service systems, most of the food is prepared in a central production area and then is conveyed in bulk or in portions, in food trucks with heated and unheated compartments, to serving pantries on the floors. In the serving pantry, the trays are assembled for delivery, individually or by small truck, to the patient rooms. Coffee, toast, eggs, and special items are prepared in the serving pantry, which may be equipped with hot plate, microwave or convection oven, coffee maker, toaster, cabinet for heating dishes, and refrigerator. The trays are returned to these pantries to be dismantled, cleaned, and stored. The dishes and flatware can be washed either in an adjacent area or in a central dishwashing room; in either case, they then are returned to the serving pantries and stored there until the next meal. A decentralized tray service requires less space in the food service department but more on the floor.

TEMPERATURE MAINTENANCE SYSTEMS

The first five delivery systems shown in figure 14 can be used with any of the production systems described in this chapter. These methods are all designed to maintain hot and cold temperatures of food cooked or reheated in the kitchen. Each delivery method has different characteristics that must be considered with regard to the physical layout and other features of the health care facility.

Insulated tray. This system uses a lightweight thermal tray with individual molded compartments that hold both hot and cold foods. Specially designed china or disposable tableware is placed in the tray compartments, and the entire tray is covered with an insulated fitted cover. An insulated cup is used for beverages. No external heat or refrigeration sources are used in delivery or holding, so foods must be at proper serving temperatures when plated. Food temperatures are maintained up to 30 minutes by the insulating properties of the tray. Meal trays are delivered to floors, either stacked or individually, on an open cart. No specialized carts are needed. There is some difficulty in washing the trays and covers in most conveyor dishwashers. Special racks may be needed. This system can be purchased or leased from the manufacturer.

Unitized pellet. This system calls for the assembly of all the hot items in a meal on a preheated plate. The plate is placed on a preheated pellet base and is covered with a stainless steel or plastic lid to retain heat and moisture. Cold items are placed on a tray simultaneously with the covered hot foods. Trays are delivered to the floor in an uninsulated cart. There is no provision for maintenance of cold temperatures, so rapid delivery and service are needed to minimize temperature changes. Maximum holding time is approximately 45 minutes. Either china or disposable tableware can be used. Careful monitoring of pellet, plate, and lid temperatures is necessary.

Hot/cold cart. This system uses a tray cart with electrically heated and refrigerated compartments to maintain proper food temperatures during delivery. Standard trays are assembled with cold food and placed in the refrigerated compartment. Simultaneously, hot foods are plated, placed on a separate smaller tray, and stored in the hot food compartment. Standard or disposable tableware is used. In another variation of this system, plated hot foods are placed in heated drawer compartments. Both versions require that personnel reassemble the tray at the point of service. Holding time prior to service can be longer because of the electrically controlled cart. These transport carts are very heavy, but can be motorized for use in facilities with ramps or in places that extend over a very large area. Considerable cart storage space is required, and more labor time is needed for cleaning and maintenance of the carts than in most other systems.

Unitray cart. This system is similar to the hot/cold cart system, with the exception that hot and cold items are loaded on opposite sections of the same tray. The trays are slotted to allow placement of one side of the tray in a heated compartment and the other side in a refrigerated compartment. Specialized carts are needed, with electrical outlets for plugging in on the floor. With this system, tray reassembly is not necessary.

Tray heater cart. This system uses specially designed disposable tableware on which hot or cold foods are placed at serving temperatures. Specially designed trays with resistance heaters built into them at the dinner plate and bowl locations are used to maintain the temperatures of hot foods. When the loaded trays are placed into the battery-powered cart, the resistance heaters are activated. Heating of individual food items is regulated by preset push-button controls. The temperatures of cold foods are not affected by the tray heaters, but no refrigeration is provided in the cart. The heaters are automatically disconnected as each tray is removed from the cart. Hot beverages are delivered in insulated containers. Cart batteries, which provide the electricity for heating and moving the cart, are recharged between uses. This system is more complex than the others described and may require more maintenance. Because specialized disposable tableware is used, operating costs may be higher than for some of the other heat-maintenance systems.

CHILL-DELIVERY/FLOOR-REHEAT SYSTEMS

The last four delivery systems illustrated in figure 14 are available for use with ready-prepared or assembly/serve production systems in which foods are portioned cold and reheated in galleys on the floor. These delivery systems are designed to maximize food quality by reheating it just prior to service, without extended hot-hold conditions required in the heat maintenance systems. There is a potential for reducing labor time and costs because of greater scheduling flexibility in portioning foods and tray assembly.

The features common to most of these systems include the transport of chilled or frozen foods on fully assembled trays to floor galleys. The types of carts used include enclosed nonrefrigerated, insulated, refrigerated, and carts on monorail. When nonrefrigerated carts are used, refrigeration is provided in the floor galley.

Several types of specialized equipment can be used for reheating foods: convection oven, microwave oven, infrared oven, or conduction oven. Microwave is the most common reheating method currently used. In any of these systems, service personnel must be trained in the proper reheating procedures in order to attain optimal food quality. A more sophisticated system in this group uses a specially designed dish that provides an electrical contact with a conductor rail in the heating module. Therefore, the need to transfer foods to an oven in the floor galley is eliminated.

DELIVERY SYSTEMS

Several factors should be evaluated in selecting a tray delivery system for an existing facility or a new facility. Among these are:
- Capability for maintaining desired level of food quality
- Compatibility of equipment with existing production system and layout of facility
- Workhours and level of skill or training needed for labor to operate the system
- Space requirements and transportability of the equipment
- Initial equipment, replacements, maintenance, and leasing costs
- Costs associated with purchase of any specialized and disposable tableware
- Costs for renovation of existing facility to accommodate a specific delivery system
- Flexibility of delivery system to accommodate a change in production system, number of meals served, or menu pattern
- Energy requirements of the system

DINING ROOM SERVICE

The social aspects of group dining areas are of particular importance in extended care facilities or rehabilitation centers where there are a significant number of ambulatory residents. One or several dining rooms may be desirable, depending on the needs and capabilities of residents. Several types of service can be used, each with certain advantages and limitations.

Cafeteria service is common in situations in which residents have relatively high mobility levels. Some waiter or waitress assistance may be needed for physically disabled persons who have difficulty in carrying filled trays to tables. With cafeteria service, attractive display of foods and temperature and portion control are possible. Also, clientele can make their own selections of desired foods. In some situations, buffet service, which has similar characteristics, is used.

Table service using waiters or waitresses is another option for dining room service. This system presents some difficulties when a selective menu is offered, but restaurant-style menus may be used. Because foods are portioned in the kitchen or service area, clientele may not be able to modify portion sizes or sauces, gravies, and so forth as easily as in a cafeteria. Unless portion sizes are carefully tailored to clientele needs, plate waste may be higher than expected.

Family-style service is rarely used and is not recommended for several reasons. Portion control is difficult, considerable handling of foods at the table increases microbiological hazards and danger of burns or spills from hot serving dishes, and food waste can be significant. More tableware is needed because bulk serving bowls and platters are used and dishwashing is increased. More labor is needed in the dining room to clear tables than in the other options.

NONPATIENT MEALS

In most hospitals and many nursing homes, employees outnumber patients. Meal service for employees therefore becomes a major part of the work of the food service department. The most common type of service system used for employees is the cafeteria, which may be designed as a traditional straight-line or modified version of a freeflow system, in which individuals serve some food items themselves. The rate of customer flow in the cafeteria is affected by the number of menu choices, physical layout of equipment, serving speed, number of lines, and number of cashiers. If large numbers of people are to be served in a limited period, special attention to line speed is necessary. Additional lines, fewer choices, line-skipping, and more cashiers may be advisable.

Food pricing is a critical management responsibility if the cafeteria is to operate profitably or at a break-even level. Whether employee meals are considered as a fringe benefit or are paid for individually, prices charged should cover food, labor, supply, and other operating costs. In cafeterias that serve the public as well as employees, a two-tiered pricing system can be used, providing employee meals at or slightly above cost.

For many years, limited operating hours for the employee cafeteria have been standard in most institutions. However, some institutions have seen the profit potential in a cafeteria-snack bar operation that provides varied menu choices for employees and visitors over an extended period. With this kind of cafeteria operation, many of the traditional special function activities could be eliminated, along with staff dining rooms. The cafeteria should offer high-quality, attractively merchandised items. It also can incorporate quick-serve foods often sold in hospital coffee shops. Consolidation and streamlining of nonpatient food services within the facility can eliminate excessive overhead and space costs and maximize managerial control over all food activities.

The trend in most hospitals toward greater emphasis on ambulatory and outpatient care has implications for the food service department. How can the food service department appropriately respond to the nutritional needs of such patients? In most communities, low-income and elderly persons are those most in need of outpatient services. In reviewing cafeteria operations in the institution, it is appropriate to consider the modified diet needs of these patients, as well as the general food requirements. Accessibility of the cafeteria to ambulatory patients, appropriateness of menu offerings, price range of foods, and hours of operation should be evaluated. If the cafeteria is viewed as a profit center as well as a service center, the needs of all persons using the health care facility on a nonpatient basis can be met in an economically responsible manner.

VENDING OPERATIONS

Vending operations have become an acceptable alternative for meeting the needs of personnel, guests, and clients on a 24-hour-a-day basis in many hospitals and nursing homes. Equipment can be owned, rented, or leased from vending companies. Food may be supplied and stocked by the food service department or by the vending company.

In many hospitals, the vending operation is run by the hospital auxiliary. Vending companies can provide selections ranging from snacks and hot and cold beverages to full-scale operations offering hot canned foods, preplated convenience foods, sandwiches, pastries, snacks, frozen desserts, and beverages. Wherever foods are vended in a chilled or frozen state, microwave ovens are usually provided for reheating.

Food quality, equipment operation and maintenance, and vending area sanitation are major concerns with most vending operations. Planning is of great importance in setting up a vending operation, and several factors must be considered, such as space and electrical sources, ease of restocking, suitable environment for persons using the machines, and disposal of paper and food waste. Sanitation of the vending area is essential and must be assigned to an appropriate department or handled by the vending company.

MOBILE MEAL PROGRAMS

Many food service departments have become aware that providing good health care for their communities involves off-premise meal service for elderly or convalescent individuals and for persons requiring special diets who cannot provide nutritional meals for themselves. In most communities, hospitals and nursing homes are perceived as the best source to meet this need.

One meal per day, which provides one-half to two-thirds of the adult daily requirements 5 days a week, is the most common service provided. A cold meal for later use also may be delivered at the same time as the hot meal. Meals are preplated in the food service department, using disposable insulated tableware in most situations. Bulk food shipping to centers is another possibility, but may involve problems in return of tableware and in cost of disposable bulk-food pans. Portion control at service time is more difficult to achieve, and special diets are hard to provide. Insulated carriers or carts for maintaining food temperature during transport are needed unless delivery can be made within a very short time. Assembly of meals and loading of delivery vehicles must be carefully planned within the department's total work schedule.

Transport and delivery is often provided by volunteers or other community agencies to client homes or to community centers. When this is the case, training for the volunteers is required. They need to know policies of the meal service program, special diet details, food handling procedures, how to deal with emergency situations, and how to note any apparent changes in a client's physical or mental condition. Home-delivered meal programs not only provide nutritional benefits for recipients but also play an important role in providing social contact for isolated persons and in serving as a check on their well-being.

Prices for the meals must be carefully determined in order to cover food, labor, and supply costs, yet remain affordable for the clientele. In many communities, additional funding is available from federal, state, or local sources, but prices and extent of service are contracted in advance.

SHARED FOOD SERVICE SYSTEMS

During an inflationary period, with high food costs and substantial labor cost increases, food service administrators find it increasingly difficult to stay within a set budget and to forecast realistically for the following year. There is constant pressure to contain current costs and at the same time improve the quality of dietary services. As a result, more and more food service administrators are expressing interest in shared food service systems as a method of providing high-quality food for patients and staff at a reasonable cost.

A shared service system can be categorized by the amount of control and responsibility exercised by the participating institutions. Thus, shared services are classified as referred service, purchased service, multiple-sponsored service, or regional service. Shared food service systems are usually either a purchased service or a multiply sponsored service. A purchased service is one that the institution pays for directly. The institution obtaining the service acts as an intermediary between the patient and the provider and therefore assumes some responsibility for the quality of the service. A multiply sponsored service is one in which a group of institutions jointly control and operate the service. Control can be established through an agreement among the institutions or through a separate corporation or cooperative. Although the nature and extent of shared food services vary, the major types of sharing are in professional and managerial expertise, food purchasing, and shared food production systems.

The sharing of professional and managerial expertise is of major importance to small or rural hospitals and extended care facilities. The opportunity to use the services of highly trained personnel on a part-time basis allows the health care institution to provide patient services that it otherwise could not afford. Although large hospitals seldom share dietetic and other professional food service personnel with other large institutions, they sometimes do so with small institutions. Usually, the fees for this service are paid directly to the large hospital, which pays the shared personnel their salary, with additional compensation for travel when necessary. The shared personnel usually are required to submit reports to the administrators of both institutions involved, to meet accreditation requirements, and to evaluate the shared program.

Shared management services are similar to shared professional personnel services. Management services that can be shared include menu planning, financial record keeping, data processing for food service functions, payroll operations, in-service training and education, and policies and procedures planning.

Shared food purchasing systems are the most common of the shared services. Standardized and least perishable items are most often purchased through shared systems, but dairy products, frozen meat, poultry, fish, frozen entrees, and nonfood supplies are frequently available through group systems. Agreement on product specifications among participating institutions is essential in attaining greatest cost savings in shared purchasing arrangements. Sharing food purchasing also implies sharing ideas about food quality, processing techniques, consumer acceptance data, and high-quality information on new products. Management time is saved in shared purchasing arrangements because the buyer in the participating institution does not have to negotiate prices or see as many vendors.

Shared food production systems are feasible, provided that a comprehensive planning and evaluation procedure is used in the developmental stages. The food service administrators should plan in conjunction with the chief executive officers of the institutions involved to identify and clarify long-range goals in level of service, quality, nutritional counseling, bacteriologic control, menu variety, system flexibility, and adaptability to changing circumstances.

The decision to enter a shared production system or to maintain independent status should be documented. One method of documentation is to survey patients, medical staff, employees, and outpatient customers about availability, quality, and level of service currently being provided or desired. Opportunities for sharing often involve a shift to a different food production/service system. Careful consideration of the food service systems described earlier in this chapter will help identify the strengths and weaknesses of the present or proposed system. Data to be collected include capital investment requirements, operating costs, quality and comprehensiveness of services, acceptability of services to client groups, and legal considerations such as taxes and contracts.

DISASTER PLANNING

Hospitals are required to have comprehensive plans that cover emergencies arising from both external and internal disasters. Specifications for these plans are stated in the JCAH *Accreditation Manual for Hospitals*:

Disaster plans. The role of the dietetic department/service in the hospital's internal and external disaster plans shall be clearly defined. The dietetic department/service shall be able to meet the nutritional needs of patients and staff during a disaster, consistent with the capabilities of the hospitals and community served. For requirements of the hospital's disaster plans, reference is made to the Functional Safety and Sanitation section of this *Manual*.

One of the major JCAH standards that applies to the food service department states:

The disaster plan should make provision, within the hospitals, for . . . availability of adequate basic utilities and supplies, as well as essential medical and supportive materials. The hospital should be essentially self-sustaining in these areas for a minimum of one week. This may include preestablished mechanisms for immediate supply of certain major critical items such as water, food, and fuel.

Water and fuel supply are concerns not only of the food service department but of the whole institution. These requirements should be provided for in the general hospital plan, which is developed by a committee composed of representatives from each department within the hospital and other technical experts. The primary concern of the food service director is to serve food that meets the needs of patients and staff and is within the capabilities of the hospital.

The food service director is responsible for setting policies for the disaster plan and, with the assistance of staff, developing procedures to implement each policy. Several alternative procedures or plans, based on the various situations that may occur, may be needed for each policy. For example, written plans must include provisions for the various situations in which:

- All employees are present and all equipment is operating
- All employees are present and no equipment is operating

- Few employees are present and all equipment is operating
- Few employees are present and no equipment is operating

In each situation, some modifications in the normal operating procedures will probably be necessary and can concern the following:

- Availability of alternate 1-week patient and nonpatient menus that can be prepared with or without prepreparation or cooking equipment
- Provision for reducing the types, the number, and the complexity of modified diets
- Changes in food delivery schedules and procedures; identification of alternative food supply sources; and sufficiency of food on hand, or at least available nearby, for production of emergency menus
- Provision for maintaining refrigerated and frozen food in a safe condition during a power failure while using an alternative power supply or dry ice
- Availability of sufficient preparation equipment that can be operated manually, such as manual can openers and food cutting, chopping, and slicing equipment, when mechanical equipment cannot be used
- Partial or total arrangement of meals on disposable ware when the power supply is off
- Plans for transport of food and meals when elevators or other electrically operated systems are not functioning
- Provisions for waste disposal in a sanitary manner
- Specific procedures for notifying the food service director and other management staff during the regular operating day or when off-duty (A list of names and telephone numbers of all key personnel should be available)
- Assignments of staff responsibilities, such as contacting off-duty personnel, reassigning employees' work activities, supervising employees, and performing other responsibilities as required
- Provision for changes in servicing procedures of nonpatient meals, with consideration given to the system of making and recording meal charges and cash control
- Security procedures for access to the department in order to protect food, supplies, and people

Developing an effective disaster plan requires careful analysis of the resources of the department, the hospital, and the community. The plan requires periodic testing or drills, with revisions made as necessary. All personnel in the department must be thoroughly trained in emergency procedures. In-service sessions, quarterly drills for internal disasters, semiannual drills for external disasters, and quarterly review of plans, with revisions as needed, should help the manager meet the disaster plan requirements.

Food Protection Practices

All employees in health care facilities have the responsibility of protecting the public from illness, as well as doing their best to cure the illnesses that bring patients to the institution. For the food service department, the responsibilities are clear-cut and fundamental: the department must protect people from the hazards of foodborne illness, as well as provide for their nutritional needs. This responsibility rests on all employees who handle food, not just on management. However, as most food service employees have little or no prior knowledge of sanitation requirements, it is up to the food service manager to see to it that such requirements are met. The responsibilities of the food service manager therefore are:

- To provide clean and properly equipped storage and work areas that meet state and local health department standards
- To purchase wholesome food from sources that comply with regulatory agency procedures; and to receive and store such foods under conditions that maintain wholesomeness and minimize risk of contamination by microorganisms, insects, rodents, or other toxic materials
- To develop written policies and procedures for personal hygiene and for daily operations in the safe preparation and service of food
- To develop written policies and work procedures for cleaning and sanitizing equipment, utensils, and work areas

- To properly dispose of waste materials according to sanitation principles and local health department regulations
- To develop programs for training and supervising employees to ensure application of policies and procedures established by the department and approved by the administration of the facility

An effective food protection program demands that managers and all employees understand the nature of potential hazards that cause foodborne illness, apply procedures that minimize those hazards, and engage in a continuing program of self-inspection and compliance.

MICROBIOLOGICAL HAZARDS

The environment literally teems with microscopic life—organisms so small that they are invisible to the naked eye—such as bacteria, yeasts, molds, parasites, and viruses. Although these microorganisms cannot be seen, the results of their growth in foods can be observed. Many kinds of beneficial organisms are responsible for the characteristic qualities of foods. Specific bacteria are responsible for producing the flavor and texture of natural cheeses, for fermenting pickles and sauerkraut, for coagulating milk to form cultured buttermilk and yogurt, and for producing vinegar from alcohol. The presence of specific actively growing yeasts are necessary in the manufacture of bread, wine, beer, and some cheeses. Molds are needed to ripen some varieties of cheese and to produce oriental foods like soy sauce.

Although we need these beneficial and valuable microorganisms, other microorganisms cause spoilage of foods, such as souring of milk, molding of breads, and putrefying of meat and other proteins. A relatively small proportion of microoganisms can produce diseases and are a constant hazard to humans, plants, and animals. The diseases or illnesses result from the growth of microorganisms on or in tissues or by the toxins they produce in foods that are consumed.

All of the changes in food products that are caused by microorganisms result from their survival and growth. These changes, either desirable or undesirable, can be controlled by applying what is known about the conditions that will either prevent or favor growth.

BACTERIA

The largest group of microorganisms is bacteria. They are small, single cells that vary in shape: round, rod, spiral, comma, or filamentous. Growth of bacteria takes place by cell division rather than by increasing size of individual cells. One cell becomes two, two become four, and so forth. The rate at which growth occurs varies among different bacteria and is affected by many factors:

Temperature. Bacteria grow over a wide temperature range. Even though the majority of bacteria grow best in a range of 80 to 90°F. (27 to

32°C.), many can and do grow between 60 to 120°F. (15 to 49°C.). Some even grow at higher temperatures in the 110 to 150°F. (43 to 65°C.) range, whereas others live and multiply under refrigeration. By varying temperatures, bacterial growth can be increased, inhibited, or stopped. The growth of most bacteria can be inhibited, but not totally stopped, by reducing the temperature of foods to 45°F. (7°C.) or lower. This makes quick cooling and adequate refrigeration an important means of preventing the hazards of bacterially caused food illness. Growth can be completely stopped by raising the temperature of food to a point that will destroy pathogenic bacteria (pasteurization), or to a point at which all bacteria are killed (sterilization). At temperatures above 110°F. (43°C.), many bacteria begin to die or are injured. More are killed as food temperatures are increased. Because most bacteria are destroyed at 140°F. (60°C.), that temperature is recommended as a *minimum* temperature for cooking or holding foods. However, certain bacteria develop a resistant form as they grow. This form, known as a spore, increases the organism's capacity to survive under unfavorable conditions. Spores are so much more resistant that very high temperatures, such as those used for canning low-acid foods (240°F. [115°C.]), are required for their destruction. Under proper conditions, spores can become actively growing cells once again.

Moisture. In general, bacteria need water to grow. Food for bacteria dissolves in water and provides energy for the cells. The amount of water available to bacteria is lessened in the presence of relatively high concentrations of sugar or salt, which explains some of the preservative effects of sugar or salt solutions. When foods are frozen, water is unavailable to support bacterial growth. Drying of foods also reduces the moisture content to levels that cannot support growth of most bacteria, although spores may survive the drying process.

Food. Bacteria require food for energy, cell structure, and metabolism. Various bacteria have markedly different food needs: some can grow on glucose, ammonium salts, water, and certain mineral ions; others require complex foods including vitamins, minerals, and proteins. The bacteria that cause foodborne illnesses thrive well in many foods we eat, especially in foods containing proteins.

Oxygen. Some bacteria will grow only if oxygen is present; others will grow only in the absence of oxygen. However, many can grow under either condition.

Acidity and alkalinity. Slightly acid, neutral, and slightly alkaline food materials will support growth of bacteria that cause food poisoning. These food materials include those of animal origin, such as meat, poultry, seafood, eggs, and milk, and low-acid vegetables, such as corn, peas, beets, and beans. Acid is used in food preservation to suppress bacterial growth and in some cases can be used in food preparation to inhibit bacterial growth. For example, commercial mayonnaise has sufficient acidity to suppress bacterial growth in salad mixtures when it is added early in the preparation stages. Acidity also increases the sensitivity of bacteria to heat. High-acid fruits, for example, do not require as severe a heat treatment in canning as the low-acid vegetables.

Inhibitors. Various substances can prevent bacterial growth. Many chemicals that occur naturally or are manufactured are used to prevent or restrain bacterial growth. For example, sodium nitrite, used in the curing of bacon, ham, and other sausages, is effective in preventing growth of *Clostridium botulinum* even at low levels of concentration.

Time. Bacterial multiplication takes place over a period of time. How rapidly bacteria grow depends on the conditions described above. In food service operations, the objective is to keep foods at the recommended temperatures and under other sanitary conditions for recommended periods of time to prevent bacterial growth. Foods requiring refrigeration after preparation must be rapidly cooled to an internal temperature of 45°F. (7°C.) or lower. Large quantities of such foods need to be cooled in shallow pans, in quick-chilling refrigeration, or by cold water circulation around the food container. The amount of cooling time needed to reach 45°F. (7°C.) should not be greater than 4 hours. Conversely, cold foods should be heated as rapidly as possible to an internal temperature of 140°F. (60°C.) or higher and should be held at that temperature for no more than 2 hours.

YEASTS

Yeasts are single-celled organisms that reproduce by budding. They are both beneficial and problematic to humans. Yeasts do not cause illnesses, but they are responsible for the spoilage of many kinds of foods. Most yeasts grow best at room temperature, but some grow at the freezing point. Yeast growth is inhibited or stopped above 100°F. (38°C.). Yeasts require a supply of moisture and food sources such as sugars and acids for growth. This explains abundant yeast growth in carbohydrate foods or acids such as vinegar and wine. Yeasts can be controlled by proper cleaning and sanitizing and are readily destroyed by boiling temperatures.

MOLDS

Molds are many-celled organisms that normally reproduce by spore formation. Mold spores are extremely small, very light, and are spread quite easily by air currents, insects, or animals. Under favorable conditions, spores actively produce the fuzzy, filamentous growth most of us readily recognize. As noted earlier, some molds are useful in the manufacture of foods. However, many molds spoil foods and, under proper growth conditions, can develop highly poisonous by-products called mycotoxins. Molds can grow over a wide range of conditions: moist or dry, acid or nonacid, high or low salt or sugar content, and at almost any temperature above freezing. Although mold spores and vegetative growth can be destroyed easily by heat, constant care is needed to keep work surfaces, containers, and equipment free from mold to prevent contamination of food products.

Foods that have become moldy should not be used, with the exception of natural cheeses that may form some mold on the exterior during aging. The moldy layer should be cut off, removing at least 1/2 inch, and care taken to prevent recontamination of the newly cut surface with mold spores.

PARASITES

Although illness due to parasites in food is quite rare, the food service manager should be aware of this potential hazard. *Trichinella spiralis* is a microscopic parasite that causes a disease in hogs, rabbits, and bears. When humans eat undercooked, infected meat, trichinosis can result. Hogs contract the disease by consuming infested, uncooked garbage. Because pork producers today do not feed garbage to hogs, trichinosis has become much less prevalent.

Heating pork to an internal temperature of 137°F. (58°C.) also destroys the parasite. At this temperature, pork is very rare and pink and not very palatable. Current recommendations of cooking pork to an internal temperature of 170°F. (77°C.) provide an ample margin of safety and yield a juicy, tender product. Processing temperatures for ready-to-eat hams and canned hams also render the meat free from threat of trichinosis. Frozen storage at 5°F. (-15°C.) or lower for 20 days also will destroy trichinosis.

Another parasitic infection is amoebic dysentery, which may occur if food or water is contaminated from human sewage. Approved water systems, plumbing, and personal hygiene can prevent risk of this illness.

VIRUSES

Viruses can be transmitted through food, but do not multiply in the food itself: they multiply only in the cells of their hosts. Viruses are more resistant to heat than other microorganisms and can survive very high temperatures. The virus causing infectious hepatitis has been most commonly transmitted through food. Persons recovering from hepatitis are apt to be carriers for a period of time after recovery and can contaminate foods through poor personal hygiene. Because it is difficult to effectively combat the possibility of contamination from known hepatitis carriers, they must not be permitted to work in food service operations. Sewage-polluted waters and fish or shellfish harvested from them are other sources of viruses.

FOODBORNE ILLNESSES

Thousands of cases of foodborne illnesses are reported to the U.S. Public Health Service every year, and many thousands of cases go unreported.

Foodborne illnesses are characterized by various degrees of upset stomach, nausea, vomiting, diarrhea, intestinal cramps, and fever. These illnesses are usually classified as foodborne infections, foodborne intoxications (poisoning), or chemical food poisoning.

FOODBORNE INFECTIONS

Foodborne infections are caused by the activity of the harmful micro-organism itself—bacteria, virus, or parasite—in the human digestive tract. Because illness results from the activity of large numbers of cells, the time period before onset of symptoms may be 8 to 72 hours after ingestion of infected food.

The most frequently occurring foodborne infection, salmonellosis, is caused by *Salmonella* bacteria of several different types. The bacteria are widely present in the intestinal tracts and feces of humans, animals, poultry, and shellfish from polluted waters. *Salmonella* contamination occurs in a continuous cycle; the bacteria are excreted by animals, rodents, and birds, and also by humans who have had the illness and may remain carriers for a period of time. Microorganisms are discharged into sewage and manure and may be found in contaminated soil or sewage-polluted waters. During slaughter of food animals, equipment and employees in the packing plant may become contaminated. Waste products may be made into animal feeds, and viable salmonella are transmitted back to farm animals and pets if animal feeds are improperly processed. Thus, the bacteria may be found on fresh meat, poultry, shelled or cracked eggs, shellfish from contaminated waters, or foods made from these products and contaminated during preparation. The presence of *Salmonella* bacteria in food items is not noticeable because appearance, flavor, and odor are not usually altered.

Symptoms of salmonellosis vary in severity, depending on the individual's susceptibility, the total number of cells ingested, and the bacterial strains involved. The symptoms include nausea, vomiting, abdominal pain, diarrhea, headache, chills, weakness, and drowsiness. Fever also can occur. The illness usually lasts 2 or 3 days but may linger.

Occurrence of salmonellosis can be avoided by reducing the possibility of food contamination; by adequate cooking of foods, which may be contaminated even under the best conditions; and by avoiding the possibility of cross-contamination of other foods.

FOODBORNE INTOXICATIONS

Food intoxication, or food poisoning, is caused by eating foods that contain toxins produced by multiplication of bacteria in those foods. Such toxins are not destroyed by cooking temperatures and do not change the flavor, appearance, or odor of foods containing them. Several kinds of bacteria can produce illness-causing toxins. Only those responsible for significant outbreaks in the United States are discussed here. Symptoms occur more rapidly than do the symptoms associated with food infection, and they resemble those of salmonellosis. However, symptoms persist until the toxins are eliminated from the body.

Staphylococcus aureus (*S. aureus*) bacteria are responsible for frequent outbreaks of food poisoning. The most important source of staphylococci is probably the human body. The organisms are found on skin and in the mouths, nasal passages, and throats of healthy persons. Infected pimples, sinuses, or cuts are reservoirs of the organism. The food supply and household pets also can be sources of *S. aureus*. Toxins will be produced when foods that support the growth of staphylococci are contaminated with the organism and are allowed to stand for a sufficient period at temperatures ideal for growth. Although the bacteria are killed when subjected to temperatures as low as 140°F. (60°C.) for 10 minutes, the toxin is highly resistant to heat, cold, and chemicals. Freezing, refrigerating, or heating foods to serving temperatures does not reduce the toxin significantly. The more toxin ingested, the greater the reaction by the body.

Foods high in protein readily support growth and have been involved in many outbreaks of illness. These foods include custards; meat sauces and gravies; fresh meats, cured meats, and meat products; roasted poultry and dressing; poultry or fish salads and mixtures; raw milk; puddings; and cream-filled pastries. Any food requiring a considerable amount of handling during preparation is a possible source of staphylococcus food poisoning, particularly if it is mishandled during or after preparation.

Symptoms of the illness usually occur 2 or 3 hours after eating toxin-containing food, but the time may vary from 30 minutes to 6 hours.

Clostridium perfringens bacteria have been identified as the cause of numerous cases of food poisoning in recent years. However, the apparent increase in reported outbreaks may reflect better identification techniques and increased reporting of foodborne illnesses. Foods most often involved in outbreaks are meat and poultry products that have been cooked and held for long periods of time or that have undergone prolonged slow cooling followed by reheating to improper temperatures, and, finally, by further holding.

Clostridium perfringens bacteria are commonly found in the intestinal tracts of healthy humans and animals and in soil, water, and dust. The bacteria have the ability to form spores that are difficult to destroy by heat treatments. The growing cells in food are destroyed through cooking, but because the spores are not, cooking cannot be relied upon to remove the threat of poisoning from these bacteria. The organisms can grow over a vast range of temperatures and are so widespread that it is impossible to reduce their incidence. Consequently, either the spore or the vegetative form should be assumed to be present in foods.

In relatively little time, under anaerobic conditions at temperatures for 60 to 120°F. (15 to 49°C.), large numbers can develop. An anaerobic condition is produced in meat or meat-containing liquids when air has been eliminated by heating, thus allowing surviving spores to germinate and multiply rapidly in warm foods. Large quantities of meat broths, gravies, or meat mixtures that are permitted to cool slowly provide an ideal medium for growth.

The symptoms of *Clostridium perfringens* poisoning are relatively mild but include abdominal cramps, diarrhea, occasionally nausea, and rarely fever or vomiting. Symptoms usually begin between 8 and 22 hours after eating the contaminated food but have been observed as soon as two hours.

Preventing food poisoning from *Clostridium perfringens* requires cooking high-protein foods, particularly meat and poultry, well enough to kill the vegetative forms of the organism; keeping foods hot (above 140° F. [60° C.]) until eaten, and promptly refrigerating foods in shallow containers for quick temperature reduction to retard multiplication of vegetative forms.

OTHER FOODBORNE ILLNESSES

Although the major causes of foodborne illnesses are *Salmonella, Staphylococcus aureus*, and *Clostridium perfringens*, many other microorganisms can cause serious or severe food poisoning. Illnesses caused by these microorganims include typhoid fever; paratyphoid fever; streptococcus, shigellosis, or bacterial dysentery; and amoebic dysentery. Prevention of these illnesses requires high standards of personal cleanliness, good work habits, safe water supplies, exclusion of carriers from food preparation jobs, and proper cooking, chilling, and holding temperatures.

Botulism is an almost always fatal food poisoning. It rarely occurs when commercially canned foods are used but is a threat to home canners who do not follow recommended thermal processing procedures for low-acid vegetables and meat products. It is caused by a toxin produced by various strains of *Clostridium botulinum* that grow in low-acid foods that have not been processed at temperatures high enough to destroy the bacterial spores. Food services should purchase only commercially processed vegetables, meats, and other low-acid foods.

CHEMICAL FOOD POISONING

Food poisoning can be caused by the contamination of foods with chemicals, such as those used in insect or rodent control; cleaning compounds; herbicides or pesticide residues; heavy metals such as copper, cadmium, tin, lead, and zinc; cyanide from certain fruit pits; or silver polish. To prevent the possibility of chemical food poisoning, all toxic chemicals and cleaning compounds should be labeled carefully and stored separately from food materials. Instructions should be scrupulously followed. All fruits and vegetables that might have surface pesticide residues should be thoroughly washed, even though most producers carefully follow application limitations on their use. Copper-, tin-, or zinc-coated utensils should not be used in the preparation, storage, or service of acidic foods.

SANITATION

The Food and Drug Administration developed the Model Food Service Sanitation Ordinance (1976), which has been recommended for adoption by state and local health agencies. In addition, the Joint Commission on Accreditation of Hospitals has published standards for sanitation and safety in dietary services. These revised standards became effective in January 1979. Recommendations on food purchasing, storage, preparation, handling and holding, facilities and equipment, and employee hygiene practices are intended to ensure that sanitary food is served in food service establishments. The recommendations from both agencies, summarized in this section, are a sound basis for the development of an effective sanitation program and can serve as an outline for employee orientation and continuing training in food safety.

FOOD SUPPLIES
Every effort must be made to purchase food in a safe and sanitary condition. Some things to consider are:

- Purchases should be made from supply sources that comply with all laws related to food processing and labeling. Foods that were processed in unlicensed food processing establishments should not be used.
- Fluid milk and fluid milk products must be pasteurized and must meet the Grade A quality standards. Dry milk products should be made from pasteurized milk.
- Only USDA- or state-inspected meat and meat products, USDA-inspected poultry, poultry products, egg products, and, when possible, USDC-inspected fishery products should be purchased.
- Shellfish should be purchased from a reputable dealer who complies with regulations of state and local agencies.
- Only clean whole eggs with shells intact and without cracks or checks, or pasteurized liquid, frozen, or dried egg products should be used. Commercially prepared hard-cooked peeled eggs also can be used.
- Food products that may have been contaminated by insects, rodents, or water, and foods in cans that bulge or are severely dented should not be accepted.
- All incoming food should be inspected for quality by looking for evidence of damage to cartons, packaging, or containers from filth, water, insects, or rodents. Damaged or spoiled products, or frozen foods that show evidence of thawing or refreezing should be rejected.

STORAGE

Foods must be protected from contamination, spoilage, and other damage during storage in dry, refrigerated, or frozen states.

Dry Storage

The following steps should be observed for dry storage of foods:

- Food not requiring refrigeration should be stored in a clean, cool, dry storeroom that is well ventilated and adequately lighted. A temperature range from 50 to 70° F. (10 to 21° C.) is recommended to maintain high quality. Containers of food, except those on pallets or dollies, should be stored at least 6 inches above the floor or as local ordinances require.
- Quantity lots of cased and boxed foods are more stable for handling if stacked in alternating patterns on dollies or pallets. Smaller lots of canned or packaged foods may be stored on metal shelves in or out of the case. Stock numbering or dating is recommended to rotate stock.
- Once the original container or package of dry bulk foods (flour, sugar, cereals, beans, and so forth) has been opened, remaining products should be emptied into food grade plastic or metal containers with tight-fitting covers. Containers should be labeled clearly and stored on dollies or shelving that is at least 6 inches above the floor or as local ordinances require.
- Cleaning supplies, bleaches, insecticides, and other potentially hazardous chemicals should be labeled and stored in an area entirely separate from food and paper storage and preferably under lock and key.
- Food and containers of food should not be stored under exposed or unprotected water or sewer lines except for automatic fire protection sprinkler heads that may be required by law.
- Floors, shelving, and walls of the storeroom should be kept clean and dry at all times, with cleaning scheduled at regular intervals.
- Items most frequently needed should be located near the entrance of the storeroom.
- Heavy packages should be stored on lower shelves.

Refrigerated Storage

The following steps should be observed for refrigerated storage of foods:

- Enough conveniently located refrigeration facilities should be provided to ensure the proper maintenance of food at 45° F. (7° C.) or lower during storage. Each refrigerator should be equipped with a numerically scaled indicating thermometer, accurate to ±3° F. (±1.5° C.). The thermometer should be located in the warmest part of the unit and placed where it can be easily read, preferably from outside the refrigeration unit. Temperature records must be maintained. Recording thermometers accurate to $\pm 3°$ F. ($\pm 1.5°$ C.) may be used in lieu of indicating thermometers.

- Perishable food should be kept in a refrigerator until preparation or service time.
- Potentially hazardous food requiring refrigeration after preparation should be rapidly cooled to an internal temperature of $45°$ F. ($7°$ C.) or lower within a cooling period of not more than four hours. Such foods prepared in large quantities should be rapidly cooled, utilizing shallow pans, agitation, quick chilling, or water circulation external to the food container. Ice used for cooling stored food, food containers, or food utensils must not be used for human consumption.
- In a walk-in refrigerator, all foods should be stored above the floor on easily cleaned metal shelving or on mobile equipment. Shelves should not be covered with any materials because this reduces air circulation around food and makes cleaning more difficult.
- Cooked food should be positioned on shelves above raw food to avoid contamination.
- Food stored in refrigerators should be covered or wrapped and containers labeled and dated. Open containers of canned food may be covered and stored in the original container in the refrigerator until used.
- Dairy products should be stored separately from strong-odored foods and fish. Fruits and vegetables should be checked daily for spoilage.
- Scheduled cleaning of refrigerated storage rooms at regular intervals and a preventive maintenance program for all refrigerated equipment should be established.

Frozen Storage

The following steps should be observed for frozen storage of foods:
- Frozen food should be kept frozen and stored at a temperature of $0°$ F. ($-18°$ C.) or lower. The freezer thermometer should be checked frequently and the temperature recorded.
- All frozen food packages should be labeled and dated and should be well wrapped in moistureproof and vaporproof material to prevent freezer burn.
- Shelving, walls, and floors of freezers should be kept clean at all times. Defrosting should be done as often as necessary to eliminate excessive frost build-up. Contents should be moved to another freezer when defrosting.
- Frozen foods should be thawed in a refrigerator at a temperature not exceeding $45°$ F. ($7°$ C.) or under clean running water at a temperature not exceeding $70°$ F. ($21°$ C.). Food thawed by the latter method should be in its original waterproof package. Most frozen

foods can be cooked directly from the frozen state. Frozen foods can be thawed in a microwave oven but only when the foods will be transferred immediately to conventional cooking equipment or when the entire uninterrupted cooking process takes place in the microwave oven.

- Thawed food should be used immediately or stored in the refrigerator for a short period before use. Thawing and refreezing of foods should be avoided because of the possibility of spoilage and the loss of flavor and nutritional value.
- Frozen foods that are partially thawed may be safely refrozen if they still contain ice crystals, but the quality may be somewhat reduced. The quality of fruits, vegetables, and red meats may not be as severely affected by temperature changes as that of fish, shellfish, poultry, and cooked foods.

PREPARATION

The following steps should be observed in the preparation of food:

- Food should be prepared with the least possible manual contact, with suitable utensils, and on surfaces that have been cleaned, rinsed, and sanitized to prevent cross-contamination.
- Raw fruits and vegetables should be thoroughly washed with clean water before being cooked or served.
- Potentially hazardous foods requiring cooking should be cooked to heat all parts of the food to a temperature of at least 140° F. (60°C.), except for: (1) poultry, poultry stuffings, stuffed meats, and stuffings containing meat, which should be cooked to heat all parts of the food to at least 165° F. (74°C.) with no interruption of the cooking process; (2) pork and any food containing pork, which should be cooked to heat all parts of the food to at least 150° F. (65°C). Even though this temperature is adequate to kill trichinae, a temperature of 170° F. (77°C.) for fresh pork is recommended for product palatability; and (3) rare roast beef, which should be cooked to an internal temperature of at least 130° F. (54°C.), and rare beef steak, which should be cooked to a temperature of 130° F. (54°C.).
- Reconstituted dry milk and dry milk products may be used in instant desserts and whipped products or for cooking and baking purposes. They should not be served as beverages or in beverages because of the potential for contamination in reconstituting and dispensing such products.
- Liquid, frozen, and dry eggs and egg products are pasteurized at temperatures high enough to destroy pathogenic organisms that might be present. However, because of the possibility of recontamination of these products after opening, thawing, or reconstitution, they are recommended for use primarily in cooked or baked products.
- Nondairy creaming, whitening, or whipping agents may be recon-

stituted on the food service premises only when they will be stored in sanitized, covered containers not larger than 1 gallon and cooled to 45° F. (7° C.) or lower within 4 hours after preparation.

- Potentially hazardous foods that have been cooked and then refrigerated should be thoroughly reheated rapidly to 165° F. (74° C.) or higher before being served or before being placed in hot food storage equipment. Steam tables, bains-marie, warmers, and similar hot food holding equipment are prohibited for the rapid reheating of potentially hazardous foods.
- Metal-stem numerically scaled indicating thermometers, accurate to ±2° F. (±1° C.) should be provided and used to ensure the attainment and maintenance of proper internal cooking, holding, or refrigeration temperatures of all potentially hazardous foods.
- Separate cutting boards should be provided for meat, poultry, fish, and raw fruits and vegetables. Cooked foods should not be cut on the same board as raw products. An exception may be allowed for this requirement if nonabsorbent boards are used and are cleaned and sanitized between use for raw and for cooked foods.

DISPLAY, SERVICE, AND TRANSPORT

The following steps should be observed in the display, service, and transport of food:

- Potentially hazardous food should be kept at an internal temperature of 45° F. (7° C.) or lower or at 140° F. (60° C.) or higher during holding, display, and service.
- Milk and milk products for drinking purposes should be provided to the consumer in an unopened commercially filled package not exceeding 1 pint in capacity or should be drawn from a commercially filled container stored in a mechanically refrigerated bulk milk dispenser. When a bulk dispenser for milk and milk products is not available and portions of less than 1/2 pint are required for service, the milk products may be poured from a commercially filled container of not more than 1/2-gallon capacity.
- Cream or half-and-half should be provided in an individual service container, protected pour-type pitcher, or drawn from a refrigerated dispenser designed for such service.
- Nondairy creaming or whitening agents should be provided in an individual service container, protected pour-type pitcher, or drawn from a refrigerated dispenser.
- Condiments for self-service use should be provided in individual packages, from dispensers, or from the original containers. Seasonings and dressings for self-service use should be served in the above fashion, or from counters or salad bars that are protected from consumer contamination.
- To avoid unnecessary manual contact with food, suitable dispensing

utensils should be used by employees or provided to consumers who serve themselves. Between uses, dispensing utensils should be stored in the food or stored clean and dry, in running water, or in a running water dipper well.

- Food on display should be protected from consumer contamination by the use of packaging; by the use of an easily cleaned counter or serving line; or by the use of salad bar protector devices, display cases, or other effective means. Enough hot-holding or cold-holding equipment should be available to maintain the required temperature of potentially hazardous food.
- Reuse of soiled tableware by self-service consumers returning to the service area for additional food is prohibited. Beverage cups and glasses are not covered by this requirement.
- Once served to a consumer, portions of leftover food should not be served again except for packaged food that is still packaged and in sound condition.
- Ice for consumer use should be dispensed only by employees with scoops, tongs, or other ice dispensing utensils or through automatic self-service ice dispensing equipment. Between uses, ice transfer utensils or receptacles must be stored in a way that protects them from contamination.
- Foods in original individual packages do not need to be overwrapped or covered unless the package has been torn or broken.
- During transportation, including transport to other locations for service, foods must be held under the conditions specified for cold or hot holding.

PERSONAL HEALTH AND CLEANLINESS

It is apparent that the key to a safe and sanitary food service is healthy employees who are properly trained in safe food handling and who practice good personal hygiene. A great many cases of food poisoning are traced to human contamination of food. Constant training and supervision of food service employees should stress personal health, a clean, neat appearance, and good work habits. The healthy employee is energetic and able to perform the required duties without undue fatigue. The following should be observed by all food service employees:

- Employees who handle food should have a health examination by a physician before beginning employment and at intervals specified by public health agencies and/or the institution.
- All food service employees should be clean and well groomed; clean uniforms and/or aprons are essential. If street clothes are permitted by the institution, they should be made of washable fabrics. Appropriate hair restraints are required.
- Clean hands and fingernails are very important in food handling.

Hands should be thoroughly washed before starting work, before and after handling food, after smoking, after using the toilet, or after using a handkerchief or tissue. Conveniently located hand sinks are required; other sinks should not be used for handwashing.

- Hands should be kept away from face and mouth.
- Smoking should be permitted only in designated smoking areas and not in food preparation or service areas. Hands should be washed before returning to food preparation or serving duties.
- Hands and fingers should be kept out of food, and serving and eating utensils picked up by their bases or handles. Following this procedure prior to serving food protects the person served and, after the food has been eaten, protects the employees' hands from contamination.
- Spoons or other utensils used in preparing foods should not be used for tasting. Separate spoons and forks for tasting should be washed after each use or disposables should be used.
- Employees should consume food only in designated dining areas.
- Personal belongings should be kept out of food preparation and service areas and stored in lockers located ouside of the food service department.
- Persons other than food service employees should be discouraged from entering the kitchen.
- Employees with open lesions, infected wounds, sore throats, or any communicable disease should not be permitted to work in food preparation or service areas. The department must have a method of ensuring that food service employees are free from these hazards.

ENVIRONMENTAL SANITATION

A clean environment is a prerequisite to good sanitation practices. An up-to-date food service facility includes equipment, materials, and a layout design that facilitates easy cleaning with hot water, detergents, and sanitizing agents. Floors should be constructed with materials that do not absorb grease or moisture. An adequate number of drains, conveniently located, facilitate washing. Walls, ceilings, and ventilation equipment must be designed and constructed for frequent, thorough cleaning.

In the purchase and placement of equipment, sanitation features should be a major consideration. Equipment should be installed in a manner that allows easy removal of soil, food materials, or other debris that collects between pieces of equipment or between the equipment and walls or floor. Although older institutions may not have the advantages of new design and equipment, the food service department can be maintained effectively by careful planning, training, and supervising. Cleaning of equipment must be regularly scheduled to prevent accumulation of dirt and spilled food. Effective cleaning reduces the possibility of food contamination by microorganisms and is of particular importance in pest control.

The following practices are recommended to maintain high environmental sanitation standards:

- All work and storage areas must be clean, well lighted, and orderly.
- Overhead pipes should be eliminated or covered by a false ceiling. They are a hazard in food preparation areas because they collect dust and might leak, thus leading to possible contamination of food.
- Walls, floors, and ceilings in all areas must be cleaned routinely.
- Ventilation hoods should be designed to prevent grease build-up or condensation that collects on walls and ceilings or drips into food or on food-contact surfaces. Filters or other grease extracting equipment should be readliy removable for cleaning and replacment if they have not been designed for easy cleaning in place.
- To prevent cross-contamination, kitchenware and food-contact surfaces of equipment should be washed, rinsed, and sanitized after each use and after any interruption of operations during which contamination could occur. Manufacturers' instructions should be followed for cleaning of all equipment.
- Food-contact surfaces of grills, griddles, and similar cooking equipment plus the cavities and door seals of microwave ovens should be cleaned at least once a day. This does not apply to deep-fat cooking equipment or filtering systems. Surfaces that do not come into contact with food should be cleaned as often as necessary to keep the equipment free from accumulation of dust, dirt, food particles, and other debris.
- A ready supply of hot water (120 to 140° F. [49 to 60°C.]) must be available.
- An adequate number of containers for garbage and refuse disposal must be available, kept covered, cleaned frequently, and insectproof and rodentproof. Disposal of such materials should be in accord with local ordinances.
- At least 20 footcandles of light should be provided on all food preparation surfaces and at equipment or utensil washing stations. Protective shields to prevent broken glass from falling on to food should be provided for all lighting fixtures located over, by, or within food storage, preparation, service, and display areas, and in areas where equipment or utensils are washed and stored.
- Effective measures to minimize the presence of rodents and insects are required. The premises must be kept in a condition that prevents harboring or feeding insects and rodents. Outside openings should be protected against the entrance of insects by tight-fitting, self-closing doors, closed windows, screening, controlled air currents, or other means.

Valuable information about the operation, cleaning, and care of equipment can be obtained from manufacturers or local distributors. A file of such reference information should be maintained in the food service department and utilized in development of equipment cleaning procedures and in training employees.

Most manufacturers recommend that equipment be cleaned with mild detergent and hot water. A solution of ammonia and water is an effective means of removing grease. Heavier or burned-on soil may require use of commercial cleaners. Selection of these cleaners should be appropriate for the type of metal used in the construction of the piece of equipment. All equipment must be thoroughly rinsed with clear water to remove all traces of cleaning agents. Some generalized instructions that can be used as a guide in developing cleaning procedures for specific equipment follow:

Open-top gas range

- Wash range daily. After top grids are entirely cooled, soak them in water and a good grease solvent; remove encrusted material with a blunt scraper.
- Boil grates and burners in a solution of sal soda or other grease solvents; clean clogged burner ports with a stiff wire.
- Wash back apron and warming-oven top with a hot detergent solution to remove grease.
- Wipe iron parts with an oiled cloth to prevent rusting.

Closed-top gas range

- Wash range daily. After top plates have cooled, rub vigorously with heavy burlap or steel wool.
- Remove any grease or dirt lodged under flanges, lids, rings, or plates.
- Wash back apron and warming-oven top with a hot detergent solution to remove grease.
- Wipe iron parts with an oiled cloth to prevent rusting.

Electric range

- Wash range daily after it has cooled; use warm water and a mild detergent to remove greasy film; rinse with clear water and dry. Take care that water does not get into the electrical elements.
- Wipe surfaces made of iron with an oiled cloth to prevent rusting.

Ovens

- Do not clean oven until it is cool.
- If racks and shelves are removable, take out and clean. Remove encrusted material from them and from inside of oven with a blunt scraper or wire brush.
- Clean heat control, but do not loosen or remove dials.
- Clean outside of oven; the method will depend on the finish.

Broilers

- Allow broiler to cool before cleaning.
- Wash grid and tray after each use with hot sudsy water; remove encrusted material with a blunt scraper, wire brush, or other abrasive; rinse with clear water and dry.
- Rub with an oiled cloth to prevent rusting.

Deep-fat fryers

- Strain fat to remove sediment. Pour fat into a container, cover tightly, and store in a cool place.
- Fill fryer with a hot soap solution and boil 10 minutes. Drain off part of the solution; use the rest for cleaning the inside of the fryer with a stiff brush and scraper, if necessary. Wash baskets and strainer in sink with hot detergent solution.
- Rinse with hot, clear water to which vinegar has been added; rinse again with clear water, and dry thoroughly.
- Cover fryer when not in use.

Steam kettles

- Wash immediately after each use. If this is not possible and food particles have hardened on the surface of the kettle, close drain valve and fill with cool water; let stand until food particles are softened.
- Wash inside and outside with hot water and detergent, scour when necessary, rinse with clear water, and dry thoroughly.

Compartment steamers

- Clean daily; do not allow accumulations of food particles or hard-water scale to collect in pan.
- Wipe out water pan and interior, flush drain lines, remove shelves, and clean slides.
- To prolong gasket life, always leave compartment door ajar when steamer is not in use.
- Keep wheel screws clean; lubricate frequently but not excessively.

Mixing machines

- Wash bowl and beater after each use.
- If the material in the bowl is an egg or flour mixture, soak bowl in cold water before washing; after washing and rinsing, dry beater and bowl; store in proper place.
- Clean beater shaft and body of the machine with warm water and mild soap. Hard scrubbing and harsh soaps might remove the paint.
- Oil motor and fill grease cups as directed by manufacturer.

Food grinders

- Wash after each use.

- Remove adjustment ring, knife, and plate; wash in hot, soapy water; rinse and dry thoroughly.
- Wash, rinse, and dry other parts of grinder.

Food slicer

- Clean slicer after each use. (Caution: disconnect from power source.)
- Clean knife blade carefully, wiping away from the cutting edge of the knife and guarding it from contact with another metal surface, which could dull or nick it.
- Use hot water, mild soap, and a clean cloth to wash thoroughly the parts that have been in contact with food. Wash or wipe other parts of the machine with a damp cloth; dry thoroughly. Avoid excessively hot water or steam; too much heat can burn up the lubricants on the friction points.
- Apply special tasteless oil to all moving parts.

Vegetable peeler

- Clean daily.
- Flush inside with water to remove all parings; empty and clean the peel trap. Remove the disk and rinse the base thoroughly.
- Wipe the outside of the machine with a damp cloth.
- Inspect and oil motor and mechanical parts regularly, and make adjustments as needed.

Coffee urns

- Remove urn bag as soon as coffee is made. Wash in cold water, leaving it to soak in cold water until it is to be used again.
- Empty urn after each meal; rinse thoroughly with clear, hot water; scour with a good detergent, special urn cleaner, or baking soda to remove discoloration; rinse thoroughly, first with hot water, then with cold.
- Clean gauges once a week with a special brush.
- Keep the outside surface shiny with a good metal polish. Apply as directed and rub with a soft flannel cloth.

Toasters

- Remove crumbs from crumb tray daily, and wipe toaster case with a soft, damp cloth; if case is greasy, use a nonabrasive cleaning compound. Take care to prevent water or cleaning compound from getting into electrical elements or on conveyor chains.
- Oil mechanisms as directed by manufacturer.

Hot-holding units

- Remove containers; wash and dry.
- Clean inside and outside of each unit of hot food table; use hot water and a washing compound; rinse and dry thoroughly.

- If unit is heated by steam, drain water and remove top sections to clean.
- If unit is heated by electricity, be careful not to get water into the electrical elements.

Refrigerators
- Clean regularly at least twice a week.
- Wash shelves and walls, using warm water and a detergent; if necessary, scour with a stiff brush, rinse with a weak solution of baking soda or borax; dry thoroughly.
- Mop walk-in refrigerator floors daily. Remove drain pipes, and flush with hot water and soda frequently.
- Defrost refrigerator regularly.

Dishwashing machines
- Clean machine after each washing period, cleaning the inside thoroughly at least once each week.
- Drain water from the machine and flush the inside; remove strainer trays and clean with a stiff brush. Do not allow scraps from the trays to get into the pump. Clean the wash and rinse sprays daily; remove bits of food and sediment caught in the openings.
- Leave machine open when not in use.
- Wash dish tables with a neutral soap solution; rinse and dry after each period of use. Avoid the use of coarse abrasives that will scratch the surface of the metal.
- Consult local health officer for sanitary regulations of the locality.

CLEANING AND SANITIZING UTENSILS AND SERVICE WARE

Food protection efforts can be fruitless if the dishes, equipment, and utensils that come into contact with food are improperly cleaned and sanitized. Effective cleaning procedures must be established, employees must be well trained, and equipment must be properly operated to achieve adequate sanitation of food production equipment and service ware.

Mechanical Ware-Washing

Dishes should be prescraped or preflushed in the prerinse section of the machine or as a separate operation and pans or dishes presoaked as needed. When dishwashing machines are available, they should be used for as many pots, pans, and other cooking utensils as possible.

Spray or immersion dishwashers or devices must be installed properly and maintained in good repair. Utensils and equipment placed in the machine must be exposed to all cycles. Automatic dispensers for detergents, wetting agents, and liquid sanitizers must be properly installed and maintained. The following also should also be observed for nonmedical cleaning and sanitizing:

- The pressure of the final rinse water must be at least 15 psi (pounds per square inch) but not more than 25 psi in the waterline immediately adjacent to the final rinse control valve. The data plate attached to the machine will state the recommended pressure for that particular dishwasher.
- Machine or waterline mounted indicating thermometers must be provided to show the water temperature of each tank within the dishwasher and the temperature of the final rinse water.
- Rinse water tanks must be protected by baffles, curtains, or some other means to minimize entry of wash water into the rinse tank. Conveyors need to be timed to ensure adequate exposure times in wash, rinse, and drying cycles.
- Equipment and utensils should be placed in racks, trays, baskets, or on conveyors in such a way that food-contact surfaces are exposed to an unobstructed application of detergent wash and clean rinse waters and that also allows free draining.
- When hot water is used for sanitizing, the following temperatures must be maintained:
    a. *Single-tank, stationary rack, dual-temperature machine.* Wash temperature 150° F. (65° C.); final rinse temperature 180° F. (82° C.)
    b. *Single-tank, stationary rack, single-temperature machine.* Wash temperature and final rinse temperature 165° F. (74° C.)
    c. *Single-tank conveyor machine.* Wash temperature 160° F. (71° C.); final rinse 180° F. (74° C.)
    d. *Multitank conveyor machine.* Wash temperature 150° F. (65° C.); pumped rinse 160° F. (71° C.); and final rinse 180° F. (82° C.)
    e. *Single-tank, pot, pan, and utensil washer (stationary or moving rack).* Wash temperature 140° F. (60° C.); final rinse 180° F. (82° C.)
- When chemicals are used for sanitizing in a *single-tank, stationary-rack spray machine and glass washer*, the following minimum temperatures should be maintained: wash temperature of 120° F. (49° C.), final rinse with chemical sanitizer at 75° F. (24° C.) or not less than the temperature specified by the machine's manufacturer.
- All dishwashing machines must be thoroughly cleaned at least once a day or when necessary to maintain a satisfactory operating condition.
- When chemicals are used for sanitizing, they should be of a type approved by the health authority and should be automatically dispensed in such concentration and for a period that provides effective bactericidal treatment according to the manufacturer's specifications.
- After sanitization, all equipment and utensils must be air-dried. Drain boards of adequate size for handling of soiled and clean tableware should be provided. Mobile dish tables are permitted for these uses.

Manual Ware-Washing

The following points should be observed for manual cleaning and sanitizing:

- A sink with not fewer than three compartments must be used for manual washing, rinsing, and sanitizing of utensils and equipment. Compartments should be large enough to permit accommodation of the equipment and utensils. Hot and cold water should be provided for each compartment.
- Drain boards or easily movable dish tables of adequate size should be provided for proper handling of soiled utensils prior to washing and for cleaned utensils after sanitizing.
- Equipment and utensils should be preflushed or prescraped and, when necessary, presoaked to remove gross food particles. (Note: A fourth sink compartment with disposer is very useful for these purposes.) A fourth compartment sink should be included in plans for facilities being renovated or under new construction.
- Except for fixed equipment and utensils too large to be cleaned in sink compartments, the following sequence should be used:
  a. Wash equipment and utensils in the first sink compartment with a hot detergent solution that is changed frequently to keep it free from soil and grease.
  b. Rinse equipment and utensils with clean hot water in the second compartment, changing water frequently.
  c. Sanitize equipment and utensils in the third compartment, using one of the following methods: (1) Immersion for at least 30 seconds in clean hot water maintained at 170°F. (77°C.). A heating device is needed to maintain this temperature. A thermometer should be used to check the temperature frequently. Dish baskets should be used to immerse utensils completely. (2) Immersion for at least 1 minute in a clean solution containing at least 50 ppm (parts per million) available chlorine as a hypochlorite and at a temperature of at least 75°F. (24°C.). (3) Immersion for at least 1 minute in a clean solution containing at least 12.5 ppm available iodine and having a pH not higher than 5.0 and at a temperature of at least 75°F. (24°C.). (4) Immersion in clean solution containing any other chemical sanitizer approved by health authorities that will provide the equivalent bactericidal effect of a 50 ppm chlorine solution at 75°F. (24°C.) for one minute.
  d. All utensils and equipment should be air-dried after sanitizing.
- Equipment that is too large to immerse can be sanitized by treatment with clean steam, provided the steam can be confined within the piece of equipment. An alternative method is to rinse, spray, or

swab with a chemical sanitizing solution mixed to at least twice the strength required for immersion sanitization.

Equipment and Utensil Storage

For proper equipment and utensil storage, the following points should be observed:

- Cleaned and sanitized equipment and utensils should be handled in a way that protects them from contamination of the parts that will be used in eating or will come in contact with food.
- Cleaned and sanitized utensils and equipment should be stored at least 6 inches above the floor in a dry, clean location in a way that protects them from contamination by splashes and dust. Stationary equipment also should be protected from contamination.
- Glasses and cups should be stored in an inverted position. Other stored utensils should be covered or inverted wherever practical. Storage containers for tableware should be designed to present the handle to the employee or consumer.

SELF-EVALUATION PROGRAM

A continuous program in self-evaluation of sanitary conditions and practices is necessary to ensure day-to-day protection of all clientele served by the food service department. The major benefit from such a program is to make both management and employees aware of the advantages of maintaining a safe and sanitary operation before a serious health hazard can arise. The checklist shown in figure 15, next page, can be used as a guide to develop such a program. Local health departments can also be consulted for all questions about food sanitation for specific localities.

SANITATION CHECKLIST

Checked by: _____   Date: _____

STANDARD	Deficiency	Comments	Date Corrected
PERSONNEL			
1. Head and facial hair is covered with hairnet, cap, or other adequate restraint			
2. Uniforms and aprons are clean and neat			
3. Fingernails are short, clean, and unpolished			
4. Employees are clean, neat, and well groomed			
5. Employees are free from colds, other communicable diseases, and infected cuts or burns			
6. Employees smoke or eat only in designated areas			
7. Employees wash hands frequently at conveniently located hand sinks			
8. Disposable gloves are properly used by food handlers			
9. Medical examination schedule for employees is followed			
10. Employees wear minimal amount of jewelry			
RECEIVING			
1. Immediately upon receipt, food is inspected for spoilage or infestation			
2. Nonfood supplies are immediately inspected for infestation			
3. All food supplies are promptly moved to proper storage areas			
4. Receiving area is clean and free of food debris, boxes, cans, or other refuse			
5. Outside doors are equipped with self-closing devices and are kept closed			
6. Door openings are screened or equipped with fly fans			
DRY STORAGE			
1. Shelves are placed high enough to permit floor cleaning and to abide by local ordinances			
2. Walls, floors, and shelves are clean			

FIGURE 15. Example of a Sanitation Checklist.

STANDARD	Deficiency	Comments	Date Corrected
3. All food is stored off the floor			
4. Storage area is dry and well ventilated, and temperature is maintained lower than 70° F. (21° C.)			
5. Shelves are placed away from walls to permit ventilation and easy cleaning			
6. Opened bulk-food supplies are stored in labeled plastic or metal containers with tight-fitting lids			
7. Nonfood supplies are stored separately			
8. Potentially harmful chemicals and cleaning supplies are stored separately			
9. A properly functioning thermometer is kept in the area			
10. Empty cartons and trash are removed from the area			
11. Storage area is free from uninsulated steam and hot water pipes or other heat-producing or moisture-producing devices			

REFRIGERATOR AND FREEZER STORAGE

STANDARD	Deficiency	Comments	Date Corrected
1. Walls, floors, and shelves are constructed of easily cleaned materials			
2. Walls, floors, and shelves are free of spills and debris			
3. Properly functioning thermometers are located in each unit			
4. Proper temperatures are maintained: 45° F. (7° C.) or lower in refrigerators and 0° F. (-18° C.) or lower in freezers			
5. Foods are arranged to permit air circulation			
6. All foods are stored off the floor			
7. Cooked foods are stored above raw foods			
8. Foods are properly wrapped or covered			
9. Frost buildup is kept to a minimum			
10. Foods are dated and rotated according to standard procedures			

STANDARD	Deficiency	Comments	Date Corrected
FOOD PRODUCTION			
1. Floors, walls, and ceilings are clean			
2. Ventilation hoods are provided where needed and are free from grease and dust			
3. Adequate light fixtures are provided, guarded, and kept clean			
4. Equipment and utensils are constructed to meet National Sanitation Foundation (NSF) standards			
5. Equipment is placed to allow easy access for cleaning			
6. Inside and outside surfaces of all cooking equipment and utensils are cleaned and sanitized regularly			
7. Utensils and equipment are stored in clean, dry places at sufficient height from the floor and are protected from flies, dust, and other contaminants			
8. Foods are stored in production areas in clean, tightly closed containers			
9. Sanitary procedures are used for handling foods during processing			
10. Adequate clean cloths for production and cleaning purposes are provided			
11. Soiled towels and cloths are properly stored			
12. Dropped items or spills are picked up or cleaned up immediately			
13. Frozen foods are defrosted under refrigeration or in cold water—not at room temperature—in original wrapping			
14. If recommended by local health ordinances, disposable gloves are used to handle food			
15. After each use, preparation equipment is cleaned and sanitized			
16. After each meal, can openers are cleaned and sanitized			
17. Adequate garbage or trash			

FIGURE 15. *Continued*

STANDARD	Deficiency	Comments	Date Corrected
receptacles are conveniently located, frequently emptied, and kept clean			
18. Separate sinks are used for washing raw foods, hands, and utensils			
19. Hot-holding equipment is used to maintain food at or higher than 140° F. (60° C.)			
20. Cold-holding equipment is conveniently located and kept clean			
21. Potentially hazardous foods are not allowed to stand at room temperature longer than absolutely necessary during preparation			
22. Metal, stem-indicating thermometers are available and are used to check food temperatures during preparation and holding			
23. Pesticides, cleaning supplies, and other potentially hazardous chemicals are located to avoid possible contamination of foods			
24. Disposable ware for tasting foods, as required during production, is used by employees			
TRANSPORT			
1. Transport equipment is constructed according to NSF standards			
2. Transport containers and carts are regularly cleaned and sanitized			
3. Proper temperatures are maintained during transport: 45° F. (7° C.) or lower for cold foods and 140° F. (60° C.) or higher for hot foods			
4. Transport carts and containers for food and nonfood supplies are covered or tightly closed			
5. Cargo area for motor vehicles used for food transport is clean and free from debris and potentially hazardous materials			
DISPLAY AND SERVICE			
1. Holding equipment and service equipment are constructed according to NSF standards			
2. Equipment is cleaned and sanitized			

STANDARD	Deficiency	Comments	Date Corrected
3. Service and dining area floors and walls are clean			
4. Tables are washed and sanitized after each use			
5. Food on display is protected from contamination by packaging, protector devices, or other effective means			
6. Potentially hazardous food is held at lower than 45° F. (7° C.) or higher than 140° F. (60° C.)			
7. Temperatures are checked periodically during meal service			
8. Employees handle food with utensils or disposable gloves			
9. Suitable dispensing equipment for trays and other tableware is used			
10. Condiments for self-service use are protected from consumer contamination			
11. Milk and milk products are served in unopened, commercially filled containers or from sanitary bulk dispensers			
12. An adequate amount of tableware is provided for self-service			
13. Leftover foods are not served again			
14. Ice is properly dispensed by employees or through self-service equipment			
15. Adequate means are provided for the removal of soiled tableware by consumers or employees			
WARE-WASHING			
1. Dishwashing machines and sinks are constructed according to NSF standards			
2. Prior to washing, tableware and utensils are scraped and flushed			
3. Properly operating thermometers for each dishwasher compartment are provided			
4. Proper wash and rinse temperatures during dishwashing are maintained			
5. Proper temperatures for manual ware-washing are maintained			
6. Automatic detergent and sanitizer			

STANDARD	Deficiency	Comments	Date Corrected
dispensers operate properly			
7. Liquid sanitizers, in the proper concentration, are used where necessary			
8. All tableware and utensils are air-dried after sanitizing			
9. Employees use proper methods for handling sanitized tableware and utensils			
10. Equipment too large for immersion is sanitized by steam and chemical sanitizers			
11. Cleaned and sanitized tableware and utensils are properly stored			
12. Dishwashers and sinks are thoroughly cleaned after use			
GARBAGE, TRASH DISPOSAL, HOUSEKEEPING			
1. Adequate nonabsorbent trash/garbage containers are provided throughout the facility			
2. Containers are emptied frequently			
3. Containers are regularly washed and sanitized			
4. Garbage or trash storage area is protected from insect or rodent infestation			
5. In accordance with local ordinances, garbage and/or trash is frequently disposed			
6. Proper storage is available for brooms, mops, and other cleaning utensils outside of food production and service areas			
EMPLOYEE FACILITIES			
1. Adequate locker and rest room facilities are provided			
2. Locker areas and rest rooms are kept clean and free from odor			
3. Sanitary equipment is operational and clean			
4. Adequate supplies for rest rooms are provided			
5. Adequate receptacles for waste materials and soiled linens are provided			

Financial Management

Fiscal responsibility and accountability are a significant part of the management function in health care facilities. Because all departments are faced with providing high-quality care while controlling rising costs, a sound system of financial planning and control is essential for the operation of an efficient and effective food service department.

Such a system requires written statements of the department mission and objectives, with orderly procedures for attaining them. Furthermore, a system of records and reports is needed for timely documentation, evaluation, and control of the departmental activities and costs. Although there are many techniques for keeping records, it is essential that procedures be standardized sufficiently to permit comparison of actual departmental costs with the operating budget, both within the institution and with other institutions. As difficult economic conditions prevail, the challenge of containing costs while providing expected services will require managers to place top priority on the financial management function.

BUDGET PREPARATION

Financial management is based on the development and use of one or more organized plans. These plans, or budgets, provide administrators with useful tools for making decisions and controlling costs. Several types of budgets are used in health care institutions. These include the operating budget, the cash budget, and the capital budget for physical facilities and equipment. The operating budget is the most essential for financial management of the food service department.

Before the operating budget can be planned, clear and specific objectives about the extent and quality of service to be provided to patients and nonpatients must be established. These objectives must be compatible with and contribute to the accomplishment of the mission and objectives of the health care institution. For example, if the hospital's goals are to expand its outpatient clinic services and extend its services to the community in other ways, then the food service department must plan for provision of meals to ambulatory outpatients and develop educational programs in normal nutrition and diet modifications. After each objective has been identified, the food service administrator must analyze them within financial parameters. Resources needed to provide these services and the costs associated with each are allocated to meet department goals.

The operating budget is not only a plan of operation, but is also used as a control device for measuring actual operations against performance forecasts based on units of service. When a variance occurs between the operating budget and actual performance, management must determine the problem, identify the cause, and take the appropriate corrective action.

Financial planning demands that considerable time and resources be available. Therefore, a timetable should be established for the budgeting process. A budget developed under the pressure of time may not be accurate enough to guide operational decisions. All food service managers should have the opportunity to participate or advise in developing the budget.

Historical data used in budget preparation must be reliable for accurate forecasts of future activities and projected costs. The record keeping and reporting system may be simple or complex, depending on the amount of detailed information desired. An excellent method for budget development and the source documents needed for collection of information are described in *Preparation of a Hospital Food Service Department Budget*, developed by the American Society for Hospital Food Service Administrators and published by the American Hospital Association.

The major purpose of a well-prepared operating budget is to guide management decisions about departmental activities. Therefore, a detailed plan of work and spending projections must be outlined and broken down into monthly schedules. An example of such a schedule is shown in figure 16, next page. Data needed to complete these schedules include the following:

- Forecasted patient days and outpatient clinic visits

ANNUAL FOOD SERVICE DEPARTMENT BUDGET REPORT, 19___

	JANUARY			FEBRUARY			ANNUAL TOTAL		
	Patient (1)	Nonpatient (2)	Total (3)	Patient (4)	Nonpatient (5)	Total (6)	Patient (11)	Nonpatient (12)	Total (13)
1 Patient Days Section									
2 Patient days	2250		2250	2050		2050	22,500		22,500
3 Clinic visits		4000	4000		4100	4100		50,000	50,000
4 Meal Count Section									
5 Patient meals	6300		6300	5240		5240	77,000		77,000
6 Cafeteria meals		3,500	3,500		3,250	3,850		40,995	40,995
7 Stipend meals		600	500		405	405		6,650	6,650
8 Special-function meals		750	750		700	700		9,000	9,000
9 Other meals	-0-	-0-	-0-	-0-	-0-	-0-	-0-	-0-	-0-
10 Total meals	6300	4750	11,050	5240	4425	10,165	77,000	56,625	133,625
11 Operating Expenses Section									
12 Salary and benefit expenses	$ 6,010	$ 2,563	$ 8,573	$ 6,426	$ 2,389	$ 7,863	$ 73,458	$ 30,550	$ 104,008
13 Food expenses	6,151	4,145	10,296	5,604	3,861	9,465	73,195	44,941	124,586
14 Supply expenses	901	669	1,570	821	623	1,444	11,011	2,923	18,994
15 Other expenses	392	161	553	358	150	508	4,799	1,920	6,712
16 Total operating expenses	$ 13,454	$ 7,538	$ 20,992	$ 12,259	$ 2,021	$ 1 80	$ 164,441	$ 81,954	$ 234,295
17 Less: cash receipts	-0-	8,000	8,000	-0-	2,400	2,400	-0-	95,750	95,250
18 Net expenses of dietary operation	$ 13,454	$ (462)	$ 12,992	$ 12,259	$ (379)	$ 1,980	$ 164,441	$ (5,890)	$ 158,545
19 Statistical Indicators/Cost									
20 per Meal									
21 Salary and benefit expenses	$ 9540	$ 5396	$ 7258	$ 9540	$ 6394	$ 7735	$ 9540	$ 5395	$ 7784
22 Food expenses	.9763	.8726	.9318	.9763	.8726	.9311	.9763	.8726	.9324
23 Supply expenses	.1430	.1408	.1421	.1430	.1408	.1421	.1430	.1408	.1421
24 Other expenses	.0623	.0339	.0500	.0624	.0339	.0500	.0623	.0339	.0503
25 Total operating expenses	$ 2.1356	$ 1.5869	$ 1.8997	$ 2.1357	$ 1.5869	$ 1.8967	$ 2.1356	$ 1.5868	$ 1.9051
26 Less: cash receipts	-0-	1.6848	.7240	-0-	1.6723	.2280	-0-	1.6909	.7166
27 Net cost per meal	$ 2.1356	$ (0.0975)	$ 1.1757	$ 2.1357	$ (0.0854)	$ 1.1687	$ 2.1356	$ (0.1041)	$ 1.1865
28 Net cost per patient day	$ 5.98	$	$ 5.97	$ 5.98	$	$ 5.90	$ 5.98	$	$ 500
29 Productivity Indicators									
30 Meals per hours — paid	5.00	8.80	6.14	4.99	8.30	6.02	4.99	8.78	6.09
31 Meals per hours — worked									
32 Meals per patient day	2.8			2.8			2.8		
33									
34									
35									

FIGURE 16. Example of a Food Service Department Operating Budget

- Forecasted patient meals and nonpatient meal equivalents (units of service)
- Total wage, salary, and fringe benefit expense for food service department employees
- Total patient and nonpatient food expense, broken out into major food purchase categories
- Total cost of supplies
- Total of all other direct and/or allocated expenses

In order for these data to be meaningful and useful in measuring department performance, unit-of-service costs have to be calculated. These unit-of-service costs include the labor, food, supply, and any other costs per patient meal and nonpatient meal equivalent.

As the budget is prepared, projected costs should be adjusted to reflect predicted inflationary pressures on labor, food, supply, and other expenses. During the actual budget period, projections also may need to be revised if economic conditions fluctuate from forecasted performance. This does not reduce its value as a basis for control, rather it indicates that management is aware of operational performance and business trends.

BUDGET CONTROL

If the service and financial goals described in the budget are going to be attained, managers need to implement controls throughout every aspect of the food service operation. Because the menu affects the total operation, it is the starting point for financial control. In the menu, food variety, form, and quality are determined. The combination of menu items and their complexity affect labor costs. Equipment use and, to some extent, the cost of equipment operation are also affected by the menu.

The budget provides the manager with the estimated average food cost per meal. That estimated cost is the target figure to use in menu planning. Although it is not usually possible to have the cost of each meal match the target, the average cost of meals for the menu planning period should match the budgeted food cost as closely as possible. In order to balance the costs of planned menus, it is necessary to use precosted standard recipes that are kept up to date with price changes. Cycle menus also save management time in menu planning and control processes (see chapter 6).

Purchasing control procedures emphasize the use of the planned menu and meal forecasts to determine quantities of food needed, the use of specifications in buying all food products, and competitive bid purchasing. Thorough receiving procedures and adequate records are needed to verify receipt of the ordered quantity and quality of items. Methods for providing inventory security and for controlling food issues to the kitchen are essential components of the total control system. Food spoilage during storage can be decreased or prevented by ensuring proper storage conditions and rotating stock. The financial losses resulting from ineffective receiving and poor storage can be prevented but very often are overlooked (see chapter 7).

Food production is another key area for cost and quality control. A common cause of increased food costs is overproduction of food, which results in leftovers that may not be acceptable for service at a later time. Accurate forecasting is vital and can be aided by the use of cycle menus. The use of a central ingredient room or ingredient area where all food ingredients are weighed or measured in the quantities needed for the day's production has been very successful in preventing overproduction or underproduction. Daily production schedules that assign preparation tasks to specific employees and state amounts of each food item to be prepared make it possible to balance work load and use labor skills to their best advantage. Production schedules can aid in protecting and enhancing food quality by scheduling cooking times in a manner that avoids excessive holding of foods. Standard recipes and procedures must be used for effective control of the production processes. Prior to serving the food, supervisory personnel should check the quality and temperature of all products against the departmental standards. Also, effective portion control procedures should be used (see chapter 8).

Personnel utilization is another key element in a financial control system. Employees need to be trained and motivated to follow procedures management has established for cost and quality control. Employees can learn to be cost conscious if they are trained in the ways to eliminate unnecessary waste, in the use of standardized recipes, in the use of scales and other measuring equipment, and in portion control. They should have cost information on the products with which they work so they can appreciate the economic value of each item. Involving employees in developing more efficient work methods, streamlining time-consuming jobs, and evaluating product quality helps build a spirit of teamwork and acceptance and at the same time increases department productivity. Staffing and scheduling patterns that make the best use of labor time are important means of controlling labor costs (see chapter 2).

Operating and maintenance costs merit attention by management, particularly in the energy cost area. Energy conservation programs are being set up in many health care institutions. Reducing energy waste in the food service department may require retraining of employees, rescheduling of activities, improved equipment maintenance, and retrofitting or replacement of older equipment. Such efforts can result in a long-range decrease in energy use and a slower increase in utility cost. The interaction of equipment and space usage with labor efficiency should be carefully reviewed, with productivity considerations in mind. Careful review of equipment maintenance costs may indicate the need for equipment replacement, more emphasis on proper equipment operation, or a more effective preventive maintenance program (see chapter 9).

FINANCIAL RECORDS AND REPORTS

Successful financial management requires a system of records and reports that present information in the best possible way. A health care facility cannot afford any more record keeping than is absolutely necessary in order to inform management of its financial status at any given time. The system selected should meet the specific needs of the individual institution and should provide usable information for evaluating and controlling department expenditures.

The types and numbers of records needed in order to determine food service costs and the methods for allocating these costs to the various services provided by the food service department must be determined. The American Society for Hospital Food Service Administrators suggests the following system for accurately determining and allocating costs to patient and nonpatient activities.

Several kinds of data must be generated and recorded on a daily, weekly, and/or monthly basis by the food service department. Although the actual monthly performance reports may be prepared by the accounting department, they should be verified for accuracy by the food service administrator. The information needed for completing the reports includes:

- Records of meals served to patients and nonpatients
- Purchasing, receiving, inventory, and issuing records
- Production forecasts and usage records
- Labor records
- Overhead, supply, and miscellaneous cost records
- Revenue from patient and nonpatient sources

DAILY CENSUS OF MEALS SERVED

All institutions should keep a daily count of the number of meals served to patients and nonpatients. The nonpatient meal count can be broken down into other subgroups, such as staff, employees, special functions, catered meals, and so forth, depending on the system of charges for meals served. The most accurate method of obtaining the number of patient meals served is to actually count the number of trays prepared each meal and the total for the day. However, because this can be time-consuming, a survey can be conducted over time to determine an average of the number of trays served. This average is then multiplied by the midnight census less newborns to find the total number of patient meals served for a day. The averaging method is the least accurate for cost allocation but may be used for budget preparation.

The methods used for obtaining the number of nonpatient meals served each day vary from one institution to another, depending on whether they are on a cash system or, as in some facilities, whether employees purchase a monthly meal card. The suggested method for a pay cafeteria is to determine the average selling price of a full noontime meal that would include meat, potato, vegetable, salad, beverage, and dessert (see Drake reference in Bibliography). When a selective menu is offered, the average price of each meal component should be used in the calculation. Once this has been determined, the average price per meal can be divided into the total cash sales to determine the daily meal equivalent.

FOOD COSTS

Purchasing, receiving, inventory, and issuing records are used to determine monthly raw food costs. Data needed from these records are the cost of foods purchased and the value of physical inventories at the beginning and end of the month. Adding the invoices together gives the total cost of purchases for the month; the physical inventory figures are needed to determine the food actually consumed. The following steps are involved in determining the total cost of food used during the month:

1. Total the value of the beginning-of-the-month inventory (including that in storage and in the kitchen).
2. Add total purchases during month (total of invoices paid during month).
3. Subtract value of inventory at end of month (total physical inventory plus stock in kitchen).

The value of the kitchen inventory may be eliminated if the amount on hand is fairly small, has a frequent rate of turnover, or is just too time-consuming to calculate. Although other methods of food cost accounting can be used, time and accuracy are two important factors to consider.

Once the total food cost has been determined, it can be expressed as food cost per meal equivalent, as shown by the daily census of meals served. However, this calculation only indicates the average cost of all meals served. Management should be concerned with the cost per meal for each group served; thus, a method is needed to allocate costs easily and accurately. The simplest method is based on patient and nonpatient meal count information. A ratio of the two types of meals served should be determined and the cost assigned accordingly.

In addition to total food costs, management also may want them broken down into food group categories such as meat, fish, poultry, and eggs; dairy products; fresh produce; frozen goods; bakery goods; and groceries. These cost breakdowns are useful in evaluating the nutritional contributions for dollars spent and for detecting month-to-month fluctuations that may need corrective action. For example, a decrease in the average amount spent for meat, fish, and poultry items may indicate that meals served were low in these foods. A considerable increase might reflect a rise in market prices, over which the manager had no control, or the too frequent use of expensive meat cuts. Small month-to-month variations are normal, but wide divergences point to a need for investigation by management for possible corrective action.

Sometimes it is desirable to have food costs calculated more often than once a month. If day-to-day figures are wanted, the form shown in figure 17, below, can be kept. The value of these figures should be considered in relation to the time and effort expended in keeping them and the fact that daily costs are even less exact than weekly or monthly costs because of variations in patterns for purchases and usage. However, the record does reflect the approximate costs per day and provides monthly total purchase and cost figures that can be used in preparing the monthly performance report, which is then compared with the budget. Computer-assisted inventory and accounting systems can provide weekly or even daily food cost data with relative ease.

	Total Purchases				Issues from Storeroom	Net Food Cost		
							To Date	
Day	To Kitchen	To Storeroom	Cost Today	Cost To Date		Today (2 + 6)	Actual	Budgeted
(1)	(2)	(3)	(4)	(5)	(6)	(7)	(8)	(9)
1								
2								
3								
4								
30								
31								
Total								

DAILY FOOD COSTS

Month _____ Year _____

FIGURE 17. Example of a Form for Daily Food Costs, by Month.

Other aspects of food costs that should not be overlooked are the cost of food stocked on patient floors and nourishments served from the kitchen. Periodically, a count of all items sent to patient floors should be recorded and costs assigned. Total costs of these items is then divided by patient days for that period to determine the average cost of floor-stocked food per patient day. The costs of other nourishments not stocked on patient floors are usually considered a part of the patient food cost and are not treated separately in the accounting process.

LABOR COSTS

Payroll records can povide a convenient source of labor cost data. A form such as the one illustrated in figure 18, next page, can be used to record labor hours worked and paid on a monthly basis. In some cases, institutions may prefer reporting by week or by pay period; either offers the advantage of a fixed number of days, so that comparisons of labor hours and costs are simpler. However, monthly reporting has the chief advantage of relating labor costs to the other costs that are reported and summarized by month. Figure 18 also provides a convenient record of overtime, sick days, and absenteeism.

Labor costs must be distributed to patient and nonpatient meals, using, in most cases, the same ratio used to allocate food costs. It will be possible to allocate the hours and costs of some employees directly to either function if their work time is exclusively spent in that area. Periodic time studies can be used to verify the accuracy of ratio apportionment of labor costs expended in combined patient and nonpatient functions.

Analysis of labor costs not only is necessary to determine total cost per meal and per patient day but also can indicate areas of inefficiency and possibilities for improvement in the operation. The efficiency of labor utilization can be more precisely evaluated by calculating productivity statistics each month and comparing them with those for past months or for other institutions. Productivity statistics may include:

- Patient trays served per patient day
- Labor minutes per patient meal
- Labor minutes per nonpatient meal equivalent
- Revenue generated per full-time equivalent employee assigned to nonpatient meal service
- Number of customer transactions for each full-time equivalent employee assigned to nonpatient meal service
- Total department employee work hours per patient day
- Total department employee work minutes spent to produce a unit of service (patient trays plus nonpatient meal equivalents)

Changes in productivity statistics may indicate the need to change operating procedures or staffing. When such indicators are calculated on a regular monthly basis and analyzed promptly, management can effect the indicated changes in a timely fashion while keeping the operation moving toward accomplishment of financial goals.

SUPPLY COSTS

Expenses for nonfood supplies, such as china, glassware, eating utensils, kitchen utensils, disposables, cleaning compounds and equipment, printed forms, and other office supplies, and for replacement of minor equipment can be controlled to some extent. Procedures for purchasing, requisitioning, inventory, and stock control are the same for these items as for food

Labor Hour and Cost Record

Date _____

Number of Working Days _____

Employee Classification and Number	Total Hours					Total Pay ($)			
	Worked		Not Worked			Worked		Not Worked	Fringe Benefits
	Regular	O/T	Sick	Vac.	Hol.	Regular	O/T		
Tray-Line Employees (701)									
Smith	112	11	8		8	364.00	53.63	52.00	91.00
Johnson	104	—	4		8	338.00	—	39.00	84.50
First Cook (900)									
Jensen	160	—	—	12	—	880.00	—	66.00	220.00
Monthly Total									
Daily Average									

FIGURE 18. Example of a Form for Labor Cost Analysis.

supplies. Cost and quantities used are also determined in the same way, using beginning inventory, purchases, and closing inventory. If desired, records can be kept and information reported by types of commodities rather than by total supplies only.

Whenever possible, all supply costs should be distributed directly to the unit that uses them. The same ratio used to determine patient and nonpatient costs for food and labor can be used. For some supplies, such as cleaning compounds, the distribution can be based on a ratio of square footage.

REVENUES

Revenue sources for the food service department are patient meals, usually handled by a noncash transfer in the institution's business office, and cash receipts from nonpatient meals served in the cafeteria, catered events, and vending operations.

Whenever cash is handled in the department, careful control procedures must be used. Basic control principles when handling cash include the following:

- Cash is frequently collected from registers and cashiers and is deposited in a safe by a designated supervisor.
- Receipts are banked daily.
- Cash receipts, as shown on the cash register, are matched with the cash on hand at frequent, specified intervals by a person other than the cashier. (Recommendations include not allowing the cashier to see the beginning and ending register readings and making surprise additional audits.)
- An electronic or electric register that is sufficiently sophisticated to provide sales data on specific items or groups of items is used. (The greater capabilities of electronic registers for analysis and control make them highly desirable for large operations.)
- Catering income is controlled through the use of appropriate documentation of orders and charges, along with proper handling of receipts.

In some institutions, vending machines are used to provide food and beverage service on a 24-hour basis. Although ownership and operation of the machines are frequently handled by an outside contractor, there is potential for substantial profit to the institution by self-operation. Managing a vending machine operation should be carefully explored by the food service administrator.

All revenues generated through patient charges, nonpatient sales, and so forth must be accounted for using approved reporting techniques of the institution. Revenue and expense data are prepared so that unit-of-service costs and profit or nonprofit figures can be analyzed to determine whether patient costs are subsidizing nonpatient meals.

FOOD SERVICE PERFORMANCE REPORT

Hospital: __MEMORIAL__
Period: __W/E 1-25-1978__
Prepared by: __MRS. GREEN__

Meal count		Current week	Percentage (7) of total	Year-to-date meals
Patient meals	(1)	5848	60 %	$
Cafeteria meals	(2)	2754	%	
Free meals	(3)	477	%	
Special-function meals	(4)	606	%	
Other meals	(5)	-0-	%	
Total meals	(6)	9485	%	

Labor cost

		Patient service	Nonpatient service	Other	Total labor	Year-to-date labor
Patient service direct	(8)	$3,584	$ 954		4,538	$
Nonpatient service direct	(9)	1,500	1,000		2,600	
Allocated labor	(10)					
Total labor cost	(11)	$5,084	1,954		$7,038	$
Total labor hours	(12)	1,136	437		1,573	

Total
full-time equivalents (13) 39.3
Total labor hours = 39.3
1,573 ÷ 40 hours = 39.3

Food and supply costs

Food costs

		Meat, fish, and poultry	Fresh produce	Frozen	Groceries	Milk and dairy	Bakery	Total food	Year-to-date food
Beginning inventory	(14)	$ 2,070	$	$1,095	$2,259	$	$	$8,944	$
Purchases	(15)	1,988	242	1,563	3,018	741	531	8,063	
Ending inventory	(16)	1,485		894	2,667			10,038	
Gross cost	(17)	$2,563	$242	$1,774	$3,610	$741	$531	$8,459	$
Percentage	(17a)	31 %	2 %	21 %	31 %	9 %	6 %	100%	%

Less nourishments (18) 455
Less transfers (19) 245
Net food cost (20) 8,751

Supply costs

	Disposables	Cleaning supplies	China, silver and utensils	Other	Total supplies	Year-to-date supplies
Beginning inventory	$ 1,337	$ 306	$ 2,093		$3,736	$
Purchases	213	350	50		613	
Ending inventory	535	483	2,087		3,103	
Gross cost	$1,017	$173	$56		$1,246	$
Percentage	81 %	14 %	5 %	0 %	100 %	%

Less transfers (19a) 20
Net supply cost (21) $1,226

Net food cost × __60__ % Patient meals and nourishments = Patient food cost = (22) $ __5,106__   Net supply cost × __60__ % Patient meals = Patient supply cost (23) $ __736__

Recap

	Patient costs					Nonpatient costs				
	This period	Cost per meal	Budget cost per meal	Year-to-date total	Year-to-date cost per meal	This period	Cost per meal	Budget cost per meal	Year-to-date total	Year-to-date cost per meal
Labor	(24) $	$	$	$	$	$	$	$	$	$
Food	(25)									
Supplies	(26)									
Total	(27) $	$	$	$	$	$	$	$	$	$
Less revenue received	(28)									
Net cost	(29) $	$	$	$	$	$	$	$	$	$

Patient meals/man-hour _____ (30)   Nonpatient meals/man-hour _____ (31)

Remarks

FIGURE 19. Example of a Performance Report Form for Cost Summarization.

MONTHLY PERFORMANCE REPORT

After all the individual cost categories have been determined for the month, it is helpful to prepare a summary form, which includes all pertinent operational data, for management analysis. The food service performance report shown in figure 19, opposite page, is an example of a comprehensive and useful monthly summary that provides a means for comparing current costs from one month to the next against budgeted goals. If cost allocations have been properly made, the true costs of patient and nonpatient meals will be shown. Variances in month-to-month costs and revenues should be carefully analyzed. Differences not explained by similar changes in patient census or nonpatient meal counts should be carefully reviewed. Some changes can be controlled; others cannot. For example, a decrease in patient meals served without changes in labor hours worked will result in an increased labor cost per meal. This may be an uncontrollable cost difference over the short run. However, if this persists, management should seek ways to decrease labor hours.

The specific figures illustrated in this chapter are shown only as examples. Each institution can adapt them to suit its own needs. However, it will be easier to compare operating data among institutions if consistent reporting forms are used. For that reason, the procedures and forms developed by the American Society for Hospital Food Service Administrators are highly recommended.

Managing
a
Nutrition
System

The reason for the existence of a food service department in a health care facility is to provide a system for supplying nutritionally adequate and appetizing meals to patients or residents. And not only is mealtime a time to receive nutrients, but, perhaps more important, it is an anticipated event that plays a big part in the morale of clientele. Many food service departments also place a high priority on providing appealing food to personnel as a convenience and to increase morale and productivity. Furthermore, a good food service department can be a strong positive force for effective public relations inside and outside the institution.

Within the food service department's general objectives are several objectives that are more specific:

- To meet the nutritional needs of patients or residents as appropriate for their specific health conditions
- To provide nutrition education and encourage positive attitudes toward nutrition
- To provide meals that enhance the patients' or residents' satisfaction with the institution
- To carry out regulations of voluntary and regulatory agencies, state and federal agencies, and other voluntary organizations as appropriate

How the operation accomplishes these objectives depends on how informed management is and how coordinated the use of its resources are. To survive and succeed in today's social and economic setting, the food service department not only must contribute to the institution's overall health care goals but also must stay within budget allocations. Planning a good menu is the first step toward reaching these goals. One of the key factors in planning menus for health care facilities is the food service manager's knowledge of both normal and therapeutic nutrition.

NUTRITION AND HEALTH

Most Americans take eating for granted. Emphasis is on choosing foods that taste good or are fun to eat, rather than on eating to survive. Without the right foods, however, good health cannot be maintained for long; nutrition is important to health. Few babies would be born healthy if their mothers were malnourished. The babies born might not grow to their full potential if they were not fed properly. Malnourished children and adults would probably suffer from frequent infections or other illnesses, the expected life span would decrease, and productivity of the population would diminish. Fortunately, most Americans do have a choice of many foods that provide good nutrition. However, they must make the right choices.

Nutrients are the basic components of food that our bodies need to remain healthy and food can supply all these nutrients. Menus should be planned carefully so that the foods listed meet the nutritional needs of the persons served. The major nutrients in food are fats, proteins, carbohydrates, minerals, vitamins, and water. The amount of each nutrient required varies with a person's age and sex. A brief description of the function of these major nutrients and some of their chief food sources follows.

Fats provide energy to the body for physical activity and also for vital body functions such as breathing and maintaining a normal temperature. Fats are a component of certain tissues in the body. Fats are composed of units called fatty acids. One of these fatty acids, linoleic acid, cannot be manufactured by the body and must be obtained from food. For this reason, it is called an essential fatty acid.

A layer of fatty tissue under the skin helps to insulate the body, and the fatty tissue surrounding the heart and kidneys provides a cushion that protects them from physical injury. Good sources of fats are butter, cream, margarine, vegetable oil, lard, meat fat, poultry fat, fish fat, nuts, and chocolate. The energy from fats is measured in calories. Fats yield 9 calories per gram (30 g.=1 oz.).

Proteins are basic materials of every cell in all body tissues—muscles, bone, skin, blood—and are vital for growth, repair, and maintenance of these tissues. Protein also can be used for energy if the body is short of energy from other sources. Protein requirements are high during the periods of rapid growth in childhood and adolescence. During pregnancy, a woman needs extra protein to build the tissues of the unborn child. Breast milk is high in protein, so during lactation a woman requires additional protein. During convalescence, especially after surgery or injury, the body requires extra protein for building new tissues or repairing damaged ones.

Proteins are made up of units called amino acids, which are linked together. Amino acids can be compared to letters in the alphabet. The body links amino acids in a specific sequence to form a specific protein tissue in the body just as letters are arranged to form words. The body must have the right amino acids in the right amounts to form the protein for specific body tissues. If the amino acids are not available, a protein cannot be formed just as a word cannot be formed if all the letters are not available.

The body can make some amino acids by using the chemical components of carbohydrate and fat, but the body must get other amino acids preformed from food. These amino acids are called indispensable, or essential, amino acids. If a food provides a variety of indispensable amino acids in a substantial amount, then it is considered high-quality protein. Good sources of high-quality protein are animal products, such as milk, eggs, lean meat, poultry, fish, and cheese. Dried peas, beans, nuts, peanut butter, enriched cereals, flour, breadstuffs, and baked goods offer some protein, but of lesser quality because they are missing some of the indispensable amino acids. These foods can be used in addition to the high-quality protein that must be included in the diet. If used for energy, proteins yield 4 calories per gram.

Carbohydrates also supply energy. Chief sources of carbohydrates are sugar, honey, syrup, flour, cereals, and potatoes. Secondary sources are beans, peas, lentils, fruits, and vegetables, which contain carbohydrates in various amounts. Carbohydrates provide 4 calories per gram.

Minerals are essential to life and health because they are needed in the chemical reactions that allow the body to get energy from carbohydrates, fats, and proteins, as well as in other body functions. Many are needed in trace amounts only and are provided by a diet adequate in other nutrients. Careful planning may be required, however, to ensure sufficient amounts of calcium and iron, two of the minerals that are deficient in the diets of many Americans. Calcium is needed for proper bone and tooth formation, muscle function, and blood clotting. Iron is an important part of the red blood cells. It is found primarily in hemoglobin, the oxygen-carrying protein of the blood.

Two minerals that may be deficient in the diet are iodine and fluorine. Both of these minerals are found mainly in sea water. They are abundant in any soil that is near or was at one time under sea water. A deficiency of iodine causes goiter, an enlargement of the thyroid gland at the front of the neck. Iodine deficiency can cause mental retardation, stunted growth in children, and slowed metabolism at all ages. Areas of the United States that border the St. Lawrence Seaway and the Great Lakes have soil that is deficient in iodine. Therefore, it is recommended that iodized salt be used by persons living in those regions. At one time, goiter was common in those areas, but today, it is rarely seen as the result of iodine deficiency. This is due not only to the use of iodized salt but also to the fact that seafood and other foods grown in soil rich in iodine are transported and readily available all over the United States.

Fluorine is necessary for proper bone formation and to prevent tooth decay. It is found naturally in some water supplies but not in many foods. Because it is not found in many sources, it is best added to a medium consumed by everybody. Fluoridation of community water supplies is the method most widely used in the United States since the 1940s.

Other essential minerals are zinc, selenium, manganese, copper, molybdenum, cobalt, and chromium. These minerals are needed only in extremely small amounts and are rarely lacking in the normal or balanced diet of a typical American.

Sodium is important for maintaining muscle function and correct chemical composition of blood. However, sodium is one of the few nutrients Americans often must limit in their diet. Americans often have too high an intake of sodium because they have learned to like the taste of table salt. Table salt used in cooking or added to food at the table is usually the most important source of sodium. Sodium is found in most foods in varying amounts. Some physical conditions require a reduced intake of sodium. In these cases, salt and foods high in sodium content are reduced in the diet.

Vitamins are the essential components of food that aid in the regulation of body processes, in the conversion of fat into energy, and in the formation of body tissues. There are several vitamins that may be lacking in the diet of typical Americans. They are vitamins A, C, and the B complex (thiamin, riboflavin, and niacin) vitamins. Vitamin A is needed to keep skin and eyes healthy. It also helps to keep mucus-secreting tissues, such as those lining the mouth and nose, healthy. A lack of vitamin A may mean eyes cannot adjust when going from bright to dark places. This is called night blindness because the problem is most noticeable at night.

Vitamin C helps keep connective tissue in the body healthy. Bleeding gums and bruising easily are the most common signs of a lack of vitamin C.

Thiamin, riboflavin, and niacin work as a team in the chemical reactions that release energy from carbohydrates, proteins, and fats. A lack of these vitamins can cause a combination of symptoms. Skin may become dry, dark in color, and sensitive to the sun. Tissue in and around the mouth may become inflamed and sore. Because these also are symptoms of other medical problems, care must be taken to identify the true cause of the symptoms. In many cases, they are not at all related to nutrition.

Vitamin D is an unusual substance. It functions with calcium to help maintain strong bone and tooth structure. A few foods are natural sources of the vitamin, but the most important sources are fortified foods. The body also has a chemical substance similar to vitamin D in the skin that can be converted to vitamin D by exposure to direct sunlight. Recent scientific research has shown that there are several chemical compounds that may act like vitamin D in some respects, but only the chemical compound labeled vitamin D_3 can function in all the activities of vitamin D. This compound is the form that should be listed on the label of fortified foods.

Table 1, next page, lists various food sources of minerals.

Water is often the forgotten nutrient. Our bodies can usually regulate water intake well through the thirst mechanism. Thirst is the body's signal that it needs more fluid. We satisfy that need by drinking some sort of fluid until we are no longer thirsty. Water is important to the body for several reasons: it is involved, along with other nutrients, in the chemical reactions in the body; it helps to maintain the proper chemical composition of blood and is necessary for eliminating waste products from the body through the kidneys; and it regulates body temperature by its intake and loss from evaporation through the skin (sweating or perspiration).

Water balance can be a problem if a person cannot respond to thirst normally. This may be true in infants, very young children, and the elderly. Certain medical problems also cause a problem with water balance. Vomiting and diarrhea may cause excessive water (fluid) loss. If a person's kidneys are not functioning properly, they often retain fluid. Some persons may have to restrict fluid intake if their hearts are unable to pump the normal fluid load in blood. Certain medication, such as diuretics, also may change water balance.

Normally about 500 milliliters of fluid are lost through perspiration every 24 hours. Another 1 to 2 liters of urine are produced in the same period. To maintain normal fluid balance, intake should equal the combined losses, or 1,500 to 2,500 milliliters, which is equivalent to about 8 cups of fluid per day.

VARIATION IN NUTRIENT NEEDS

Everyone needs the same nutrients, although the amounts needed vary according to age and sex. The needs of children and teenagers per pound of body weight are higher than those of adults, because of the growing process. Similarly, nutrient needs of pregnant or nursing women are high in order to provide for the needs of the growing fetus or infant. As growth ends in adulthood, nutrient needs, and especially caloric needs, decrease.

Scientists from the Food and Nutrition Board of the National Research Council, National Academy of Sciences, have evaluated research on the

TABLE 1: FUNCTIONS AND FOOD SOURCES
OF VITAMINS AND MINERALS

Nutrient	Function	Food Source
Calcium	Helps maintain bone and tooth structure, blood clotting properties, and muscle function.	Dairy products, such as milk (whole, 2% or skim, evaporated), cheese, ice cream, yogurt. Less important sources are leafy green vegetables (collard greens, spinach, dandelion greens).
Iodine	Aids normal function of thyroid gland.	Ocean fish, vegetables grown in soil close to an ocean, and iodized table salt.
Fluorine	Helps maintain bone and tooth structure.	Fluoridated water.
Sodium	Maintains correct chemical composition of blood, muscle function, and bone structure.	Table salt, seasoned salt, canned soup, snack foods (potato chips, pretzels, and corn chips), cured meats, canned vegetables, mustard, catsup, Worcestershire sauce, and steak sauce. Note: Almost all foods contain some sodium. Many are preserved with a sodium-containing compound.
Vitamin A	Aids normal adaptation of eye to darkness and maintains normal skin and mucous secreting tissues.	Deep green and yellow fruits and vegetables, such as carrots, yellow squash, tomatoes, cantaloupe, dandelion greens, collard greens, sweet potatoes; vitamin A fortified milk; and liver.
Vitamin C	Maintains normal connective tissue.	Citrus fruits (oranges, grapefruit, lemons, limes), broccoli, collard greens, mustard greens, cauliflower, cantaloupe, strawberries, orange juice, grapefruit juice, and tomato juice.
Thiamine Riboflavin Niacin	All participate in chemical reactions that release energy from proteins, fats, and carbohydrates.	Meats, poultry, fish, dried peas and beans, nuts, whole grain and enriched bread, cereals, and flour. Pork is particularly high in thiamine. Milk is particularly high in riboflavin.
Vitamin D	Aids good bone and tooth formation and is important in body's use of calcium.	Vitamin D fortified milk, eggs, liver, and fish liver oil. These foods contain limited amounts of vitamin D.

nutrient needs of the human body. As a result of their work, the Recommended Daily Dietary Allowances (RDAs) have been published. The RDAs are specific amounts of energy (calories), proteins, vitamins, and minerals recommended to meet the daily needs of practically all healthy persons in the United States. (The phrase *practically all healthy persons* is used because statistically there is always a chance that someone in the population is unique and requires slightly different amounts of nutrients.) The RDAs are revised approximately every five years as new research is completed. Table 2, pages 124-127, shows the RDAs for 1980.

Because it would be very time consuming to evaluate a menu by calculating the nutrient content of each food item and then comparing the total amount of each nutrient in the menu with the RDA, nutritionists have devised a simpler system for evaluating nutrient intake. Most foods can be grouped into one of five different categories according to the nutrient content of the food. The four groups usually referred to as the *basic four* are: meat, milk, fruits and vegetables, and breads and cereals. A fifth food group includes foods high in calories, such as fats and sweets, which are low in essential nutrients. This grouping system could be called the recommended daily guide to good eating.

Table 3, page 129, summarizes how many servings persons of different age groups should have and includes recommendations for pregnant and lactating women. If this guide is followed, nutrient needs should be met. Nutritionally adequate menus can be planned using this system for various age groups. The milk and dairy product group provides calcium, vitamin D, thiamin, riboflavin, niacin, and protein; the meat and meat substitute group supplies protein, fat, B-vitamins, and iron; the fruits and vegetables group provides the major sources of vitamins A and C; and breads and cereals provide a major source of carbohydrates, iron, and B-vitamins. The fifth group is labeled *other* and includes foods that are high in calories but low in nutrients (empty calorie foods). In order to meet nutrient needs, foods should be chosen from the first four (basic four) good groups in adequate amounts before foods from the fifth group are added to meet energy needs.

There is a difference in the number of servings from the milk group recommended for various ages and for pregnant and lactating women. This corresponds to the increased needs for protein, calcium, and vitamin D during periods of growth. If the minimum number of servings is chosen from the basic four food groups, the total calorie count will be 1,000 to 1,500 per day. This is a rather low calorie level and would be a good basis for a nutritionally adequate weight reduction diet.

PLANNING THE NORMAL DIET

Many persons in health care institutions and long-term care facilities follow an unrestricted diet. Such a diet is often called a general, regular,

TABLE 2. RECOMMENDED DAILY DIETARY ALLOWANCES,[a] REVISED 1980

Category	Age, years	Weight kg.	Weight lb.	Height cm.	Height in.	Protein, g.	Vitamin A, µg. RE[b]	Vitamin D, µg.[c]	Vitamin E, mg. αTE[d]
						Fat-Soluble Vitamins			
Infants	0.0-0.5	6	13	60	24	kg. × 2.2	420	10	3
	0.5-1.0	9	20	71	28	kg. × 2.0	400	10	4
Children	1-3	13	29	90	35	23	400	10	5
	4-6	20	44	112	44	30	500	10	6
	7-10	28	62	132	52	34	700	10	7
Males	11-14	45	99	157	62	45	1000	10	8
	15-18	66	145	176	69	56	1000	10	10
	19-22	70	154	177	70	56	1000	7.5	10
	23-50	70	154	178	70	56	1000	5	10
	51+	70	154	178	70	56	1000	5	10
Females	11-14	46	101	157	62	46	800	10	8
	15-18	55	120	163	64	46	800	10	8
	19-22	55	120	163	64	44	800	7.5	8
	23-50	55	120	163	64	44	800	5	8
	51+	55	120	163	64	44	800	5	8
Pregnant						+30	+200	+5	+2
lactating						+20	+400	+5	+3

[a]Source: Food and Nutrition Board, National Academy of Sciences-National Research Council. The allowances are intended to provide for individual variations among most normal persons as they live in the United States under usual environmental stresses. Diets should be based on a variety of common foods in order to provide other nutrients for which human requirements have been less well defined.

[b]RE = retinol equivalent. 1 RE = 1 µg. retinol or 6 µg. carotene.

[c]As cholecaloiferol. 10 µg. cholecaloiferol = 400 IU vitamin D.

[d]αTE = α tocopherol equivalent. 1 αTE = 1 mg. d-α-tocopherol.

Category	Age, years	Weight kg.	lb.	Height cm.	in.	Vitamin C, mg.	Thiamin, mg.	Riboflavin, mg.	Niacin, mg. NE[e]	Vitamin B6, mg.	Folacin[f], µg.	Vitamin B12, µg.
						Water-Soluble Vitamins						
Infants	0.0–0.5	6	13	60	24	35	0.3	0.4	6	0.3	30	0.5[g]
	0.5–1.0	9	20	71	28	35	0.5	0.6	8	0.6	45	1.5
Children	1–3	13	29	90	35	45	0.7	0.8	9	0.9	100	2.0
	4–6	20	44	112	44	45	0.9	1.0	11	1.3	200	2.5
	7–10	28	62	132	52	45	1.2	1.4	16	1.6	300	3.0
Males	11–14	45	99	157	62	50	1.4	1.6	18	1.8	400	3.0
	15–18	66	145	176	69	60	1.4	1.7	18	2.0	400	3.0
	19–22	70	154	177	70	60	1.5	1.7	19	2.2	400	3.0
	23–50	70	154	178	70	60	1.4	1.6	18	2.2	400	3.0
	51+	70	154	178	70	60	1.2	1.4	16	2.2	400	3.0
Females	11–14	46	101	157	62	50	1.1	1.3	15	1.8	400	3.0
	15–18	55	120	163	64	60	1.1	1.3	14	2.0	400	3.0
	19–22	55	120	163	64	60	1.1	1.3	14	2.0	400	3.0
	23–50	55	120	163	64	60	1.0	1.2	13	2.0	400	3.0
	51+	55	120	163	64	60	1.0	1.2	13	2.0	400	3.0
Pregnant						+20	+0.4	+0.3	+2	+0.6	+400	+1.0
lactating						+40	+0.5	+0.5	+5	+0.5	+100	+1.0

[e]NE = niacin equivalent. 1 NE = 1 mg. niacin or 60 mg. dietary tryptophan.

[f]The folacin allowances refer to dietary sources as determined by Lactobacillus casei assay after treatment with enzymes (conjugases) to make polyglutanyl forms of the vitamin available to the test organism.

[g]The RDA for vitamin B_{12} in infants is based on average concentration of the vitamin in human milk. The allowances after weaning are based on energy intake (as recommended by the American Academy of Pediatrics) and consideration of other factors such as intestinal absorption.

TABLE 2. Continued

Category	Age, years	Weight kg.	Weight lb.	Height cm.	Height in.	Calcium, mg.	Phosphorus, mg.	Magnesium, mg.	Iron, mg.	Zinc, mg.	Iodine, µg.
						Minerals					
Infants	0.0-0.5	6	13	60	24	360	240	50	10	3	40
	0.5-1.0	9	20	71	28	540	360	70	15	5	50
Children	1-3	13	29	90	35	800	800	150	15	10	70
	4-6	20	44	112	44	800	800	200	10	10	90
	7-10	28	62	132	52	800	800	250	10	10	120
Males	11-14	45	99	157	62	1200	1200	350	18	15	150
	15-18	66	145	176	69	1200	1200	400	18	15	150
	19-22	70	154	177	70	800	800	350	10	15	150
	23-50	70	154	178	70	800	800	350	10	15	150
	51+	70	154	178	70	800	800	350	10	15	150
Females	11-14	46	101	157	62	1200	1200	300	18	15	150
	15-18	55	120	163	64	1200	1200	300	18	15	150
	19-22	55	120	163	64	800	800	300	18	15	150
	23-50	55	120	163	64	800	800	300	18	15	150
	51+	55	120	163	64	800	800	300	10	15	150
Pregnant						+400	+400	+150	h	+5	+25
lactating						+400	+400	+150	h	+10	+50

hThe increased requirement during pregnancy cannot be met by the iron content of habitual American diets or by the existing iron stores of many women. Therefore, the use of 30-60 mg. of supplemental iron is recommended. Iron needs during lactation are not substantially different from those of nonpregnant women, but continued supplementation of the mother for 2 to 3 months after parturition is advisable in order to replenish stores depleted by pregnancy.

Mean Heights and Weights and Recommended Energy Intake

Category	Age, years	Weight kg.	Weight lb.	Height cm.	Height in.	Energy Needs (with range) kcal	millijoule
Infants	0.0-0.5	6	13	60	24	kg. x 115 (95-145)	kg. x .48
	0.5-1.0	9	20	71	28	kg. x 105 (80-135)	kg. x .44
Children	1-3	13	29	90	35	1300 (900 - 1800)	5.5
	4-6	20	44	112	44	1700 (1300 - 2300)	7.1
	7-10	28	62	132	52	2400 (1650 - 3300)	10.1
Males	11-14	45	99	157	62	2700 (2000 - 3700)	11.3
	15-18	66	145	176	69	2800 (2100 - 3900)	11.8
	19-22	70	154	177	70	2900 (2500 - 3300)	12.2
	23-50	70	154	178	70	2700 (2300 - 3100)	11.3
	51-75	70	154	178	70	2400 (2000 - 2800)	10.1
	76+	70	154	178	70	2050 (1650 - 2450)	8.6
Females	11-14	46	101	157	62	2200 (1500 - 3000)	9.2
	15-18	55	120	163	64	2100 (1200 - 3000)	8.8
	19-22	55	120	163	64	2100 (1700 - 2500)	8.8
	23-50	55	120	163	64	2000 (1600 - 2400)	8.4
	51-75	55	120	163	64	1800 (1400 - 2200)	7.6
	76+	55	120	163	64	1600 (1200 - 2000)	6.7
Pregnant						+300	
lactating						+500	

The data in this table have been assembled from the observed median heights and weights of children together with desirable weights for adults for the mean heights of men (70 inches) and women (64 inches) between the ages of 18 and 34 years as surveyed in the U.S. population.

The energy allowances for the young adults are for men and women doing light work. The allowances for the two older age groups represent mean energy needs over these age spans, allowing for a 2% decrease in basal (resting) metabolic rate per decade and a reduction in activity of 200 kcal/day for men and women between 51 and 75 years, 500 kcal for men over 75 years, and 400 kcal for women over 75. The customary range of daily energy output is shown for adults in parentheses, and is based on a variation in energy needs of ±400 kcal at any one age, emphasizing the wide range of energy intakes appropriate for any group of people.

Energy allowances for children through age 18 are based on median energy intakes of children of these ages followed in longitudinal growth studies. The values in parentheses are 10th and 90th percentiles of energy intake, to indicate the range of energy consumption among children of these ages.

house, or normal diet. These persons should be served nutritionally adequate meals that meet their food preferences. The nutrient-rich foods shown in table 4, pages 130-131, offer a variety of items from each of the four basic food groups that will help ensure adequate daily nutrient intake. The food offered also should meet the recommended number of servings from these food groups for the ages being served. Additional foods and desserts can be included to meet caloric needs.

Although a standard meal pattern may be used in an institution, nutritionally it makes no difference if a hamburger is served for breakfast and cereal is served for dinner. Nutritious foods that are acceptable and appealing to the appetites of those being served are important. It does little good to serve foods that meet the nutritional needs of a group or individual but are so unpalatable or disliked that they are not eaten. In order to meet nutritional requirements, milk, bread, and a fruit or vegetable should be offered at each meal. A 2- to 3-oz. serving of meat or other food high in protein can be offered at lunch and dinner. Good snack choices include milk, fruit (fresh, canned, or frozen), cheese, peanut butter and crackers, raw vegetables, or eggnog.

Those persons following an unrestricted diet may eat their daily meals according to their individual preferences. However, it is usually not desirable to let more than 15 hours pass between meals. Meals at frequent intervals help ensure an adequate nutrient intake for persons who are unable to tolerate a large amount of food at one time. For example, well-distributed daily meals would include breakfast at 8 a.m., lunch at noon, dinner at 5:30 p.m., and a snack later in the evening.

Ethnic or regional food habits should be considered when planning menus. Children and the elderly often prefer plain foods that are not highly seasoned. It also is important to provide foods that can be easily eaten by those with chewing problems.

MODIFIED DIETS

At times, it may be necessary to change the consistency or types of food eaten in order to treat some medical problems. The most common types of modified diets are clear-liquid, full-liquid, soft, mechanically soft, sodium-restricted, and calorie-controlled (diabetic/weight reduction) diets. All modified diets should be planned so that they are as nutritionally adequate as possible. The recommended daily guide to eating, shown in table 3, and the RDAs can be used to evaluate adequacy. However, these guides are not designed for meeting nutritional requirements during illness. A brief description of the purpose of each of these diets mentioned above and the foods allowed follows.

CLEAR-LIQUID DIET

The clear-liquid diet is usually used in preparation for certain tests when

TABLE 3. RECOMMENDED DAILY GUIDE TO GOOD EATING[a]

Food Group	Recommended Number of Servings					
	Child	Teenager	Adult	Pregnant Woman	Lactating Woman
Milk 1 cup milk, yogurt, or **calcium equivalent:[b]** 1½ slices (1½ oz.) cheddar cheese[c] 1 cup pudding 1¾ cups ice cream 2 cups cottage cheese[c]	3	4	2	4	4
Meat 2 ounces cooked, lean meat, fish, poultry, or **protein equivalent:[b]** 2 eggs 2 slices (2 oz.) cheddar cheese[c] ½ cup cottage cheese[c] 1 cup dried beans, peas 4 tbs. peanut butter	2	2	2	3	2
Vegetable-Fruit ½ cup cooked or juice 1 cup raw Portion commonly served, such as a medium-size apple or banana	4	4	4	4	4
Grain, whole grain, fortified, enriched 1 slice bread 1 cup ready-to-eat cereal ½ cup cooked cereal, pasta, grits	4	4	4	4	4

Courtesy of National Dairy Council.

[a]The recommended daily guide to good eating provides the foundation for a nutritious, healthful diet. The servings from the four food groups for adults supply about 1,200 calories. The table gives recommendations for the number and size of servings for several categories of people.

[b]Others complement but do not replace foods from the four food groups. Amounts should be determined by individual caloric needs.

[c]Count cheese as serving of milk or meat, not both simultaneously.

TABLE 4. NUTRIENTS FOR HEALTH[a]

Nutrient	Important Sources of Nutrient	Some Major Physiological Functions		
		Provide energy	Build and maintain body cells	Regulate body processes
Protein	Meat, Poultry, Fish; Dried beans and peas; Eggs; Cheese; Milk	Supplies 4 calories per gram	Constitutes part of the structure of every cell, such as muscle, blood, and bone; supports growth; and maintains healthy body cells	Constitutes part of enzymes, some hormones and body fluids, and antibodies that increase resistance to infection
Carbohydrate	Cereal; Potatoes; Dried beans; Corn; Bread; Sugar	Supplies 4 calories per gram; Major source of energy for central nervous system	Supplies energy so protein can be used for growth and maintenance of body cells	Unrefined products supply fiber—complex carbohydrates in fruits, vegetables, and whole grains—for regular elimination; assists in fat utilization
Fat	Shortening, Oil; Butter, Margarine; Salad dressing; Sausages	Supplies 9 calories per gram	Constitutes part of the structure of every cell and supplies essential fatty acids	Provides and carries fat-soluble vitamins (A, D, E, and K)
Vitamin A (Retinol)	Liver; Carrots; Sweet potatoes; Greens; Butter, Margarine		Assists formation and maintenance of skin and mucous membranes that line body cavities and tracts, such as nasal passages and intestinal tract, thus increasing resistance to infection	Functions in visual processes and forms visual purple, thus promoting healthy eye tissues and eye adaptation in dim light
Vitamin C (Ascorbic Acid)	Broccoli; Oranges; Grapefruit; Papayas; Mangos; Strawberries		Forms cementing substances, such as collagen, that hold body cells together, thus strengthening blood vessels, hastening healing of wounds and bones, and increasing resistance to infection	Aids utilization of iron

Nutrient	Food Sources	Some Major Physiological Functions	
Thiamin (B₁)	Lean pork Nuts Fortified cereal products	Aids in utilization of energy	Functions as part of a coenzyme to promote the utilization of carbohydrates; promotes normal appetite; contributes to normal functioning of nervous system
Riboflavin (B₂)	Liver Milk Yogurt Cottage cheese	Aids in utilization of energy	Functions as part of a coenzyme in the production of energy within body cells; promotes healthy skin, eyes, and clear vision
Niacin	Liver Meat, Poultry, Fish Peanuts Fortified cereal products	Aids in utilization of energy	Functions as part of a coenzyme in fat synthesis, tissue respiration, and utilization of carbohydrate; promotes healthy skin, nerves, and digestive tract; aids digestion and fosters normal appetite
Calcium	Milk, Yogurt Cheese Sardines and salmon with bones Collard, kale, mustard, and turnip greens	Combines with other minerals within a protein framework to give structure and strength to bones and teeth	Assists in blood clotting; functions in normal muscle contraction and relaxation and normal nerve transmission
Iron	Enriched farina Prune juice Liver Dried beans and peas Red meat	Aids in utilization of energy Combines with protein to form hemoglobin, the red substance in blood that carries oxygen to and carbon dioxide from the cells; prevents nutritional anemia and its accompanying fatigue; increases resistance to infection	Functions as part of enzymes involved in tissue respiration

Courtesy of National Dairy Council.

[a] When a nutrient is added or a nutritional claim is made, nutrition labeling regulations require listing the 10 leader nutrients on food packages. These nutrients appear in the table above with food sources and some major physiological functions.

the gastrointestinal tract must be empty. It also is used immediately after surgery, when the patient is unable to tolerate solid foods. Any foods that are clear of all particulate matter and are liquids at body temperature can be used. These include clear broth, consomme, plain gelatin, and strained or clear fruit juices, tea, coffee, carbonated beverages, and sugar. This diet should be used only for a few days because it is lacking in essential nutrients and calories.

FULL-LIQUID DIET

The full-liquid diet is used as part of the progression from the clear-liquid diet to a regular diet or whenever solid foods are not tolerated. Any liquid or solid foods that have been liquefied in a blender can be used. If carefully planned, a full-liquid diet can be nutritionally adequate. Eggnog and vegetables should be included frequently because they greatly add to the nutrient content of the diet. Pureed meat may be added to broth in some circumstances, but meat is usually omitted from the full-liquid diet. Table 5, below, lists a sample basic food pattern for a full-liquid diet. Figure 20, next page, shows a sample menu for a full-liquid diet.

SOFT DIET

The soft diet is one that includes liquid foods and those solid foods that contain a restricted amount of indigestible fiber and connective tissue. Spices and condiments are usually eliminated, and any other foods that

TABLE 5. BASIC FOOD PATTERN FOR FULL-LIQUID DIET

Food Group	Recommended Daily Quantity
1. Milk and milk products	Whole milk, 2 quarts; or 1½ quarts plus 1 cup nonfat dry milk
2. Meat and meat alternates	Strained meat, 2 oz., available in baby foods, may be added to soups; 1 oz. liver should be substituted several times weekly
	Eggs, 3, in soft custard or in beverages prepared in blender, with chocolate or vanilla flavoring
3. Vegetables and fruits	Any vegetable puree or juice may be used in soups, citrus juices (1 cup)
4. Breads and cereals (whole grain or enriched), potatoes, and legumes	Strained cereals, ½ cup; riced or mashed potatoes, ½ cup, in soup
Fats and sweets	Can be used as flavorings for soups gruels, cocoa, milk, custards, etc., as desired or needed to fulfill caloric requirement

---

Sample Menu

BREAKFAST

Orange juice (½ cup)
Oatmeal gruel (½ cup with milk)
Cocoa (1 cup with 2 tbs. nonfat dry
milk added)

10:00 a.m.

Eggnog (1 cup milk, powdered
pasteurized eggnog mix with
flavoring and sweetening as
desired)

NOON

Cream of tomato soup (with 1 oz.
liver and 2 tbs. nonfat dry milk
added)
Milk shake (1 cup milk, 4 tbs.
nonfat dry milk, pureed banana,
and ice cream)

3:00 p.m.

Tomato juice (½ cup)
Soft custard (with 2 tbs. nonfat
dry milk added)

NIGHT

Cream of potato soup (with 1 oz.
beef added)
Cherry-flavored gelatin
Milk (1 cup with 2 tbs. nonfat dry
milk added)

8:00 p.m.

Apricot milk shake (1 cup milk, 2
tbs. nonfat dry milk, pureed
apricots, and ice cream)

FIGURE 20. Sample Menu for a Full-Liquid Diet.

are not well tolerated also should be avoided. Table 6, page 134, lists a sample basic food pattern for a soft diet.

MECHANICALLY SOFT DIET

The mechanically soft diet is used for persons who are unable to chew regular food adequately. Usually, foods are pureed or strained, and very soft and liquid foods without tough skins or seeds are included. Because individuals may tolerate food consistency differently, it is best to consult the person to find which foods are acceptable.

Tube feedings may be necessary for patients who are unable to take foods orally. Food must then be blenderized so it can be administered through a small tube that is inserted through the nose and mouth into the stomach or directly into the stomach.

At one time, tube feedings were prepared by blenderizing foods in the dietary department. A recipe was developed by the dietitian according to patient tolerance. In some facilities, when tube feedings are used infrequently, this procedure may still be followed. In most facilities, however, commercially prepared tube feedings are now used. These products are sterilized and can be chosen to meet patient tolerance. They are more convenient for facilities that use tube feedings routinely. There are also commercial products that have been modified to meet the special needs of patients with digestion and absorption abnormalities or special caloric needs. Current nutrient information is available from the manufacturer.

TABLE 6. ADAPTATION OF BASIC FOOD PATTERNS FOR SOFT DIET

Food Groups	Recommended Daily Quantity	Foods Included
1. Milk and milk products	Whole milk, 1 pint	Whole milk, 1 pint, or evaporated milk, 1 cup, or buttermilk, 1 pint, or dry whole milk, ½ cup
	Protein supplement: nonfat dry milk, ½ cup	Nonfat dry milk may be added to the whole milk or used in cereal, soup, mashed potato, or desserts
2. Meat and meat alternates (3 servings)	Meat, poultry, fish, 1 serving	Prepared any way except fried, 3-oz. edible portion
		Note protein supplement in milk group
	Meat alternates, 2 servings cheese; peanut butter; eggs (4 or 5 per week)	Additional meat, 1 oz., or cheddar cheese, 1 oz., or cottage cheese, ½ cup, or peanut butter, freshly ground, 2 tbs., or 1 egg prepared any way except fried
3. Vegetables and fruits (4 or more servings)	3a. Dark green, deep yellow, or leafy vegetables, 1 serving	Cooked vegetables in groups 3a and 3b; asparagus, beans (green or wax), beets, carrots, peas, spinach, squash, peeled and strained tomatoes
	3b. Other vegetables, 1 or more servings	The following strong-flavored cooked vegetables may be used if tolerated: broccoli, brussels sprouts, cabbage, cauliflower, onions, rutabagas, turnips
		Vegetables may be pureed if further reduction in fiber is necessary; however, pureed vegetables are not well accepted by many patients
	3c. Citrus fruits and other sources of vitamin C, 1 serving	Juice only, ½ cup
	3d. Other fruits, 1 or more servings	Bananas; cooked and peeled apples, apricots, peaches, and pears; fruits with seeds omitted (the trend is toward more liberal use of raw and cooked fruits)

TABLE 6. *Continued*

Food Groups	Recommended Daily Quantity	Foods Included
4. Breads and cereals (whole grain or enriched), potatoes, and legumes	4 or more servings	Enriched white or rye bread; enriched farina, cornmeal, hominy grits, puffed wheat, puffed rice, wheat flakes, cornflakes. If whole grain cooked cereals are served, they should be strained
		Potatoes in any form; rice, macaroni, spaghetti, and noodles may be served as alternates to potatoes
Fats and sweets	Butter or fortified margarine, 3 servings	1 pat=1 tsp
	Sweets as needed to satisfy caloric requirement and appetite	Sugar, jelly, honey, syrup. Desserts of all types, but without coconut, raisins, or nuts

Cost may be a factor in the use of these products. Careful comparison of the nutrients contained in each of the products may demonstrate that the lower-cost product contains the same or only slightly different amounts of nutrients than the one that is more costly.

SODIUM-RESTRICTED DIET

Patients with medical problems related to body fluid balance often must restrict sodium from their diet. This is because sodium must be maintained in a narrow range of concentration in body fluid. If it is too high, extra body fluid will be retained to dilute the sodium concentration. Medical problems for which sodium intake may need to be restricted because excess body fluid aggravates the condition include hypertension (high blood pressure), heart disease, and kidney disease.

Sodium-restricted diets can be ordered in specific milligrams or milliequivalents (1 meq.=23 mg.). This is the most precise way of ordering the diet. A sodium-restricted diet also can be ordered by title, such as "No added salt" or "Low-sodium diet." If titles are used, the medical staff and dietitian of each facility must define what is meant in terms of food items or sodium intake for the diet. The sodium-restricted diets most often used are 3,000 mg., 2,000 mg., and 1,000 mg. Choosing a recommended number of servings from each of the four food groups will ensure that the sodium limit per day is not exceeded. Some facilities prefer to assign points to commonly eaten foods. One point is usually equal to one milliequivalent. Thus, a 45-point sodium diet is equal to 45 meq., or 1,000 mg., of sodium.

TABLE 7. BASIC FOOD PATTERN FOR MILD LOW-SODIUM DIET[a]

Food Group	Food Suggestions	Foods to Avoid
1. Milk and milk products	2 to 3 cups of the following: Whole, skim, or unsalted buttermilk as a beverage and in food preparation Yogurt	Cultured buttermilk
2. Meat and meat alternates	2 or more 2-oz. servings of the following: Baked, broiled, roasted, stewed, or fried meat, fish, or poultry Cheddar cheese, Swiss cheese, cottage cheese, or cream cheese Eggs Dried beans and peas Peanut butter Unsalted nuts	Any meat, fish, or poultry that is smoked, brine cured, salted, dried, canned, or salted and soaked; frankfurters; corned beef; chipped dried beef; luncheon meats; ham; salt pork; sausage; salted codfish; sardines; herring; anchovies; caviar; other cheeses; salted nuts
3. Vegetables and fruits	4 or more servings of the following: Asparagus, beets, broccoli, brussels sprouts, cabbage, carrots, green and wax beans, green peppers, lettuce, mushrooms, potatoes, pumpkins, spinach, sweet potatoes, tomatoes, winter squash Apples, apricots, blackberries, boysenberries, cantaloupe, cherries, grapefruit, honeydew melons, lemons, oranges, peaches, pears, pineapples, plums, raspberries, strawberries, tangerines, and so forth Include at least one fruit or vegetable that is a good source of vitamin A every other day or combine selected foods to meet the RDA for vitamin A	Olives, pickles (dill and sweet), potato chips, sauerkraut

[a]2-3 gr., 2000-3000 mg., or 87-130 mEq. sodium. This is a normal diet with *mild* restriction of certain foods that have an excessively high salt content. Iodized salt may be used in preparing foods, but no salt is allowed on the tray or at the table.

If no source of iodine (such as an iodized salt substitute) is included, the diet will be deficient in iodine. Salt substitutes should not be used without permission of the patient's physician.

TABLE 7. *Continued*

Food Group	Food Suggestions	Foods to Avoid
	Include at least one fruit or vegetable that is a good source of vitamin C daily, *or* combine selected foods to meet the RDA for vitamin C	
	All other vegetables and fruits not listed in foods to avoid	
4. Breads and cereals (whole grain or enriched), potatoes, and legumes	4 or more servings of the following:	
	Whole grain, enriched, or restored breads	Breads, rolls, or crackers with salted tops; pretzels
	Unsalted crackers	
	Cereals	
	Noodles, macaroni, spaghetti, rice	
Fats	Moderate (no more than 6 tsp.) amounts of salted butter, margarine, lard, cream vegetable shortenings, salad oils, mayonnaise, and French dressing	Bacon, bacon fat, and salad dressings, such as Roquefort and Thousand Island
Sweets	As desired	
Seasonings	Small amounts of iodized salt in food preparation	Table salt, flavored salt, monosodium glutamate
Other foods	1 or more servings of the following:	
	Coffee, decaffeinated coffee, tea, cocoa, carbonated beverages, homemade cream soups, unsalted popcorn, canned low-sodium soups	Bouillon cubes, canned or prepared soups, olives, pickles, relishes, salted popcorn, soy sauce

Adapted and reprinted, with permission, from the Wisconsin Department of Health and Social Services (see Bibliography).

The points from all food items selected have to be totaled as they are eaten in order to ensure that the sodium restriction is not exceeded before the end of the day. Tables 7, opposite, and 8, page 138, show sample basic food patterns for sodium-restricted diets.

Some patients on sodium-restricted diets have a low calorie intake because of poor appetite or the need to lose weight. When calorie intake is decreased to approximately 1,500 or fewer calories, the sodium intake also is decreased because the amount of food eaten is less. Patients may

TABLE 8. BASIC FOOD PATTERN FOR 1,000-MG. SODIUM DIET[a]

Food Groups	Recommended Daily Quantity	Description
1. Milk and milk products	1 pint	Whole, skim, or buttermilk (unsalted) or ½ pint evaporated milk or ⅔ cup nonfat dry milk
2. Meat and meat alternates	5 oz. lean meat	1 oz. lean meat, fish, or poultry (cooked weight, edible portion—not counting bone and excess fat) equals: 1 egg (limit is 3 per week for cardiac patients) or 1 oz. low-sodium dietetic cheese or 2 tbs. low-sodium dietetic peanut butter
3. Vegetables and fruits	5 or more ½-cup servings with no sodium added in freezing, canning, or cooking	1 serving of a dark green or deep yellow vegetable for vitamin A 1 serving citrus fruit (1 orange, ½ grapefruit, ½ cup orange or grapefruit juice, or 1 cup special low-sodium dietetic tomato juice) for vitamin C 3 servings other vegetables and fruits
4. Breads and cereals (whole grain or enriched), potatoes, and legumes	6 to 8 servings	3 slices regular bread daily; additional slices should be low-sodium bread 1 serving equals 1 slice bread or ½ cup cooked cereal or ¾ cup puffed rice, puffed wheat, or shredded wheat or ½ cup cooked macaroni, noodles, rice, or spaghetti or ½ cup white potato or ¼ cup sweet potato or ⅓ cup corn (without sodium) or ½ cup cooked dried beans or peas
Fats and sweets	Calories should be kept low enough to keep patient at a low normal weight	Salt-free butter or margarine, oil, or shortening (omit butter and shortening for cardiac patients) Sugar, jam, jelly, honey, or syrup

[a]The 1,000-milligram sodium diet contains approximately 1,300 calories without the fats and sweets food group. Each teaspoon of butter, margarine, or oil would add 45 calories. Each level teaspoon of sugar, jelly, or honey would add 20 calories.

then increase their use of salt in food preparation or use of regular salted foods to keep their sodium intake at the level prescribed. In such instances, actual estimates of the patients' sodium intake, using an average sodium value for the foods as listed in table 9, below, is desirable.

Sodium and salt are important flavor components of food. When they are eliminated from the diet, alternative flavorings should be used, such as:

For *beef*—dry mustard, marjoram, nutmeg, onion, sage, thyme, pepper, bay leaf

For *lamb*—mint, garlic, rosemary, curry, pineapple, lemon juice, oregano

For *veal*—bay leaf, ginger, marjoram, curry, currant jelly, apricots

TABLE 9. SHORT FORM FOR CALCULATION OF SODIUM (Na) CONTENT

Food	Portion	Average Sodium
Milk, nonfat	8 oz.	125 mg.
Milk, whole	8 oz.	120 mg.
Milk, sodium restricted	8 oz.	5 mg.
Meat, fish, poultry	1 oz.	25 mg.
Egg	1	60 mg.
Fruit or juice	1 small serving or ½ cup	2 mg.
Vegetables, unsalted[a]	About ½ cup	9 mg.
Bread, regular	1 slice	120 mg.
Bread, sodium restricted	1 slice	5 mg.
Rice, spaghetti, noodles (unsalted)	½ cup	5 mg.
Potato	1 small	5 mg.
Cooked cereals, unsalted	½ cup	5 mg.
Butter, regular	1 tsp.	50 mg.
Butter, sodium restricted	1 tsp.	Negligible
Oil or shortening, unsalted	1 tsp.	Negligible

One-half cup of most all vegetables (fresh, frozen,[a] and dietetic canned) have from 4-9 mg. of sodium, except the following:

Artichokes	86 mg.
Beet greens	76 mg.
Beets	43 mg.
Carrots	33 mg.
Celeriac root	100 mg.
Celery	88 mg.
Chard, Swiss	86 mg.
Collards	25 mg.
Dandelion greens	44 mg.
Kale	43 mg.
Mustard greens	18 mg.
Radishes	18 mg.
Sauerkraut	747 mg.
Spinach	50 mg.
Turnips, white	34 mg.

Adapted and reprinted, with permission, from the Wisconsin Department of Health and Social Services (see Bibliography).

[a]The label on frozen vegetables should be checked for salt or sodium (Na) because some vegetables, such as peas, lima beans, and mixed vegetables, have been stored in a brine (salt) solution.

For *chicken*—paprika, mushrooms, thyme, sage, parsley, cranberry sauce

For *fish*—dry mustard, paprika, curry, bay leaf, lemon juice, mushrooms, sherry

For *eggs*—pepper, green pepper, mushrooms, dry mustard, paprika, pineapple

For *vegetables*—lemon juice, marjoram, nutmeg, dill seed, mustard, parsley, onion, mace, ginger, basil, oregano

CALORIE-CONTROLLED DIET

Many Americans are concerned about being overweight not only for social reasons, but also, and perhaps more important, for medical reasons. Our energy needs are determined by our weight, age, sex, and activity level. These factors determine what the body's daily energy output is. The food we eat determines what the body's energy intake is. Food provides energy in the form of proteins, fats, and carbohydrates. To maintain body weight, energy output must equal energy intake. When energy intake is greater than energy output, energy is stored in the form of fat, and weight is gained.

The only way to lose weight is to shift the energy balance so that stored energy (fat) is used up. This is done by decreasing energy intake and maintaining or increasing energy output. Decreasing calorie (food) intake is the most common way of shifting the balance so that stored energy is used. Calorie-controlled weight reduction diets are used to help overweight persons achieve their ideal body weight.

The food exchange system is usually used for calorie-controlled diets. This system was developed by the American Dietetic Association and the American Diabetes Association in 1950 and revised in 1976. The exchange system classifies foods into one of five food groups, as is shown in table 10, pages 141-145. Each food within a group, in the portion size stated, provides approximately the same amount of proteins, fats, carbohydrates, and calories as any other food within the same group. A meal pattern is outlined indicating how many servings from each group should be chosen at each meal to maintain a certain calorie level.

For persons with diabetes, it also is important to monitor the carbohydrate intake at each meal. This can easily be done with the exchange system. Persons with diabetes are unable to utilize carbohydrates normally. This is usually due to a lack of the hormone insulin. Insulin is necessary for cells to obtain energy from carbohydrates. In some diabetic patients, insulin is injected into the blood stream at certain times during the day as prescribed by a physician. Insulin remains active for several hours. Carbohydrates ingested by the diabetic person must be divided between each meal to match insulin activity. The meal pattern for a diabetic diet uses

TABLE 10. FOOD EXCHANGE LIST

Food Groups	Composition	Exchange
1. Milk and milk products	One exchange of milk contains 12 gr. of carbohydrate, 8 gr. of protein, a trace of fat, and 80 calories	*Nonfat fortified milk* Skim or nonfat milk, *1 cup* Powdered (nonfat dry, before adding liquid), *⅓ cup* Canned, evaporated skim milk, *½ cup* Buttermilk made from skim milk, *1 cup* Yogurt made from skim milk (plain, unflavored), *1 cup* *Low-fat fortified milk* 1% fat-fortified milk (omit ½ fat exchange), *1 cup* 2% fat-fortified milk (omit 1 fat exchange), *1 cup* Yogurt made from 2% fortified milk (plain, unflavored) (omit 1 fat exchange), *1 cup* *Whole milk (omit 2 fat exchanges)* Whole milk, *1 cup* Canned, evaporated, whole milk, *½ cup* Buttermilk made from whole milk, *1 cup* Yogurt made from whole milk (plain, unflavored), *1 cup*
2. Meat and meat alternates	One exchange of lean meat (1 oz.) contains 7 gr. of protein, 3 gr. of fat, and 55 calories	Beef: baby beef (very lean), chipped beef, chuck, flank steak, tenderloin, plate ribs, plate skirt steak, round (bottom, top), all cuts rump, spareribs, tripe, *1 oz.* Lamb: leg, rib, sirloin, loin (roast and chops), shank, shoulder, *1 oz.* Pork: leg (whole rump, center shank), smoked ham (center slices), *1 oz.* Veal: leg, loin, rib, shank, shoulder, cutlets, *1 oz.* Poultry: meat without skin of chicken, turkey, cornish hen, guinea hen, pheasant, *1 oz.* Fish: any fresh or frozen, *1 oz.* canned salmon, tuna, mackerel, crab, and lobster, *¼ cup* clams, oysters, scallops, shrimp, *5 or 1 oz.* sardines, drained, *3* Cheeses containing less than 5% butterfat, *1 oz.* Cottage cheese, dry and 2% butterfat, *¼ cup* Dried beans and peas (omit 1 bread exchange), *½ cup*

TABLE 10. Continued

Food Groups	Composition	Exchange
	For each exchange of medium-fat meat omit ½ fat exchange	Beef: ground (15% fat), corned beef (canned), rib eye, round (ground commercial), 1 oz.
		Pork: loin (all cuts tenderloin), shoulder arm (picnic), shoulder blade, Boston butt, Canadian bacon, boiled ham, 1 oz.
		Liver, heart, kidney, and sweetbreads (these are high in cholesterol), 1 oz. Cottage cheese, creamed, ¼ cup
		Cheese: mozzarella, ricotta, farmer cheese, Neufchatel, 1 oz. Parmesan, 3 tbs.
		Egg (high in cholesterol), 1 Peanut butter (omit 2 additional fat exchanges), 2 tbs.
	For each exchange of high-fat meat omit 1 fat exchange	Beef: brisket, corned beef (brisket), ground beef (more than 20% fat), hamburger (commercial), chuck (ground commercial), roasts (rib), steaks (club and rib), 1 oz.
		Lamb: breast, 1 oz.
		Pork: spareribs, loin (back ribs), pork (ground), country-style ham, deviled ham, 1 oz.
		Veal: breast, 1 oz.
		Poultry: capon, duck (domestic), goose, 1 oz.
		Cheese: cheddar types, 1 oz.
		Cold cuts, 4½″ x ⅛″ slice
		Frankfurter, 1 small
3. Vegetables and fruits	One exchange of vegetables contains about 5 gr. of carbohydrate, 2 gr. of protein, and 25 calories	Cooked vegetables, ½ cup
		Asparagus
		Bean sprouts
		Beets
		Broccoli
		Brussels sprouts
		Cabbage
		Carrots
		Greens:
		mustard
		spinach
		turnip
		Mushrooms
		Okra
		Onions

Cauliflower
Celery
Cucumbers
Eggplant
Green onions
Green pepper
Greens:
  beet
  chards
  collards
  dandelion
  kale

Rhubarb
Rutabaga
Sauerkraut
String beans
Summer squash
Tomatoes
Tomato juice
Turnips
Vegetable juice cocktail
Zucchini

Raw vegetables, as much as desired

Chicory
Chinese cabbage
Endive
Escarole

Lettuce
Parsley
Radishes
Watercress

Fruits

One exchange of fruit contains 10 gr. of carbohydrate and 40 calories

Apple, *1 small*
Apple juice, *1/3 cup*
Applesauce (unsweetened), *1/2 cup*
Apricots, fresh, *2 medium*
Apricots, dried, *4 halves*
Banana, *1/2 small*
Berries:
  blackberries, *1/2 cup*
  blueberries, *1/2 cup*
  raspberries, *1/2 cup*
  strawberries, *3/4 cup*
Cherries, *10 large*
Cider, *1/3 cup*
Cranberries, without sugar, *as desired*
Dates, *2*
Figs, fresh, *1*
Figs, dried, *1*
Grapefruit, *1/2*
Grapefruit juice, *1/2 cup*
Grapes, *12*

Grape juice, *1/4 cup*
Mango, *1/2 small*
Melons:
  cantaloupe, *1/4 small*
  honeydew, *1/8 medium*
  watermelon, *1 cup*
Nectarine, *1 small*
Orange, *1 small*
Orange juice, *1/2 cup*
Papaya, *3/4 cup*
Peach, *1 medium*
Pear, *1 small*
Persimmon, native, *1 medium*
Pineapple, *1/2 cup*
Pineapple juice, *1/3 cup*
Plums, *2 medium*
Prunes, *2 medium*
Prune juice, *1/4 cup*
Raisins, *2 tbs.*
Tangerine, *1 medium*

TABLE 10. Continued

Food Groups	Composition	Exchange
4. Breads and cereals (whole grain or enriched), potatoes, and legumes	One exchange of bread contains 15 gr. of carbohydrate, 2 gr. of protein, and 70 calories	*Bread* White (including French and Italian), *1 slice* Whole wheat, *1 slice* Rye or pumpernickel, *1 slice* Raisin, *1 slice* Bagel, small, ½ English muffin, small, ½ Plain roll, bread, *1* Frankfurter roll, ½ Hamburger bun, ½ Dried bread crumbs, *3 tbs.* Tortilla, 6", *1* *Cereal* Bran flakes, ½ *cup* Other ready-to-eat unsweetened cereal, ¾ *cup* Puffed cereal, unfrosted, *1 cup* Cereal, cooked, ½ *cup* Grits, cooked, ½ *cup* Rice or barley, cooked, ½ *cup* Pasta, cooked spaghetti, noodles, macaroni, ½ *cup* Popcorn, popped, no fat added, *3 cups* Cornmeal, dry, *2 tbs.* Flour, 2½ *tbs.* Wheat germ, ¼ *cup* *Crackers* Arrowroot, *3* Graham, 2½" sq., *2* Matzoth, 4" x 6", ½ Oyster, *20* Pretzels, 3⅛" long x ⅛" dia., *25* Rye wafers, 2" x 3½", *3* Saltines, *6* Soda, 2½" sq., *4*	*Dried beans, peas, and lentils* Beans, peas, lentils (dried and cooked), ½ *cup* Baked beans, no pork (canned), ¼ *cup* *Starchy vegetables* Corn, ⅓ *cup* Corn on cob, *1 small* Lima beans, ½ *cup* Parsnips, ⅔ *cup* Peas, green (canned or frozen), ½ *cup* Potato, white, *1 small* Potato, mashed, ½ *cup* Pumpkin, ¾ *cup* Winter squash, acorn or butternut, ½ *cup* Yam or sweet potato, ¼ *cup* *Prepared foods* Biscuit 2" dia., *1* (omit 1 fat exchange) Corn bread, 2" x 2" x 1", *1* (omit 1 fat exchange) Corn muffin, 2" dia., *1* (omit 1 fat exchange) Crackers, round butter type, *5* (omit 1 fat exchange) Muffin, plain, small, *1* (omit 1 fat exchange) Potatoes, French fried, length 2"–3½", *8* (omit 1 fat exchange) Potato or corn chips, *10* (omit 2 fat exchanges) Pancake, 5" x ½", *1* (omit 1 fat exchange) Waffle, 5" x ½", *1* (omit 1 fat exchange)

| Fats and sweets | One exchange of fat contains 5 gr. of fat and 45 calories | Margarine, soft, tub or stick,[a] *1 tsp.*
Avocado (4″ in diameter),[b] *1/8*
Oil, corn, cottonseed, safflower, soy, sunflower, *1 tsp.*
Oil, olive,[b] *1 tsp.*
Oil, peanut,[b] *1 tsp.*
Olives,[b] *5 small*
Almonds,[b] *10 whole*
Pecans,[b] *2 large whole*
Peanuts[b]
   Spanish, *20 whole*
   Virginia, *10 whole*
Walnuts, *6 small*
Nuts,[b] other, *6 small*
Margarine, regular stick, *1 tsp.*
Butter, *1 tsp.*
Bacon fat, *1 tsp.*
Bacon, crisp, *1 strip*
Cream, light, *2 tbs.*
Cream, sour, *2 tbs.*
Cream, heavy, *1 tbs.*
Cream cheese, *1 tbs.*
French dressing,[c] *1 tbs.*
Italian dressing,[c] *1 tbs.*
Lard, *1 tsp.*
Mayonnaise,[c] *1 tsp.*
Salad dressing, mayonnaise type,[c] *2 tsp.*
Salt pork, *3/4-inch cut* |

Adapted from Exchange Lists for Meal Planning, prepared by committees of the American Diabetes Association, Inc. and The American Dietetic Association in cooperation with the National Institute of Arthritis, Metabolism, and Digestive Diseases and the National Heart and Lung Institute, National Institutes of Health, Public Health Service, U.S. Department of Health, Education, and Welfare.

[a] Made with corn, cottonseed, safflower, soy, or sunflower oil only.
[b] Fat content is primarily monounsaturated.
[c] If made with corn, cottonseed, safflower, soy, or sunflower oil, can be used on fat-modified diet.

the exchange system. This ensures that the person gets sufficient calories as well as proper carbohydrate distribution. The meal pattern for a diabetic should not be changed from one day or meal to the next because of the need to have a specific amount of carbohydrates available at each meal.

FAT-RESTRICTED DIET

A fat-restricted diet is used primarily to treat the symptoms of gallbladder stones or infection of the gallbladder (cholecystitis). The gallbladder stores bile, which is made in the liver and is used to help digest fat. The gallbladder contracts to release bile as fat enters the intestine and is digested. If there are stones in the gallbladder or if the gallbladder is infected, contraction of the organ becomes very painful. When fat intake is restricted, gallbladder contraction is decreased and the patient suffers less discomfort. Fat from the diet is restricted to 45 or fewer grams a day. Table 11, below, lists some of the foods allowed on a fat-restricted diet.

TABLE 11. BASIC FOOD PATTERN FOR FAT-RESTRICTED DIET[a]

Food Groups	Food Suggestions	Foods to Avoid
1. Milk and milk products	2 or more cups of the following:	
	Skim milk or skim buttermilk as beverage or in food preparation	Whole milk, whole milk products, 2% milk
	Yogurt made from skim milk	
2. Meat and meat alternates	2 or 3 servings of the following (limit to 6 oz. daily):	
	Baked, roasted, broiled, or stewed meat, fish, and poultry; lean beef, veal, lamb, pork, and ham; whitefish, shrimp, water-packed tuna, oysters, and salmon; chicken and turkey	Fried foods, fish canned in oil, duck, goose
	Cottage cheese	All other cheeses, peanut butter, nuts
	Eggs limit to 1 per day; egg whites as desired	
	Dried beans and peas	
3. Vegetables and fruits	4 or more servings of the following:	
	Asparagus, beets, broccoli, brussels sprouts, cabbage, carrots, green and wax beans, green peppers, lettuce, mushrooms, potatoes, pumpkins, spinach, sweet potatoes,	Any vegetables or fruits not tolerated
		Avocados, potato chips, fried vegetables

[a]This diet is nutritionally adequate. Fats are restricted to approximately 40-45 gr. of fat or 25% of the total calories per day.

TABLE 11. *Continued*

Food Groups	Food Suggestions	Foods to Avoid
	tomatoes, winter squash	
	Apples, apricots, black-berries, boysenberries, cantaloupe, cherries, grapefruit, honeydew melons, lemons, oranges, peaches, pears, pineapples, plums, raspberries, strawberries, tangerines	
	Include at least one fruit or vegetable that is a good source of vitamin A every other day, *or* combine selected foods to meet RDA for vitamin A	
	Include at least one fruit or vegetable that is a good source of vitamin C daily, *or* combine selected foods to meet RDA for vitamin C	
4. Breads and cereals (whole grain or enriched), potatoes, and legumes	4 or more servings of the following:	
	Whole grain, enriched, or restored breads and plain rolls; saltines, soda crackers, graham crackers	Sweet rolls, coffee cake, doughnuts, other crackers
	Cereals	
	Noodles, macaroni, spaghetti, rice	
Fats	No more than 3 tsp. of butter, margarine, or salad oil per day	Bacon
Sweets	1 or more servings of the following:	
	Puddings and gelatin desserts made with allowed foods; ices and sherbets; fruit whips made with egg whites; angel food cake; arrowroot or vanilla wafers; sugars, jellies, jams, syrups, honey	Pies and pastries; desserts made with fats, whole eggs, whole milk, cream, chocolate, coconut, nuts
Seasonings	As tolerated	
Other foods	1 or more servings of the following:	
	Pickles; coffee, tea, cocoa; carbonated beverages; fat-free broths, soups, and gravies made with allowed foods	Chocolate; greasy broths, soups, gravies; olives

Adapted and reprinted, with permission, from the Wisconsin Department of Health and Social Services (see Bibliography).

Other gastrointestinal abnormalities may cause fat to be digested and absorbed improperly. These problems also may require a fat-restricted diet. A physician should prescribe a specific amount of fat to be allowed in the diet. A 45-g.-per-day fat diet is often adequate.

DIET FOR MANAGEMENT OF HYPERLIPOPROTEINEMIA

Excess serum lipids (fats) have been shown to be risk factors for developing cardiovascular disease. Serum cholesterol and serum triglycerides are the lipid components of the blood that can easily be measured. If serum levels of either are elevated, the patient has a greater than average chance of having a myocardial infarction (heart attack), cerebral hemorrhage (stroke), and generally decreased circulation. Efforts to decrease serum cholesterol and triglyceride levels help prevent cardiovascular abnormalities. In most cases, the necessary decrease is achieved by both diet and drug treatment.

Cholesterol and triglycerides are carried through the blood in several different molecules made up of lipids and proteins. Detailed laboratory tests are sometimes done to determine exactly which lipoprotein molecules are elevated. These tests indicate which type of hyperlipoproteinemia the patient has so that precise treatment can be used. Results are classified as type I, type IIa or b, type III, type IV, or type V.

Elevated serum cholesterol levels can be decreased by restricting cholesterol and saturated (hydrogenated) fat intake from the diet. Elevated serum triglyceride levels respond to a decreased intake of carbohydrate and weight reduction. Tables 12, 13, and 14, pages 149, 151, and 154, list some of the foods allowed for management of hyperlipoproteinemia.

NUTRITIONAL STATUS ASSESSMENT

Nutritional care of patients must go beyond simply planning nutritionally adequate menus in order to be successful. It must include an evaluation of the patient's actual nutritional status. Nutritional status assessment consists of evaluating food intake records for nutritional adequacy, making some physical measurements, and completing certain laboratory tests. The persons responsible for nutritional assessment may vary from one facility to another. In most instances, the physician will work together with at least one of the following: dietitian, dietetic technician, food service supervisor, or nurse. The actual procedure for nutritional assessment also will vary, depending on the available staff and the type of patients or residents involved. The evaluation can be relatively simple if the patient appears to be healthy. It should be carried out more thoroughly for patients with chronic debilitating medical problems or acute illness or injury that increase nutritional needs or hinder food intake.

The first step in assessing nutritional status is to gather information about the food habits of a patient. Such dietary information includes:

TABLE 12. BASIC FOOD PATTERN FOR TYPE IIa
HYPERLIPOPROTEINEMIA DIET[a]

Food Groups	Food Suggestions	Foods to Avoid
1. Milk and milk products	2 or more cups of the following: Skim buttermilk; yogurt made with skim milk, evaporated skim milk, or regular skim milk	Whole milk, whole milk products, 2% milk
2. Meat and meat alternates	2 or more servings of the following: Limit to 3 oz., 3 times per week of lean beef, lamb, ham, or pork; fish, clams, scallops, oysters, crabs, lobster; chicken, turkey, veal, dried or chipped beef; or the following:	Regular ground beef or hamburger, fatty meats, cold cuts, sausages,[c] goose, duck, poultry skin, shrimp, fish roe, all organ meats, convenience foods containing saturated fats
	Skim milk cottage cheese, specially prepared cheeses high in polyunsaturated fat or containing up to 1% fat	Creamed cheese and all other cheeses made from cream or whole milk
	Egg whites only or egg substitutes[b] containing no cholesterol	Egg yolk
	Dried beans and peas that are prepared with permitted fats	Pork and beans Canned chili con carne
	Soy-protein meat substitutes; nonhomogenized peanut butter	
3. Vegetables and fruits	4 or more servings of the following: Any fresh, frozen, or canned vegetables without added fat or sauces	Buttered, creamed, or fried vegetables unless prepared with allowed fat
	Any fresh, canned, frozen, or dried fruit or juice; avocado in small amounts	
4. Breads and cereals (whole grain or enriched), potatoes, and legumes	4 or more servings of the following: Whole wheat, white, rye, pumpernickel, Italian, French, oatmeal or raisin breads; English muffins; matzo, saltines, graham crackers; and pretzels	Baked goods and products containing egg yolk and whole milk, egg or cheese bread, commercial biscuits, sweet rolls

[a]Low cholesterol, increased polyunsaturated fat diet. This diet meets the Recommended Dietary Allowances of the National Research Council in all nutrients except iron.
[b]Commercial egg substitutes, which are low cholesterol, are allowed.
[c]Meat alternates made from textured vegetable protein in the form of bacon, sausage, and so forth, are allowed.

TABLE 12. *Continued*

Food Groups	Food Suggestions	Foods to Avoid
	Baked goods made with allowed fats and containing no whole milk or egg yolk	waffles, muffins, French toast, cheese-flavored and other flavored crackers
	All cereals and grain products, such as rice, macaroni, spaghetti, and flour	Egg noodles
Fats	For each ounce of meat eaten, 1 tsp. of one of the following:	
	Corn oil, safflower oil, soft safflower margarines[d] prepared from polyunsaturated oils; whipped toppings made with polyunsaturated oils; commercial salad dressings not containing sour cream or cheese.	Other margarines, shortenings, and oils; butter, lard, salt pork, suet, bacon, and meat drippings; foods containing coconut oil or palm oil; gravies and cream sauces, unless made with allowed fat and/or skim milk
Sweets	The following as desired:	
	Fruit ices; sherbet (1-2% fat); gelatin desserts; fruit whips, meringues; angel food cake (including mix), other cakes, pies, and cookies; puddings; frosting made with allowed ingredients, such as skim milk and egg white; pure sugar candies, such as gum drops, jelly beans, and mints (not chocolate); jam, jelly, honey, and syrup (containing no fat)	Commercial cakes, pies, cookies, and mixes; ice cream and ice milk; desserts containing whole milk, saturated, or hydrogenated fat, and egg yolks
		All other candy
Seasonings	As desired	
Other foods	Olives, pickles, nuts, cocoa	Coconut, chocolate, cashews and macadamia nuts, corn chips, potato chips, and flavored snack crackers
	Bouillon, clear broth, fat-free vegetable soup, cream soup made with skim milk, packaged dehydrated soups	All other soups
	Alcohol used with discretion and with physician's permission	

Adapted and reprinted, with permission, from the Wisconsin Department of Health and Social Services (see Bibliography).

[d]If not available, check with dietitian or margarine companies for the margarine highest in polyunsaturated fat.

TABLE 13. BASIC FOOD PATTERN FOR TYPE IIb
OR TYPE III HYPERLIPOPROTEINEMIA DIET[a]

Food Groups	Food Suggestions	Foods to Avoid
1. Milk and milk products	2 or more cups of the following:	
	Skim milk, skim buttermilk, yogurt made from skim milk or evaporated skim milk	Whole milk and whole milk products
2. Meat and meat alternates	2 or more servings of the following:	
	Cooked lean beef, lamb, pork or ham, veal or poultry	All fatty meats, bacon, sausages,[c] canned
	Canned fish (oil drained); ¾ cup crab or lobster meat; 9-12 clams, oysters, or scallops	meat products, commercially prepared convenience food items, poultry skins, duck, goose,
	Specially prepared low-fat cheese, skim milk, cottage cheese, or ¼ cup creamed cottage cheese, which is equal to 1 oz. of meat	spareribs, organ meats, regular ground beef, fish roe, commercially fried
	Egg whites only or egg substitutes[b]	fish, shrimp, cream cheese and all regular cheeses and cheese
	Dried beans and peas prepared with permitted fats but limited for appropriate carbohydrate intake	spreads, egg yolks, pork and beans, chili con carne
	Soy-protein meat substitutes	
3. Vegetables and fruits	4 or more servings of the following:	
	Average servings of any fresh, frozen, or canned vegetable without added fat or sauces; limited potatoes, corn, lima beans, dried peas, and beans for appropriate carbohydrate intake	Buttered, creamed, or fried vegetables unless prepared with allowed fat
	½ cup per serving of any fresh, unsweetened, canned, or frozen fruit or juice or unsweetened dried fruit	Sweetened fruit and juice
4. Breads and cereals (whole grain or enriched), potatoes, and legumes	4 servings or more of the following if applicable for weight maintenance:	
	Enriched or whole grain bread, hamburger and hot	Butter rolls, cheese or egg breads, flavored

[a]Controlled-carbohydrate, controlled and modified-fat, low-cholesterol diet. The first step is to attain and maintain ideal body weight. The second step is to control carbohydrates and the kind of fat in the diet. This diet may not meet the Recommended Dietary Allowances of the National Research Council for all sex-age groups in iron.
[b]Commercial egg substitutes, which are low cholesterol, are allowed.
[c]Meat alternates made from textured vegetable protein in the form of bacon, sausages, and so forth are allowed.

TABLE 13. *Continued*

Food Groups	Food Suggestions	Foods to Avoid
	dog buns, hard rolls, graham or soda crackers, matzo or melba toast, biscuits, muffins, pancakes, and waffles made with allowed ingredients	crackers, commercial biscuits, muffins, sweet rolls, waffles, pancakes, sugar-coated cereals
	½ cup cooked or ¾ cup ready-to-eat cereal, pasta, rice	
Fats	Number of servings of the following depends on caloric level desired. A serving consists of:	
	1 tsp. polyunsaturated vegetable oil or special margarine prepared from oils, 1 tsp. nuts, 1 tbs. commercial salad dressings containing no sour cream or cheese, ⅛ avocado, 5 small olives, 2 tsp. peanut butter, whipped toppings made from unsaturated vegetable oils	All other fats, bacon, meat drippings, butter and butter products, coconut and coconut oil, palm kernel oil, hydrogenated vegetable shortenings, animal fats, and sauces unless made with allowed fat
Sweets	Limit sugar as much as possible and desserts to no more than 2 servings per day. The following may be exchanged for 1 serving of bread or cereal:	
	1½-inch cube angel food cake, ⅓ cup gelatin dessert, ¼ cup sherbet or fruit ice, ½ cup plain pudding prepared with skim milk	Commercial cakes, pies, cookies, and mixes (except angel food cake)
	If desired and approved by the physician, 1 serving of the following may be substituted for dessert:	
	1 tbs. sugar, honey, molasses, syrup, jam, or jelly; ½ oz. hard candy, jelly beans, gum drops, marshmallows, and mints (not chocolate); 6 oz. sweetened soft drink	Other candies, chocolate
Other foods	If the physician approves the use of alcohol, total daily intake is limited to 2 servings per day. One serving from the following list may be exchanged for 1 serving of bread or cereal because of the effects of alcohol on blood triglycerides:	
	1 oz. gin, rum, vodka, or whiskey; 1½ oz. dessert or	

TABLE 13. *Continued*

Food Groups	Food Suggestions	Foods to Avoid
	sweet wine; 2¼ oz. dry table wine; 5 oz. beer	
	Bouillon without fat; broth; soup without rice, noodles, corn, or lima beans; homemade soup made with skim milk and allowed vegetables	Greasy soups
	1 cup popcorn without fat can be exchanged for 1 serving of bread	Potato chips, corn chips, and flavored snack chips
	Coffee, tea, club soda	
	Flavorings, herbs, spices	
	Unflavored gelatin, vinegar, mustard, rennet tablets, unsweetened pickles, olives (5 small olives may be exchanged for 1 fat serving)	

Adapted and reprinted, with permission, from the Wisconsin Department of Health and Social Services (see Bibliography).

- Past and present food habits
- Food intolerances
- Life-style (physical, psychological, socioeconomic, and religious background)
- Handicapping conditions affecting food intake and mobility (energy needs)
- Weight history and current height and weight

Some of this information may be available from the patient's medical record. Much information can be collected by interviewing the patient or a member of the patient's family. The information gathered should be summarized, evaluated, and recorded in the patient's medical chart.

Dietary information should be evaluated for poor nutrient intake or significant weight loss or gain. If nutrient intake appears inadequate, or if the relationship between weight and height is not within normal limits, further assessment should be done. A physical examination should include checking eyes, mucus membranes, hair, and skin for any obvious signs of malnutrition. Laboratory analysis may be necessary to determine serum or blood levels of various nutrients. If any laboratory values are abnormal, the reason for the abnormality should be identified. Any abnormal laboratory values that correlate with poor intake of a particular nutrient warrant changes in the food intake. For example, if the serum protein or serum albumin level is low and the person's dietary intake of protein is low, increased dietary protein intake may remedy the situation. High protein supplements also may be necessary.

TABLE 14. BASIC FOOD PATTERN FOR TYPE IV
HYPERLIPOPROTEINEMIA DIET[a]

Food Groups	Food Suggestions	Foods to Avoid
1. Milk and milk products	2 or more cups of the following:	
	Skim milk, skim buttermilk, yogurt made from skim milk	Whole milk and whole milk products, 2% milk
2. Meat and meat alternates	2 or more servings of the following if appropriate for weight maintenance:	
	Cooked lean beef, lamb, pork or ham, veal or poultry	All fatty meats, cold cuts, bacon and sausages,[c] canned meat products, commercially prepared convenience food items, poultry skins, duck, goose, spareribs, regular ground beef, organ meats, fish roe and caviar, cream cheese
	Canned fish (oil drained), clams, crab, lobster, oysters, scallops, shrimp	
	Specially prepared low-fat cheese, creamed cottage cheese (limit of 2 oz. regular cheese per week)	
	Limit egg yolks to 3 per week; no limit to number of egg whites[b]	
	Dried beans and peas prepared with permitted fats, (considered a bread exchange)	
	Soy-protein meat substitutes, peanut butter, (considered a meat exchange)	
3. Vegetables and fruits	4 or more servings of the following:	
	Average servings of any fresh, frozen, or canned vegetable without added fat or sauces; limited potatoes, corn, lima beans, dried peas, and beans for desired (or appropriate) carbohydrate intake	Buttered, creamed, or fried vegetables unless prepared with allowed fat
	½ cup per serving of any fresh, unsweetened, canned or frozen fruit or juice or unsweetened dried fruit	Sweetened fruit and juice
4. Breads and cereals (whole grain or enriched), potatoes, and legumes	4 or more servings of the following if appropriate for weight maintenance:	
	Enriched or whole grain	Butter rolls, cheese or

[a]Controlled-carbohydrate, modified-fat diet. The first step is to attain and maintain ideal body weight. The second step is to follow the maintenance diet. This diet may not meet the Recommended Dietary Allowances of the National Research Council for all sex-age groups in iron.
[b]Commercial egg substitutes, which are low cholesterol, are allowed. Two ounces of liver, sweetbreads, or heart may be substituted for one egg yolk.
[c]Meat alternates made from textured vegetable protein in the form of bacon, sausages, and so forth, are allowed.

TABLE 14. *Continued*

Food Groups	Food Suggestions	Foods to Avoid
	bread, hamburger and hot dog buns, hard rolls, graham or soda crackers, matzo or melba toast, biscuits, muffins, pancakes, and waffles made with allowed ingredients	egg breads, flavored crackers, commercial biscuits, muffins, sweet rolls, waffles, pancakes, egg noodles
	½ cup cooked or ¾ cup ready-to-eat cereal, pasta, rice	
Fats	For the following, include only the amount appropriate for weight maintenance:	
	Any vegetable oil except coconut oil, margarine made from polyunsaturated oils, commercial salad dressings containing no sour cream, nuts (except coconuts), peanut butter	All other fats including commercial whipped toppings
Sweets	Limit sugar as much as possible and desserts to no more than 2 servings per day. The following may be exchanged for 1 serving of bread or cereal:	
	1½-inch cube angel food cake, ⅓ cup gelatin dessert, ¼ cup sherbet or fruit ice, ½ cup plain pudding prepared with skim milk	Commercial cakes, pies, cookies, and mixes (except angel food cake)
	If desired and approved by the physician, 1 serving of the following may be substituted for dessert:	
	1 tbs. sugar, honey, molasses, syrup, jam, or jelly; ½ oz. hard candy, jelly beans, gum drops, marshmallows, and mints (not chocolate); 6 oz. sweetened soft drink	Other candies, chocolate
Other foods	If the physician approves the use of alcohol, total daily intake is limited to 2 servings per day. One serving from the following list may be exchanged for 1 serving of bread or cereal because of the effects of alcohol on blood triglycerides:	
	1 oz. gin, rum, vodka, or whiskey; 1½ oz. dessert or sweet wine; 2½ oz. dry table wine; 5 oz. beer	
	Bouillon without fat; broth; soup without rice, noodles,	Greasy soups

TABLE 14. *Continued*

Food Groups	Food Suggestions	Foods to Avoid
	corn, or lima beans; homemade soup made with skim milk and allowed vegetables	
	1 cup popcorn without fat can be exchanged for 1 serving of bread	Potato chips, corn chips, and flavored snack chips
	Coffee, tea, club soda	
	Flavorings, herbs, spices	
	Unflavored gelatin, vinegar, mustard, rennet tablets, unsweetened pickles, olives (5 small olives may be exchanged for 1 fat serving)	

Adapted and reprinted, with permission, from the Wisconsin Department of Health and Social Services (see Bibliography).

Nutritional assessment should not be delayed until a problem becomes obvious, because it will then be more difficult to manage the situation. The patient's height, weight, and diet history should be determined when the patient is admitted. The patient's medical condition should be reviewed for any potential nutritional problem. Table 15, next page, lists the signs indicative of malnutrition. If a nutritional problem is evident, thorough nutritional assessment should be initiated. Nutritional status should be reevaluated at appropriate intervals according to the patient's medical condition.

In long-term care facilities such as nursing homes, patient care is often subject to very gradual changes in food intake that can easily be overlooked. Food intake of these patients should be noted on a daily basis and weight should be monitored regularly. Laboratory tests should be done if there is a significant change in food intake or weight.

If nutritional assessment indicates that the patient is at nutritional risk, steps should be taken to correct the problem. A nutritional care plan should be developed and should outline what nutritional care is needed and how the care is to be provided. All of this information, that is, nutritional assessment results and nutritional care plan, should be listed on the patient's chart. This medical record serves as:

- A means of communication among all members of the treatment team
- A means of providing continuing care in different health care settings and a resource to be used in treating illness
- An important tool in determining appropriate utilization of services and quality of care
- A constant and valuable source of information for research, educational, and statistical studies

TABLE 15. PHYSICAL SIGNS INDICATIVE OR SUGGESTIVE OF MALNUTRITION

Body Area	Normal Appearance	Signs Associated with Malnutrition
Hair	Shiny; firm; not easily plucked	Lack of natural shine; dull and dry; thin and sparse; fine, silky, and straight; color changes (flag sign); can easily be plucked
Face	Skin color uniform; smooth, pink, healthy appearance; not swollen	Skin color loss (depigmentation); skin dark over cheeks and under eyes (malar and supraorbital pigmentation); lumpiness or flakiness of skin of nose and mouth; swollen face; enlarged parotid glands; scaling of skin around nostrils (nasolabial seborrhea)
Eyes	Bright, clear, shiny; no sores at corners of eyelids; membranes a healthy pink and are moist; no prominent blood vessels or mound of tissue or sclera	Eye membranes are pale (pale conjunctivae); redness of membranes (conjunctival injection); Bitot's spots; redness and fissuring of eyelid corners (angular palpebritis); dryness of eye membranes (conjunctival xerosis); cornea has dull appearance (corneal xerosis); cornea is soft (keratomalacia); scar on cornea; ring of fine blood vessels around cornea (circumcorneal injection)
Lips	Smooth, not chapped or swollen	Redness and swelling of mouth or lips (cheilosis); especially at corners of mouth (angular fissures and scars)
Tongue	Deep red in appearance, not swollen or smooth	Swelling; scarlet and raw tongue; magenta (purplish color) of tongue; smooth tongue; swollen sores; hyperemic and hypertrophic papillae; and atrophic papillae
Teeth	No cavities, no pain, bright	May be missing or erupting abnormally; gray or black spots (fluorosis); cavities (caries)
Gums	Healthy, red, do not bleed, not swollen	Spongy and bleed easily; recession of gums
Glands	Face not swollen	Thyroid enlargement (front of neck); parotid enlargement (cheeks become swollen)
Skin	No signs of rashes, swellings, dark or light spots	Dryness of skin (xerosis); sandpaper feel of skin (follicular hyperkeratosis); flakiness of skin; skin swollen and dark; red swollen pigmentation of exposed areas (pellagrous dermatosis); excessive lightness or darkness of skin (dyspigmentation); black and blue marks due to skin bleeding (petechiae); lack of fat under skin
Nails	Firm, pink	Nails are spoon-shape (koilonychia); brittle, ridged nails

TABLE 15. *Continued*

Body Area	Normal Appearance	Signs Associated with Malnutrition
Muscular and skeletal systems	Good muscle tone, some fat under skin, can walk or run without pain	Muscles have wasted appearance; baby's skull bones are thin and soft (craniotabes); round swelling of front and side of head (frontal and parietal bossing); swelling of ends of bones (epiphyseal enlargement); small bumps on both sides of chest wall (on ribs), beading of ribs; baby's soft spot on head does not harden at proper time (persistently open anterior fontanelle); knock-knees or bowlegs; bleeding into muscle (musculoskeletal hemorrhages); person cannot get up or walk properly
Internal systems		
Cardiovascular	Normal heart rate and rhythm, no murmurs or abnormal rhythms, normal blood pressure for age	Rapid heart rate (above 100 tachycardia); enlarged heart; abnormal rhythm; elevated blood pressure
Gastrointestinal	No palpable organs or masses (in children, however, liver edge may be palpable)	Liver enlargement; enlargement of spleen (usually indicates other associated diseases)
Nervous	Psychological stability, normal reflexes	Mental irritability and confusion; burning and tingling of hands and feet (paresthesia); loss of position and vibratory sense; weakness and tenderness of muscles (may result in inability to walk); decrease and loss of ankle and knee reflexes

Adapted from Nutritional Assessment in Health Programs, G. Christakis (ed.). *Am J Public Health*, 1973 (suppl), Vol. 63, No. 11.

- A proof of work done that is useful in reimbursement for provided services
- A document that can provide legal protection for the health care facility, its employees, and the patient

It is up to the individual facility to identify who should be authorized to make entries in a medical record. If a registered dietitian is not available on a regular full-time basis, dietetic technicians or dietetic assistants may be designated as authorized alternatives to record pertinent information. Documentation of nutritional care should follow the same order as the process of planning care. Therefore, the medical record should include a summary of the nutritional assessment, a statement of plans, a description of services provided, an evaluation of the plans, and a revision of plans on the basis of effectiveness.

Frequency of recording depends on the condition of the patient and the policy of the facility. Frequent progress notes may be required when the patient is critically ill or in a rapidly changing condition. A suggested policy is to include a progress note each time a nutritional care plan is revised or reviewed. A statement of the new plan or review findings should be included. The actual format used for writing progress notes depends on the policy of the individual facility. Whatever the format, information should be clear, concise, and as brief as possible without omitting pertinent information. There are usually one of two formats used for a medical record: source-oriented or problem-oriented medical record (POMR).

In the source-oriented format, entries are structured according to source of information, with entries included in order of occurrence. Dietary or nutritional care information should be included in the progress notes section. Entries are written in brief paragraph form, and incomplete sentences or key phrases may be used. The entry is signed with the name and title of the person writing it.

The POMR focuses on the patient's problems, personal profile, plans for care and education, assessment of progress, and results. An initial data base consisting of medical social history is gathered in which problems are listed and given a number. Initial treatment of these problems is recorded and progress notes are recorded as they pertain to specific problems in the problem list. A SOAP approach is used for each progress note. SOAP is the acronym used to identify the information that can be included in each progress note:

S—Subjective information: what the patient says
O—Objective information: what the facts are relating to the patient's progress, such as laboratory values, results of diagnostic tests, changes in weight, observations and examinations by health professionals, and nutrient intake calculated from diet history
A—Assessment: what the data mean

P—Plan: what should be done for the patient

More information on the topic of recording in medical records can be found in *Patient Nutritional Care in Long-Term Care Facilities* (see Bibliography). This reference provides the following illustrations of nutritional care documentation in both the source-oriented and SOAP formats:

> Mr. Allen is concerned about feeding himself. He is unable to see what is on the tray and has minimal use of his right hand. His appetite is good and he currently weighs 160 lb.
>
> Dietetic service will arrange the dishes appropriately on his tray. Self-feeding devices will be included. A plate waste study will be performed for three days, and the nutrient intake will then be evaluated. Nurses will provide encouragement and supervision during mealtime.
>
> Joan Smith, R.D.
> Consultant Dietitian

> S—Patient wants to feed himself, even though he has minimal use of right hand and is blind.
> O—Patient attempts to feed himself and asks questions about arrangement of foods on tray.
> A—Appetite is good; weight is 160 lb.
> P—Dietetic service uses self-feeding devices and appropriate tray arrangement; plate waste study for three days enables evaluation of nutrient encourage intake; nurses and supervise patient during mealtime.
>
> Joan Smith, R.D.
> Consultant Dietitian

Menu
Planning

PLANNING CONSIDERATIONS

The most important plan a food service manager makes is the menu. It should be regarded as a responsibility of top priority because it determines how the resources of the operation are going to be used. Menus should be planned with the following factors in mind:
- Food preferences and nutritional needs of group(s) being served
- Departmental budget allocation
- Personnel availability, skills, and time
- Market conditions and availability of food
- Type of production and service system
- Amount of space and type of storage, preparation, and service equipment

FOOD PREFERENCES

Nutritional needs of individuals, as discussed earlier in this chapter, differ widely. And just as important as differing nutritional needs are the personal, cultural, and regional food preferences. Menu planners too often put their own personal likes and dislikes of foods and food combinations on the menu without ever attempting to find out what the clientele really likes to eat.

Food preference biases can be avoided by using informal and formal methods to analyze and study how the patients, employees, and guests in a facility react to various foods. Informal observation in the dining room, cafeteria, patient floors, and with staff, for example, provides valuable insights. Questionnaires designed to survey food preferences and satisfaction during a patient's stay in the hospital or nursing home also are useful sources of menu planning information. Rating forms can be used that allow persons to rank their preference for various foods in relation to one another and their preferences for food combinations, for example: cranberry sauce or cranberry relish with turkey, raisin sauce or mustard sauce with ham, dumplings or biscuits with beef stew.

Food combination preferences are particularly important when a limited menu or a nonselective menu is served. In a facility in which the population changes frequently, it is important to survey food preferences frequently to keep menus current. Nutritional assessment procedures also may provide essential food habit information that can be used in planning menus for patients on regular or modified diets.

Most people do not mind being served favorite foods on a frequent basis, but less preferred foods should not be repeated within short intervals of time. Breakfast habits and preferences vary widely among different individuals. For that reason, breakfast menus should offer a range of choices in order to suit varying habits, yet be flexible enough to avoid food waste.

DEPARTMENTAL BUDGET ALLOCATION

With some effort and imagination, a skilled menu planner can design menus that offer variety, interest, and appeal and remain within almost any budget. The menu should be planned using updated, precosted recipes. If a running cost total is noted as the menu is set up, with high-cost and low-cost items balanced, the total food cost for each patient day can stay within the budget allocation. In addition, the same food cost level should be maintained from one day to another, rather than compensating for an overbudget day with an underbudget day at a level that is considerably below the desired daily average allowable cost. This approach works fairly well in controlling costs when planning nonselective menus, provided that recipe cost information is current and projected market conditions are considered when menus are planned far in advance.

When a choice of meal components is offered, a forecast of the number of portions of each item that can be selected must be determined before computing the total cost per meal or patient day. When menus are planned for both employees and guests, costs of foods and selling prices must be considered. Selling price should cover food, labor, and some overhead costs. However, it is somewhat more difficult to arrive at an accurate forecast of demand because the selling price itself will affect the demand for items. Careful histories of menu item popularity can sharpen the forecast if the same combinations of food items are offered each time.

Some facilities use the U.S. Department of Agriculture's family food plans at various cost levels (*thrifty, low cost, moderate cost,* and *liberal*) to allocate the food dollar among food groups. The food plans are designed to allocate food expenditures among food categories in order to obtain a balanced diet.

PERSONNEL AVAILABILITY, SKILLS, AND TIME

The availability and skills of production personnel must be considered when planning a menu, but need not necessarily limit the extent and quality of the menu. Products requiring considerable skill and time to prepare are widely available, with all or most of the labor provided by the food manufacturer. Menu items that cannot be produced on-premise with available labor skills or equipment can be part of the menu in most institutions if food costs fall within budget constraints.

Employees' expectations and sources of self-satisfaction in preparing food items should be considered when planning menus. Plans should be made for the average level of skill and energy, but whenever possible, challenges should be offered to employees who seek to enhance their job skills. Overloading production schedules by poor menu planning can lead to tired, frustrated employees. Menus that balance the production work load from day to day and that accommodate other essential job tasks help create positive employee attitudes.

At present, estimates of labor time requirements are intuitive, based on the judgment and past experiences of the manager. Current research now reports using industrial engineering methods to predetermine production times. Better estimates of total preparation time for each menu item could assist managers in planning the menu mix, scheduling personnel, and forecasting labor cost for menu items. But whichever method is used, menus must be planned in a manner that allows employees to produce the food in the allotted time while working at a normal pace. Most employees can adjust to occasional miscalculations but become frustrated and angry when crises become routine. Also, low productivity will result when employee time and skill are underutilized as a result of poorly planned menus or when labor time is not adjusted downward to accommodate the use of more convenience foods.

MARKET CONDITIONS

Several factors affecting the supply and price of foods in the marketplace should be considered when planning menus:

- *Weather conditions.* Sharp supply and price fluctuations for fresh produce for short periods of time commonly result from variable weather conditions. Favorable weather conditions can result in an unexpected abundance of produce at lower prices. Adverse weather conditions can result in high prices and a shortage of produce. Fruits and vegetables grown for processing also are affected and result in supply problems that may extend over several months.

- *Supply cycles.* Improvements in food processing, distribution, and storage technology have increased the availability of many foods during the entire year. However, seasonal fluctuations still occur for many fresh fruits and vegetables that are marketed in unprocessed forms. Supplies of meat animals and poultry tend to fluctuate in cycles but the time period is longer. For example, beef supply cycles fluctuate over a period of several years, whereas pork or poultry items have a much shorter cycle. Familiarity with local markets is necessary to remain informed of the current status of fresh supplies. When supplies decrease and prices increase, the frequency of use of these food items should be reevaluated and substitutions should be made. Menus should be planned to take advantage of the seasonal abundance of food products.
- *Geographic locations.* The types and quality of food products available to a facility may be limited to some degree by its location in relation to the source of supply. Improvements in transportation systems have eliminated this problem for many products. However, a variety of food products in the ready-to-serve state still may not be available to small hospitals or nursing homes in rural areas. Therefore, food service managers considering a system requiring a high degree of purchased convenience items need to investigate carefully the market availability of these items to achieve interesting menus at an acceptable cost level and still meet nutritional and quality standards.

PRODUCTION AND SERVICE SYSTEMS

In conventional production systems whereby foods are prepared, held hot or cold, and served on the same day, menus can be limited by the amount of time available for food preparation between meal periods. The menu planner should try to spread the work load as evenly as possible among employees over the workday, yet avoid holding conditions that may damage food quality.

In cook/chill or cook/freeze systems, time limits may not be as severe, because once food is produced, it is held in a chilled or frozen state until it is served. Service period deadlines do not limit the production schedules in these two systems. However, not all food items are suitable for these holding methods without extensive ingredient or process modification. Menu planners need to be completely familiar with the problems associated with certain menu items and should revise production procedures accordingly.

The critical relationship between the menu items offered and the service system selected must be considered. The method of service and the distance that trays or bulk food must be transported can limit the types of menu items that can be served successfully. For example, fried eggs, hot cakes, omelets, and ice cream may not retain proper temperature and may deteriorate in quality if too great a time passes between preparation and service. The number of sauces and casserole dishes may have to be limited in bulk food distribution because of limited space in food carts for the extra containers and because of extra handling required at point of service.

SPACE AND EQUIPMENT

A menu cannot be planned successfully unless the amount and type of space available for storing foods before, during, and after preparation is considered. Purchasing policies need to take storage space into account so that delivery schedules can be arranged to ensure that adequate amounts of needed foods are always on hand. Equipment capability also must be considered as menus are planned. A menu item cannot be produced unless the necessary equipment is available at the time needed. Unfortunately, many small food services do not have labor-saving equipment, such as mechanical slicers, shredders, choppers, peelers, and so forth, that save time and allow production of more complicated products within relatively short periods. Although this equipment is expensive, labor time and money can be saved through increased productivity while menu item variety is improved. When planning menus, demands on equipment must be balanced to avoid overloading ovens, steam equipment, or other production areas.

MENU DECISIONS

Several decisions must be made by the food service manager before planning any menus. Some of these decisions require input from other departments as well as the dietary department before policies can be established. For example, the number of meals served per day and the times at which they are served affect and are affected by the operations of the food service department and other departments.

The policies and procedures manual should state clearly the meal plan, the exact times meals are served, and the menu pattern for the facility. The menu planning responsibility for normal and modified diets also should be clearly specified.

MEAL PLAN

The meal plan is an administrative decision requiring input from other patient-care departments and the medical staff. The number of food items offered on the menu for each meal varies according to the meal plan. Three-, four-, or five-meal-a-day plans are used in health care facilities.

The three-meal plan is a traditional breakfast-lunch-dinner or break-fast-dinner-supper pattern. However, because of changing food habits and labor scheduling and availability, the other plans are being used in many facilities.

The four-meal plan, which has become popular, consists of a continental breakfast (beverage, cereal, and/or hot roll or quick bread); brunch in late morning (breakfast and/or lunch items); main meal in the late afternoon; and an evening snack of a substantial nature. Obviously, this kind of plan must have full support from nursing and medical services because the entire facility will be affected by it.

The five-meal plan consists of an early continental breakfast, a mid-morning brunch, a light early-afternoon refreshment, a main meal in late afternoon, and an evening nourishment before retiring.

Menus must be carefully planned to distribute the day's nutrients in a balanced fashion over all meals and to avoid excessive amounts of calories, particularly with the four-meal and five-meal plans. Regardless of which meal plan is used, no more than 15 hours should elapse between the last meal of one day and the first meal of the following.

TYPE OF MENU

Menus can be either nonselective or selective. A nonselective menu gives the patient no choice in what is served. Although many food service managers believe that the nonselective menu saves time, money, and waste, patient dissatisfaction can outweigh these perceived advantages. Despite careful planning and preparing of nonselective menus, many patients may be dissatisfied because the menus do not accommodate individual food likes and dislikes and forces patients to consume unwanted foods or leave them as plate waste. However, in many extended-care facilities, nonselective menus are frequently used because residents are incapable of making their own selections.

There are several obvious advantages of a selective menu: patients can choose what they want, the amount of plate waste can be lowered, and food costs can drop. This is especially true when an expensive entree is paired with an inexpensive one, thus allowing the lower-cost item to offset the higher one. When patients choose their own food, they are more likely to eat everything and may even choose fewer items than would have been served on a nonselective menu. For example, when both bread and another starchy food are offered, only one may be selected.

A selective menu requires that the food service department prepare several different menu items for each meal but in smaller quantities. Therefore, even a facility with limited equipment and personnel can offer a more diverse and interesting menu. Careful item pairing will balance work load, equipment use, and costs. Carefully planned selective menus also include options that can be used on modified diets. To help ensure that patients select a nutritionally adequate diet, menu items are often grouped in categories from which a specified number of selections are made. Use of selective menus for modified diets can be an effective educational tool in teaching patients to manage their own diets.

In some short-term care hospitals, menus with a wide number of selections are used. The menu resembles that of a restaurant in variety and number of selections and remains the same from day to day, with the exception of one or more daily specials. Many of these facilities use a cook/chill system and/or incorporate several convenience entrees and desserts in addition to items prepared in the hospital. Greater patient satisfaction is noted in these operations.

CYCLE MENUS

Menu planning in many facilities is streamlined by use of a cycle menu. This is a set of carefully planned, tested menus that are used in rotation for a specified number of weeks. During a cycle, no menu is repeated. Depending upon the average patient stay, the cycle may be three, four, or more weeks in length. Longer cycles are desirable in long-term care facilities and for employees. Short cycles are used in acute care hospitals.

Cycle menus require careful planning and can be either selective or nonselective. The first cycle can be regarded as a test period, after which adjustments should be made to increase the attractiveness of the meals, to avoid any preparation or service difficulties encountered, or to reduce cost. The cycle menus also should be adjusted with the changing seasons and market conditions. Cycle menus should be reviewed and changed periodically, particularly if clientele changes or if new food items or forms of food are introduced. Cycles should be flexible enough to feature holiday items or adjust to other social activities, particularly in extended care facilities. A balanced level of item popularity should be maintained throughout the cycle, and the beginning and end of the cycle should be sufficiently different from one another. The repetition of food items on the same day of each week should be avoided.

Once established, the cycle menu saves personnel time and labor in planning menus, in food procurement, and in food production. Purchase orders should be filed with the menus to simplify future purchasing and production forecasts, and actual selection of each item should be recorded so that greater forecast accuracy can be attained each time the cycle is repeated. The cycle menu is useful as a training device because it enables employees to become more familiar with the production of each item, and it also allows for better organization of employee time.

PLANNING RESPONSIBILITY

Although the job title of the person responsible for menu planning differs from one facility to another, the ultimate planning authority should rest with a person who has direct responsibility for supervising food production and service. In smaller operations, this may be either the food service supervisor or the dietetic technician. In such cases, regular and modified menus are checked by a consultant dietitian. In larger institutions, menus may be planned by a full-time dietitian or by a committee consisting of the food service director, dietitians, food service supervisors, and key food production personnel. When these personnel are included, they understand the importance of following the menus as planned and can contribute good ideas as well as practical advice on production matters.

MEAL PATTERN

Translating the daily food needs of patients or residents into attractive and appealing meals requires an organized approach. The normal diet—also called the regular, general, or house diet—is the starting point in planning because it is the basis for all diet modifications. Planning and producing modified diets are easier when the normal diet menu includes several foods that also can be served on modified diets. However, the variety in the general menu should not be restricted by this consideration. Only slight changes in many foods will make them suitable for the other diets. In order to meet nutritional needs, the normal diet is based upon the food patterns shown in tables 13 and 14, pages 151 and 154.

The menu planner uses the normal diet and the basic four food groups to develop the meal pattern. The meal pattern simply lists the basic components for each meal, such as:

Breakfast
Fruit or juice
Hot or cold cereal
Meat or meat alternate
Bread and butter/margarine
Beverage
Lunch or supper
Meat or meat alternate or soup and sandwich
Vegetable and/or salad
Bread and butter/margarine
Dessert or fruit
Beverage
Dinner
Appetizer
Soup or juice
Meat or meat alternate
Potato, rice, or pasta
Vegetable
Fruit or vegetable salad
Bread and butter/margarine

Dessert

Beverage

On a four-meal or five-meal plan, the individual meal components will vary from the example listed above in order to spread total food intake over all meals. On any meal plan, a selective menu offers one or more choices for each component. The number of items offered at each meal on each day should be approximately the same to ensure that the recommended number of servings from the food groups are served and to maintain an even level of food intake from day to day. It is helpful to use a menu planning form to assist in planning meals that conform to the standard for the facility.

PLANNING MENUS

In order to plan menus, a place and time for planning should be selected. Reference materials also should be gathered, including previous menus, inventory lists, standardized recipe files, market reports, popularity index of menu items previously served, trade publications, and other manuals and publications available from professional associations. (See references at the end of the book.) Using a standard menu planning form, which lists meal patterns, meals, and days of the week, the following steps should be noted when planning a normal diet menu:

1. Meat or meat alternate entrees for the main meals should be selected first for the entire cycle. Entree choices must be made first because other foods in each meal are selected to complement and enhance them. Also, because the largest portion of the food dollar is spent for these foods, the frequency of their use must be controlled. It can be helpful to make a list of possible meat or meat alternate entrees to use in menu planning, such as the one illustrated in table 16, next page. This type of list can save time and money, give variety, and prevent repetition of menus on the same day of each week.

2. The vegetables and potatoes, rice, or pasta to be served with the main dish for each meal should be selected on the basis of color, form, texture, and flavor. A colorful vegetable in whole, sliced, diced, or some other interesting form would make the meal more attractive. Crisp vegetables can complement a soft or creamy main dish.

3. Salads that will provide contrast in color, flavor, and texture to the meal should be added. Chilled salads complement hot entrees. Main dish salads, chef's salads, and cold plates that include salads also are popular entrees.

4. Different breads, such as yeast breads, quick breads, sweet dough breads, and specialty breads, complement the entree and can be varied from meal to meal.

5. Desserts should be selected to complete and balance the meal in

flavor, texture, and sometimes in caloric content. Fresh, canned, and frozen fruits are offered as alternates in many facilities.

6. Beverages are usually standardized in most institutions. In addition to coffee, tea, and other hot beverages, a variety of milks should be offered. Most people prefer a low-fat milk to whole milk, and flavored milks offer a change.

7. Breakfast menus should be planned last. Although breakfast menus are simple, they should provide interesting food variations from day

TABLE 16. MENU PLANNING SUGGESTIONS: ENTREES, VEGETABLES, SALADS AND RELISHES, DESSERTS, GARNISHES, LEFTOVER FOODS

ENTREES

Meats

BEEF:
Corned beef
Roast beef
Pot roast
Broiled steak
T-bone
Sirloin
Filet mignon
Club steak
Cubed steak
Country-fried steak
Spanish steak
Swiss steak
Steak with vegetables
Steak stroganoff
Mock drumsticks
Barbecued kabobs
Barbecued short ribs
Braised short ribs
Beef pot pie
Beef stew with
vegetables
Beef stew with
dumplings
Beef ragout
Hungarian goulash
Chop suey
Meat loaf
Swedish meatballs
Spanish meatballs
Meatballs with
spaghetti
VEAL:
Roast leg of veal
Roast veal shoulder
Baked veal chops
Veal chops in sour
cream

Breaded veal cutlets
Veal birds
Veal fricassee with
poppy-seed noodles
Veal stew with
vegetables
Veal a la king
Veal patties with
bacon
Veal paprika with
rice
Curried veal with
rice
LAMB:
Roast leg of lamb
Roast lamb shoulder
Broiled lamb chops
Lamb stew
Braised lamb riblets
Barbecued lamb
Lamb patties with
bacon
Curried lamb with
rice
Lamb fricassee with
noodles
PORK (fresh):
Baked fresh ham
Roast pork loin
Roast pork shoulder
Roast pork with
dressing
Baked pork chops
Breaded pork chops
Deviled pork chops
Barbecued pork chops
Stuffed pork chops
Breaded pork cutlets
Barbecued spareribs
Spareribs with kraut

Spareribs with
dressing
Pork birds
PORK (cured):
Baked ham
Baked ham slices
Grilled ham slices
Baked Canadian bacon
Ham loaf
Ham patties
Glazed ham balls
VARIETY MEATS:
Braised tongue
Braised liver
Liver and bacon
Liver and onions
Baked heart
Braised heart
Sweetbread cutlets
Creamed sweetbreads
MISCELLANEOUS:
Frankfurters with
kraut
Cheese-stuffed
wieners

Meat Extenders

Baked hash
Corned beef hash
Stuffed peppers
Beef roll
Beef upside-down pie
Spaghetti with
meat sauce
Creole spaghetti
Beef and pork
casserole
Spanish rice

TABLE 16. *Continued*

ENTREES (continued)

Meat Extenders (continued)

Creamed beef
Creamed chipped beef
Creamed chipped beef
  and peas
Chipped beef and
  noodles
Veal croquettes
Meat turnovers
Veal soufflé
Curried veal with rice
Creamed ham and
  celery
Ham a la king
Ham croquettes
Ham soufflé
Ham timbales
Ham and egg scallop
Creamed ham on
  spoon bread
Cold baked ham with
  potato salad
Chef's salad bowl
Russian salad bowl
Baked ham sandwiches
Ham and cheese
  sandwiches
Ham salad sandwiches
Bacon and tomato
  sandwiches
Bacon and tomato on
  bun with cheese sauce
Hamburgers on buns
Ham biscuit roll
Ham turnover with
  cheese sauce
Ham shortcake
Ham and sweetbread
  casserole
Sausage and dressing
Sausage and apple
  dressing
Sausage rolls
Sausage cakes
Fried scrapple
Bacon and potato
  omelet
Pork and noodle
  casserole
Baked lima beans
Baked lima beans
  with sausage
Boiled lima beans
  with ham
Baked navy beans

Chili con carne
Chili-spaghetti
Ranch-style beans
Baked eggs and bacon
  rings
Pizza
Cold luncheon meat
  with macaroni
  salad
Barbecued hamburgers
Wieners with meat
  sauce on bun
Hot luncheon sandwich
Hot roast beef
  sandwich
Hot roast pork
  sandwich
Barbecued ham,
  pork, or beef
  sandwiches
Western sandwich
Toasted chipped beef
  and cheese sandwich

Poultry

TURKEY:
  Roast turkey
  Baked turkey roll
  Hot turkey sandwich
  Sliced turkey sandwich
CHICKEN:
  Baked chicken
  Broiled chicken
  Fried chicken
  Barbecued chicken
  Chicken Tahitian
  Breast of chicken
    with ham slice
  Chicken a la Maryland
  Fricassee of chicken
  Chicken with dumplings
  Chicken with noodles
  Chicken pie
  Chicken or turkey loaf
  Chicken soufflé
  Chicken turnovers
  Chicken and rice
    casserole
  Chicken a la king
  Singapore curry
  Creamed chicken:
    on biscuit
    in patty shell
    on toast cups
    on chow mein noodles
    on spoon bread

Chicken croquettes
Chicken cutlets
Scalloped chicken
Chicken timbales
Chicken chow mein
Chicken biscuit roll-
  mushroom sauce
Chicken salad
Chicken salad in
  cranberry or
  raspberry mold
Chicken salad sandwich

Fish

FRESH AND FROZEN FISH:
  Fried salmon steaks
  Poached salmon
  Baked halibut steak
  Poached halibut steak
  Fried halibut steak
  Fried or baked fillets:
    haddock, perch, sole,
    whitefish, catfish
  Fried whole fish:
    whiting, smelts
  French-fried shrimp
  Creole shrimp with rice
  French-fried scallops
  Fried clams
  Fried oysters
  Scalloped oysters
  Deviled crab
  Crab casserole
  Broiled lobster
CANNED FISH:
  Salmon loaf
  Salmon croquettes
  Creamed salmon
    on biscuit
  Salmon biscuit roll
    with creamed peas
  Scalloped salmon
  Salmon and potato
    chip casserole
  Casserole of rice
    and tuna
  Tuna croquettes
  Creamed tuna:
    on toast
    on biscuit
  Tuna soufflé
  Scalloped tuna
  Tuna biscuit roll-
    cheese sauce
  Tuna-cashew casserole
  Codfish balls

TABLE 16. *Continued*

ENTREES (continued)

Fish (continued)

Tuna and noodles
Crab salad
Lobster salad
Shrimp salad
Tuna salad
Salmon salad
Cold salmon with
  potato salad
Hot tuna bun
Tuna sandwich,
  plain or grilled

Meatless Dishes

Cheese rarebit
Cheese balls on
  pineapple slice
Cheese croquettes
Cheese soufflé
Cheese fondue
Macaroni and cheese
Scalloped macaroni

Baked rice and cheese
Rice croquettes with
  cheese sauce
Chinese omelet
Rice with mushroom
  and almond sauce
Fried mush
Baked eggs with
  cheese
Curried eggs
Creamed eggs
Egg cutlets
Egg and noodle
  casserole
Noodle casserole
Hot stuffed eggs
Eggs a la king
Scalloped eggs and
  cheese
Scrambled eggs
Omelet
Spanish omelet
Vegetable casserole
  with pinwheel
  biscuits

Cauliflower casserole
Vegetable timbales
Spinach timbales
  with poached egg
Mushroom puff
Cheese puff
Spoon bread
Corn rarebit
Corn pudding
Scalloped corn
Hot potato salad
Creamed asparagus
  on toast
French toast
Plain fritters
Corn fritters
Fruit fritters
Grilled cheese
  sandwich
Egg salad sandwich
Fruit plates
Cottage cheese salad
Deviled eggs
Brown bean salad
Stuffed tomato salad

VEGETABLES

Green Vegetables

ARTICHOKES:
  With butter or
    mayonnaise
ASPARAGUS:
  Buttered or creamed
  With cheese sauce
    or hollandaise
BEANS, GREEN:
  Buttered or creamed
  Creole
  With almonds or
    mushrooms
  Southern style
BROCCOLI:
  Almond buttered
  Buttered
  With cheese sauce,
    lemon butter, or
    hollandaise
BRUSSELS SPROUTS:
  Buttered
CABBAGE:
  Au gratin
  Buttered or creamed
  Creole
  Hot slaw

CELERY:
  Buttered or creamed
CELERY CABBAGE:
  Buttered
PEAS:
  Buttered or in cream
  With carrots,
    cauliflower,
    celery, or onions
  With mushrooms or
    almonds
SPINACH:
  Buttered
  Wilted
  With egg or bacon
  With new beets

Other Vegetables

BEETS:
  Buttered
  Harvard
  Julienne
  In sour cream
  With orange sauce
  Hot spiced
  Pickled

CARROTS:
  Buttered or creamed
  Candied
  Glazed
  Lyonnaise
  Mint glazed
  Savory
  With celery
  With peas
  Parsley-buttered
  Sweet-sour
CAULIFLOWER:
  Buttered
  Creamed
  French fried
  With almond butter
  With cheese sauce
  With peas
CUCUMBERS:
  Scalloped
EGGPLANT:
  Creole
  Fried or French fried
  Scalloped
MUSHROOMS
  Broiled
  Sautéed

TABLE 16. *Continued*

VEGETABLES (continued)

Other Vegetables (continued)

ONIONS:
  Au gratin
  Baked
  Buttered
  Casserole
  Creamed
  French fried
  Stuffed
  With Spanish sauce
RUTABAGAS:
  Buttered
  Mashed
SQUASH, SUMMER:
  Buttered
  Mashed
TOMATOES:
  Baked
  Breaded
  Broiled tomato
    slices
  Creole
  Scalloped
  Stewed
  Stuffed
TURNIPS:
  Buttered
  In cream
  Mashed
  With new peas

Fruits Served as Vegetables

APPLES:
  Buttered
  Fried
  Hot Baked
BANANAS:
  Baked
  French fried

GRAPEFRUIT:
  Broiled
PEACHES:
  Broiled
PINEAPPLE RING:
  Broiled
  Sautéed

Potatoes or Substitutes

POTATOES, IRISH:
  Au gratin
  Baked
  Browned
  Buttered new
  Chips
  Creamed
  Croquettes
  Duchesse
  Fried
  French fried
  Lyonnaise
  Mashed
  O'Brien
  Potato cakes
  Potato pancakes
  Potato salad, hot
    or cold
  Rissole
  Scalloped
  Stuffed baked
POTATOES, SWEET:
  Baked
  Candied or glazed
  Croquettes
  Mashed
  Scalloped
MACARONI AND
SPAGHETTI:
  Macaroni and cheese
  Macaroni salad
  Scalloped macaroni

NOODLES:
  Buttered
  Poppy seed
RICE:
  Buttered
  Curried
  Fried rice with
    almonds
  Green rice
  Croquettes

Other Starchy Vegetables

CORN:
  Buttered
  In cream
  On cob
  Corn and tomato
  Corn pudding
  O'Brien
  Scalloped
  With celery and bacon
  With green pepper
    rings
  Succotash
LIMA BEANS:
  Buttered
  In cream
  With bacon
  With mushrooms
  With almonds
PARSNIPS:
  Buttered:
  Browned
  Glazed
SQUASH:
  Baked acorn
  Baked hubbard
  Mashed butternut
  Mashed hubbard

SALADS AND RELISHES

Fruit Salads

Apple and celery
Apple and carrot
Apple and cabbage
Cranberry relish
Cranberry sauce
Frozen fruit
Mixed fruit

Waldorf

Vegetable Salads

Beet pickles
Beet relish
Brown bean
Cabbage relish
Cabbage

Cabbage-carrot
Cabbage-marshmallow
Cabbage-pineapple
Carrot-raisin
Celery cabbage
Coleslaw

TABLE 16. Continued

SALADS AND RELISHES (continued)

Vegetable Salads (continued)		Relishes
Creamy coleslaw	Molded pear	Rhubarb
Cucumber-onion	Perfection	Strawberry
in sour cream	Molded pineapple-	Tomato
Hawaiian tossed	cheese	Watermelon
Head lettuce	Molded pineapple-	
Potato	cucumber	**Relishes**
Red cabbage	Molded pineapple-	
Salad greens with	relish	Burr gherkins
grapefruit	Molded pineapple-	Carrot curls
Stuffed tomato	rhubarb	Carrot sticks
Tossed green	Raspberry ring mold	Cauliflowerets
Tomato	Ribbon mold	Celery curls
Tomato-cucumber	Spicy apricot	Celery fans
Vegetable-nut	Sunshine	Celery hearts
	Swedish green top	Celery rings
	Tomato aspic	Cherry tomatoes
Gelatin Salads	Under-the-sea	Cucumber slices
		Cucumber wedges
Applesauce mold	**Salad Ices**	Green pepper rings
Autumn		Olives, green,
Beet	Apricot	ripe, stuffed
Bing cherry	Cherry	Onion rings
Cabbage parfait	Cranberry	Radish accordions
Cranberry ring mold	Grapefruit	Radish roses
Frosted cherry	Lemon	Spiced crabapples
Frosted lime	Lime	Spiced peaches
Grapefruit	Mint	Spiced pears
Jellied citrus	Orange	Stuffed celery
Jellied vegetable	Pineapple	Tomato slices
Jellied waldorf	Raspberry	Tomato wedges
		Watermelon pickles

GARNISHES

Yellow-Orange		
	SWEETS:	Cinnamon apples
CHEESE AND EGGS:	Apricot preserves	Cranberries
Balls, grated, strips	Orange marmalade	Plums
Rossettes	Peach conserve	Pomegranate seeds
Egg, hard-cooked	Peanut brittle,	Red raspberries
or sections	crushed	Maraschino cherries
Deviled egg halves	Sugar, yellow or	Strawberries
Riced egg yolk	orange	Watermelon cubes, balls
FRUIT:	VEGETABLES:	SWEETS:
Apricot halves,	Carrots, rings,	Red jelly, apple,
sections	shredded, strips	cherry, currant,
Cantaloupe balls	MISCELLANEOUS:	loganberry, raspberry
Lemon sections, slices	Butter balls	Cranberry glace, jelly
Orange sections,	Coconut, tinted	Gelatin cubes
slices	Gelatin cubes	Red sugar
Peach slices	Mayonnaise	VEGETABLES:
Peach halves with jelly		Beets, pickled, Julienne
Spiced peaches	**Red**	Beet relish
Persimmons		Red cabbage
Tangerines	FRUIT:	Red peppers, rings,
	Cherries	strips, shredded

TABLE 16. *Continued*

GARNISHES (continued)

Red (continued)	Parsley, sprig, chopped	Mints

Red (continued)

Pimiento, chopped, strips
Radishes, red: sliced roses
Stuffed olives, sliced
Tomato, aspic, catsup, chili sauce: cups, sections, sliced, broiled
MISCELLANEOUS:
Paprika
Tinted coconut
Cinnamon drops ("red hots")

Green

FRUIT:
Avocado
Cherries
Frosted grapes
Green plums
Honeydew melon
Lime wedges
SWEETS:
Citron
Green sugar
Gelatin cubes
Mint jelly
Mint pineapple
Mints
VEGETABLES:
Endive
Green pepper, strips, chopped
Green onions
Lettuce cups
Lettuce, shredded
Mint leaves
Olives

Parsley, sprig, chopped
Pickles:
Burr gherkins, strips, fans, rings
Spinach leaves
MISCELLANEOUS:
Coconut, tinted
Mayonnaise, tinted
Pistachios

White

FRUIT:
Apple rings
Apple balls
Grapefruit sections
Gingered apple
White raisins
Pear balls
Pear sections
VEGETABLES:
Cauliflowerets
Celery cabbage
Celery, curls, hearts, strips
Cucumber, rings, strips, wedges, cups
Mashed potato, rosettes
Onion rings
Onions, pickled
Radishes, white
MISCELLANEOUS:
Cream cheese frosting
Sliced hard-cooked egg white
Shredded coconut
Marshmallows
Almonds

Mints
Whipped cream
Powdered sugar

Brown-Tan

BREADS:
Crustades
Croutons
Cheese straws
Fritters, tiny
Noodle rings
Toast, cubes, points, strips, rings
MISCELLANEOUS:
Cinnamon
Dates
French-fried cauliflower
French-fried onions
Mushrooms
Nutmeats
Nut-covered cheese balls
Potato chips
Rosettes
Toasted coconut

Black

Caviar
Chocolate-covered mints
Chocolate sprill
Chocolate, shredded
Chocolate sauce
Olives, ripe
Prunes
Prunes, spiced
Pickled walnuts
Raisins, currants
Truffles

DESSERTS

Cakes and Cookies

CAKE:
Angel food, plain, chocolate, filled
Applesauce
Banana
Boston cream
Burnt sugar
Chiffon

Chocolate and jelly rolls
Coconut
Cupcakes
Fruit upside-down
Fudge
German sweet chocolate
Gingerbread
Lazy daisy
Marble

Pineapple cashew
Poppy-seed
Spice
White
COOKIES:
Brownies
Butter tea

TABLE 16. *Continued*

DESSERTS (continued)

Cakes and Cookies (continued)

Butterscotch
Chocolate chip
Coconut macaroon
Date bars
Oatmeal
Fudge balls
Ginger, crisp
Marshmallow squares
Peanut butter
Sandies
Sugar cookies

Pies and Pastries

ONE-CRUST PIES:
Apricot cream
Banana cream
Butterscotch
Chiffon
Coconut cream
Coconut custard
Custard
Date cream
Dutch apple
Frozen pies
Fruit-glazed cream
Pecan cream
Pineapple cream
Pumpkin
Rhubarb custard
TWO-CRUST PIES:
Apple
Apricot
Blackberry
Blueberry
Boysenberry
Cherry
Gooseberry
Mincemeat
Peach
Pineapple
Plum
Prune
Raisin
Rhubarb
Strawberry
COBBLERS, FRUIT:
(Same fruits as
for pies)

Puddings

Apple crisp

Apple dumplings
Apple brown Betty
Baked custards
Banana cream
Bavarian cream
Bread pudding
Butterscotch pudding
Caramel tapioca
Cherry crisp
Chocolate cream
Coconut cream
Cottage pudding
Cream puffs
Date cream
Date pudding
Date roll
English toffee dessert
Floating island
Fruit gelatin
Fruit whips
Fudge pudding
Icebox dessert
Lemon snow
Meringue shells
Peach crisp
Peach melba
Pineapple cream
Royal rice pudding
Shortcake
Steamed pudding
Tapioca cream
Vanilla cream

Frozen

ICE CREAMS:
Apricot
Banana
Butter brickle
Caramel
Chocolate
Chocolate chip
Coffee
Lemon custard
Macaroon
Peach
Peanut brittle
Pecan
Peppermint stick
Pineapple
Pistachio
Raspberry
Strawberry
Toffee
Tutti-frutti

PARFAITS, SHERBETS:
Apricot
Cherry
Cranberry
Green gage plum
Lemon
Lime
Orange
Mint
Pineapple
Plum
Raspberry
Rhubarb
Watermelon

Miscellaneous

CHEESE:
Assorted, with
crackers and fruit
FRUIT:
Baked or Stewed:
Apples
Fruit compote
Rhubarb
Canned or Frozen:
Apricots
Berries
Cherries
Figs
Fruit cup
Peaches
Pears
Pineapple
Plums
Prunes
Rhubarb
Raw:
Apples
Apricots
Bananas
Berries
Cherries
Figs
Grapefruit
Grapes
Melons
Oranges
Peaches
Pears
Pineapple
Plums
Prunes

TABLE 16. *Continued*

LEFTOVER FOODS

BREAD AND CRACKERS:
Bread crumbs—
for crumbing
cutlets, croquettes,
and other fried food;
thickening steamed
and other puddings
Canapes
Cinnamon toast
Croutons—as soup
accompaniment
Desserts—bread pud-
ding, brown Betty
French toast
Hot dishes—cheese
fondue; scalloped
macaroni; soufflé;
stuffing for meat,
poultry, or fish
Melba toast
Toast points—
as garnish
CEREALS:
Chinese omelet
Fried or French-fried
cornmeal mush or
hominy grits
Meatballs with cooked
cereal as extender
Rice and tuna
Rice croquettes
Rice custard
Soup with rice, spaghetti,
or noodles
CAKES AND COOKIES:
Baked fruit pudding
Cottage pudding
Crumbs to coat balls of
ice cream
Crumb cookies
Icebox cake
Spice crumb cake
EGGS:
Boiled or poached—add
to cream sauce,
mayonnaise, or
French dressing, as a
garnish for vegetables,
egg cutlets, in salad
Scrambled—potato salad,
sandwich spread
Egg whites, raw—angel
food cake, Bavarians,

fluffy or
boiled dressing,
macaroons, meringue,
prune whip, white
sheet or layer cake
Egg yolks, raw—cooked
salad dressing, custard
sauce, filling,
or pudding,
Duchesse potatoes,
Hollandaise, hot cake
batter, scrambled eggs,
strawberry Bavarian
cream pie, yellow
angel food cake
FISH:
Creamed, a la king, or
scalloped
Fish cakes or croquettes
Salad
Sandwich spread
FRUIT:
Applesauce cake
Apricot or berry muffins
Frozen fruit salad
Fruit slaw
Fruit tarts
Jellied fruit cup or salad
Jelly or jam
Mixed fruit salad or fruit
cup
Prune or apricot filling
for rolls or cookies
Sauce for
cottage pudding
MEAT:
Apple stuffed with
sausage
Bacon in sauce for
vegetable
Baked beef hash
Boiled lima beans with
ham
Chili con carne
Chop suey
Creamed ham or meat
on toast
Creamed ham in timbale
cases
Creole spaghetti
Ham or bacon omelet

Hot tamale pie
Meat croquettes
Meat pie or meat roll
Meat turnovers
Salad
Sandwiches
Scalloped potatoes
with ham
Scrapple
Stuffed peppers
**MILK AND CREAM,
SOUR:**
Biscuit brown bread
Butterscotch cookies
Fudge cake
Griddle cakes
Salad dressing
Sour cream pie
Spice coffee cake
Veal chops in
sour cream
POULTRY:
Chicken and rice
casserole
Chicken timbales
Creamed chicken in
patty cases
Chicken a la king
Croquettes
Cutlets
Jellied chicken loaf
Pot pie
Salad
Sandwiches
Soufflé
Soup
Turnovers
VEGETABLES:
Combination-carrots and
peas, corn and beans,
corn and tomatoes,
peas and celery
Fritters
Potatoes—Duchesse,
hashed-brown,
lyonnaise, cakes,
omelet, salad (hot and
cold)
Salad, in combination
(when suitable)
Soup
Vegetable pie
Vegetable timbales

Source: Fowler, S., West, B., and Shugart, G. *Food for Fifty,* 5th ed. New York: John Wiley & Sons, Inc., 1971. Reprinted by permission of John Wiley & Sons, Inc.

to day. Nontraditional items such as breakfast sandwiches should be considered when planning breakfast menus. Trade journals also can provide creative ideas for breakfast menus that are simple yet appetizing and attractive.

After the normal diet menu has been planned, the soft, liquid, and other modified diets can be planned, making only the substitutions necessary to conform to the prescribed diet as stated in the facility's diet manual. An advantage of this approach is that it keeps the number of modified diet foods at a minimum, thus eliminating many small batches of diet foods and reducing labor hours.

MENU EVALUATION

The final step in menu planning is a careful evaluation of the proposed menus to see that nutritional objectives are attained, that resources are effectively used, and that menus are appealing. The following list describes the characteristics of a good menu and can easily be used as an evaluation checklist:

1. *Menu pattern.* Each meal is consistent with the established menu pattern, including all food components specified as necessary to meet nutritional needs.

2. *Color and eye appeal.* Color combinations are pleasant and blend well. A variety of colors is used in each meal. Colorless or one-color meals are avoided. Attractive garnishes are used.

3. *Texture and consistency.* A mix of soft, creamy, crisp, chewy, and firm textured foods are included in each meal.

4. *Flavor combinations.* Food flavors are compatible yet varied. Two or more foods with strong or pronounced flavors, such as broccoli, onions, turnips, cabbage, and cauliflower, are avoided in the same meal. Other combinations, such as tomato juice and macaroni-tomato casserole or macaroni and cheese and pineapple-cheese salad, are avoided also.

5. *Sizes and shapes.* Meals include a pleasing contrast of food sizes and shapes. Too many chopped or mixed items in the same meal, such as cubed meat, diced potatoes, mixed vegetables, and fruit cocktail, are avoided.

6. *Food temperatures.* Hot and cold items are offered in each meal. Climate or season of the year is considered in selecting types of foods.

7. *Preparation methods.* Two or more foods prepared in the same manner in a meal are avoided. A balanced distribution of creamed, boiled, fried, baked, and braised foods is attained from day to day.

8. *Popularity.* Popular and less-popular foods are part of the same meal if a selection is offered. Serving popular foods in one meal

and less-popular foods at another meal is avoided.

9. *Day-to-day distribution.* Types of food offered on consecutive meals and days are varied in ingredients as well as in method of preparation. For example, the menus avoid meatloaf at noon and another ground beef entree in the evening. Variations in the foods offered the same day each week are planned. Hot dogs every Monday and chicken every Sunday, for example, are avoided.

10. *Clientele preferences.* Menus are appropriate for cultural, ethnic, and personal food preferences of clientele. Prejudices are avoided.

11. *Availability and cost of food.* Seasonal foods are used frequently. High- and low-cost foods are balanced within each day's menus and throughout the menu cycle so that budget constraints are met.

12. *Facilities and equipment.* Available equipment is adequate to produce high quality in the food selections on the menu. Equipment use is balanced throughout the day and cycle. Menu items are compatible with transport and service equipment. Number and type of serving dishes are available for attractive presentation of menu items.

13. *Personnel and time.* Adequate number and needed personnel skills are available for preparation and service. Personnel work load is balanced from day to day and week to week. Adequate time is available for production and service of foods on each menu.

14. *Menu form and presentation.* Menu item descriptions are specific, appealing, and accurate. Format follows consistent, accepted sequence.

After correcting any problems noted during the evaluation, the menus should be rechecked. This procedure should be followed each time menus are planned, but the time involved will be reduced when cycle menus are used. Whenever a menu is actually produced, any problems encountered should be noted on the master menu form and the appropriate changes made before repeating the menu in another cycle.

MENU FORMAT

After the menus for normal and modified diets have been planned, evaluated, and refined, they are written in two different styles, one for production and service personnel and the other for patients. The menu used in the kitchen provides information for production personnel, such as ingredient state, name, and number of the recipe to be used and the production forecast. Information on portion sizes, special comments about the recipe, or advance preparation needs can be added. When the menu is written in this format, it serves as a production sheet. The names of each item should be very specific. For example, the kind of fruit juice, the flavor of gelatin, the type of bread item, and so forth should be stated if not already specified in the recipe. This ensures that the balance of flavors, colors, and textures as originally planned will be prepared and served.

Selective menus distributed to patients should be informative, attractive, and easy to understand. Terminology should be used that is clear and simple, yet accurate and easy for a reader who may not be at peak alertness. Nutrition education information also can be included. Specially designed forms can be used to make menus more appealing. Menus should be consistent in format and have clear directions on how to mark choices. Meal components should be listed in expected order of consumption. Descriptive terms should be accurate—truth-in-menu is as important as accurate labeling on commercial food products.

Although foods should be described in appetizing terms, they also should live up to the adjectives. Crisp salads should be crisp, hot rolls should be hot, and homemade breads should truly be baked on-premise. Fanciful names may not be familiar to patients, who may hesitate to select such items. If such terms are used, a brief description of the item should be added, for example, under-the-sea salad (lime gelatin with pears, topped with whipped lime gelatin).

SPECIAL MENUS

Nourishing foods are essential to the normal growth and development of children. When children are hospitalized and separated from the security of parents and home, food takes on added significance. Meals not only should satisfy nutritional requirements and appetites but also should be fun to eat. The family should be consulted about the child's food preferences and eating habits. Menu items should be appropriate to the child's age and developmental stage, with modification of the physical form of the food when needed. Raw fruits and vegetables that can be eaten as finger foods are usually much more popular than traditional salads. Raw vegetables can be accompanied by nutritious dips for added appeal. Many hospitals and institutions for children use specially designed menu forms, with attractive colors and artwork. Nutrition education, particularly for children who may be on modified diets, is appealingly incorporated.

Menus for school-age children and adolescents need to be adjusted for nutrient needs and for the child's activity level. Food preferences of this age group can be distinctly different from those of adults and should be carefully considered.

The nutritional needs of the healthy older person differ from the younger adult's needs only in the number of calories. This is due to decreased physical activity and slowing of body processes. Frequently, older persons are in need of improved nutritional content of meals, particularly if they have been living alone or have some disease or ailment. Lack of motivation to prepare meals or to consume regular meals often leads to being either overweight or underweight. Planning menus to meet the needs of older persons presents many challenges, particularly on a long-term basis. When older persons enter or are placed in a long-term care facility, the change from their familiar environment to an unknown one often produces marked psychological reactions, such as feelings of rejection, insecurity, and despondency. These feelings may be expressed by complaints about the food, refusal to eat, or by an insistence for foods that are common and familiar. For this reason, a complete food habit profile is very important soon after admission. The family or friends can be helpful in providing additional information.

Principles that apply to the planning, preparation, and serving of the normal diet should be followed, but foods can be varied in quantity or form for the older person. Personal likes and dislikes should be given every consideration. Although loss of teeth or poorly fitted dentures may make chewing more difficult for some older persons, it should not be assumed that all persons with these handicaps must have their foods very soft or finely ground. A variety of food textures in each meal should be included and their acceptability evaluated. Colorful, appetizing meals that stimulate interest and appetite should be planned. Whenever possible, a selective menu should be used so that individual tastes can be satisfied. Because meals are eagerly awaited, they should always be on time.

Dining areas for ambulatory persons should be comfortable and attractive, with sufficient space for movement of wheelchairs and service personnel. In most nursing homes, table service by waiters or waitresses is advisable because many older persons have difficulty managing a tray. If table service is customary, an occasional buffet will be a pleasant variation in the routine.

Trays for persons confined to their rooms should be attractively arranged for convenience as well as for appeal. If the patient has to be fed, sufficient time should be allowed so that the person doing the feeding will not have to hurry. Staff doing the feeding should be fully acquainted with the nature of menu items so that they can answer questions and encourage reluctant eaters to consume at least some of each food item. Persons with limited vision find that eating is more enjoyable when the foods they are eating or being fed are described to them.

Nourishing between-meal snacks are desirable. Substantial snacks in the evening often can reduce the need for sedation. The time span between the last meal on one day and breakfast on the following day should be no more than 15 hours.

CAFETERIA MENUS

The menu planner should pay special attention to cafeterias that serve employees, visitors, and outpatients. Well-managed cafeterias can be a showcase for the high-quality food served in the facility as well as a profitable operation. Although it has been customary to offer most of the items on the facility's general menu, additional items are recommended when patients are served a nonselective menu. Even when selective menus are used, the cafeteria menu that includes other choices can attract additional customers. A variety of cold and hot sandwiches, salads, main dish salads, and salad plates are popular in many facilities. Depending on the facility's location, persons working in nearby clinics or other businesses may be attracted by realistically priced and quick-service items. The added menu variety is needed to keep employees from the facility interested, particularly if the general menu is on a relatively short cycle. Although many facilities use up leftover items as added choices in the cafeteria, this practice is ill-advised if high-quality standards and customer levels are to be maintained.

All foods should be attractively merchandised. Commercial cafeterias that display salads and desserts near the cafeteria entrance or toward the start of the cafeteria line enjoy increased sales of these items. One or more daily specials should be offered, and some of the items on the general menu should be combined for a one-price meal. Consideration should be given to the price mix of cafeteria menu items to ensure affordable alternatives to customers as well as a range of appeal. Keeping precise sales histories on menu items helps in forecasting demand and in eliminating items with low popularity. Observing plate waste is another good way to assess acceptance.

Cycle menus can be used in cafeterias as well as for patient service. However, the cycle should be several weeks in length if employees use the cafeteria for meals. The many advantages of cycle menus prevail, with the added advantage of balancing appeal and selling price considerations for the cafeteria.

In short-term hospitals and other facilities that have relatively large numbers of visitors and outpatients, it can be advantageous to have food available in the cafeteria, a coffee shop, or vending machines for most of the day. If a coffee shop is not available, several cold items can easily be provided in a restricted area of the cafeteria with limited staff. Sandwiches, rolls, donuts, juices, ice cream products, desserts, and beverages can be offered. Microwave ovens that are customer or employee operated are useful for quick heating of items during limited-service hours. Chapter 3 gives added information on supplemental nonresident food service.

COMPUTER-ASSISTED MENU PLANNING

Computer-assisted procedures are used for menu planning in some facilities. To take advantage of the computer's speed, accuracy, and capacity, several kinds of information are essential and must be expressed in quantitative (numerical) terms. Programs can be designed to plan menus that consider labor and raw food cost, nutrients, color, consistency, frequency, and other factors. However, the two variables of nutrients and raw food cost are the most widely used in current computer menu planning programs.

The greatest obstacle to computer-assisted menu planning has been the absence of sufficient data about each variable. The food service department must use standardized recipes for all items. Without their use, there is little point in planning menus that accurately ensure nutrient quantities and cost. Ingredients that constitute each recipe must be issued through a controlled procedure, and personnel must follow recipes exactly. Food composition data must be available for each food item. However, values for all items on the market either are not available or differ from those stated in government handbooks. Nutrient data for many products must be obtained from the manufacturer. Data must usually be developed by the food manager, specifying such things as frequency with which menu items may be served and food combinations allowed on one menu. This involves coding for ingredients, color, flavor, shape, and other factors in such a way that the computer can identify these considerations and deal with them. Menu cost is a combination of raw food and labor costs. Yet, because accurate production time data are not available for most food items and are difficult to obtain, accurate labor cost planning is impossible. These are a few of the problems involved in computer-assisted menu planning that have led many operations to continue using manual procedures. Flexibility in adjusting to special needs of clientele or incorporating new items is severely limited as well.

Food
Procurement

Competent purchasing plays a vital role in the final results of a food service operation. The food buyer must be able to make informed, accurate, and effective decisions concerning the types of food needed, the forms of food available, and the quantities and quality required by the operation to meet consumer demands. The nature of food buying, with rapidly changing market conditions, makes it difficult for the most experienced buyer to remain current. Therefore, to be effective in this role, the person responsible for food procurement must have adequate and up-to-date knowledge of the food marketing system, the structure of the wholesale markets in which purchasing will take place, market supply, and price trends. These generalized areas of knowledge have a significant impact on the cost-effectiveness of the food procurement function.

FOOD MARKETING

The food distribution and marketing system is part of the largest industrial system in the United States: the food and fiber system. Using inputs of technology, capital, machinery, fertilizer, chemicals, petroleum, and labor, farmers produce about $130 billion of basic food and fiber products each year. These basic raw materials are sold to the marketing sector of the food and fiber system.

The U.S. food marketing system serves more than 200 million Americans by getting farm products to them in the form and at the time they want them. More than 90 percent of the foods consumed domestically are produced by the U.S. farm sector. Imported foods such as coffee, tea, and others make up the remaining 10 percent. The food marketing system assembles, grades, stores, processes, packages, transports, wholesales, retails, prices, communicates, takes risks, controls quality, merchandises, exchanges ownership, brands, regulates, develops, and tests new products.

The food marketing system includes more than half a million firms that employ the equivalent of more than five million workers on a full-time basis. Among those workers, persons employed by the away-from-home eating places comprise more than 40 percent of the total. The outputs of nearly three million U.S. farms and food products from countries around the world are gathered by firms within the marketing system and are processed to some extent by more than 23,000 food manufacturing or processing firms within the system.

Food processors and manufacturers are a direct market outlet for vast quantities of raw farm products as well as the source of supplies for hundreds of thousands of distributors. This large, complex system requires great coordination to effectively overcome the problems of food perishability, seasonal availability, volume, distance, and logistics. To permit the system to be dynamic and responsive, the system must provide not only a means for product flow from producer to consumer but also a communication system for the flow of information about consumer preferences and demands.

DECENTRALIZATION

For many years, large central (terminal) markets served as a price-making center for agricultural products and a place where supply and demand forces met. However, technological changes and shifts in location of production and processing centers plus reorganization within agricultural industries have brought new patterns of marketing and price-making that do not involve assembling raw farm products at large terminal markets. The great advances in transportation, market news services, grading, and storage technologies reduced the importance of physical contact among sellers, products, and buyers afforded by terminal markets. Nevertheless, there are still more existing terminal markets in major cities, chiefly for fruits and vegetables. Fresh produce is trucked into the market, and buyers examine and purchase quantities needed from jobbers or from grower representatives.

Livestock and grain marketing provide examples of market decentralization. Half a century ago, more than three-fourths of livestock was sold through large terminal markets such as those in Chicago, Cincinnati, St.

Louis, Omaha, Denver, and Philadelphia. Today, the major proportion of livestock is sold through regional markets located close to livestock production and feeding areas, thus eliminating terminal market charges, decreasing transportation costs and losses from the transport of live animals, and providing greater efficiency in marketing a higher-quality product.

A similar trend has occurred in grain marketing, whereby subterminal or regional elevators intercept millions of bushels of grain that formerly went to huge terminal elevators. Although these marketing trends offer advantages in physical efficiency, they create some difficulties in establishing prices. In actuality, the market prices for raw agricultural products are determined by the interaction of relatively small product volumes sold through terminal markets and larger volumes sold through widely dispersed regional market transactions. Communications technology provides a means for resolving the problems of unified pricing for a commodity despite decentralized marketing, and progress is being made toward that goal.

For the most part, producers receive a residual price from products sold in the market system. As a means of reducing production risks and improving the relatively weak price-bargaining positions of small agricultural producers, some changes are taking place in the organization of the production sector. Producers of specialized fruit and vegetable, dairy, and other products have formed producer-owned marketing cooperatives in an attempt to exert more influence in achieving equitable prices for raw products. In the long run, this could exert a price-stabilizing influence, because the fluctuating prices received by producers who bear the majority of market risk tend to disrupt production plans and contribute to production cycles and variations.

Because the market prices for grains—wheat, corn, oats, and soybeans —affect the quantities and prices of animal products and many other processed food products, the food buyer should follow the cash and futures market prices for these basic commodities. A continuing upward trend in food and feed grain prices will usually result in higher prices for animal products—red meats, poultry, eggs, and dairy products—because grains make up an important portion of the animal diet. In a period of higher grain prices, producers tend to restrict the numbers of livestock raised and to market more grain products directly. Conversely, in a period of declining grain prices, it becomes more profitable to convert more grain into animal products, with a resultant increase in meat supply and decrease in market prices for such products.

The U.S. Department of Agriculture provides daily, weekly, monthly, and quarterly market trend reports through the Economic Research Service and the Statistical Reporting Service. State departments of agriculture also routinely provide market information on products produced within respective states. Price and supply information can be obtained through these agencies. They also furnish audiovisual media and reports for persons interested in maintaining current market information.

TRANSPORTATION

Although transportation is a vital link between all segments of the food marketing system, it does not contribute costs in proportion to its importance, despite rising energy and transportation costs. Approximately 8 percent of the costs of marketing food products are accounted for in intercity rail and trucking charges and in airline transport. Although the transport space occupied by many food products is high when compared with the product value, few products require more careful handling than food. The perishable nature of food products requires a maximum degree of technical knowledge and speed in transport to prevent or minimize loss of quality. The transport requirements of different perishable food commodities vary widely. The food itself may be susceptible to damage from spoilage, freezing, overheating, and contaminating during transit.

Many food products require refrigeration. Fresh fruits and vegetables, even after harvest, continue to generate and give off heat by respiration. At lower temperatures, less heat is generated from this source and the decay and aging processes proceed more slowly. Over the years, several cold-storage methods have been used in trucks and rail cars, including ice, ice and salt, dry ice, and mechanical refrigeration, which is the most common.

More recently, cryogenic refrigeration systems using liquid nitrogen or liquid carbon dioxide have been developed. When interior trailer temperatures reach a preset point, the liquid gas is sprayed into the air, removing heat. The use of these refrigerants requires careful control to prevent high levels of nitrogen or carbon dioxide from adversely affecting the quality of some products. Moderate concentrations of carbon dioxide, however, are successfully used to retard decay and ripening of fruits and vegetables as well as to retard microbial growth on fresh meats and meat products during transport storage.

Many fruits and vegetables, including asparagus, bananas, avocados, beans, cucumbers, lettuce, and many citrus fruits, however, also must be protected against damage from chilling. For many fresh and frozen produce, air circulation is needed during transport to maintain even temperatures throughout the load. For fresh fruits and vegetables, humidity control is needed.

Because speed and efficiency are important in getting foods to their destination at reasonable cost, there has been a rapid application of palletization in loading food products. Bags or cartons of products are stacked on wooden pallets that can be moved by forklifts. Containerization, which takes palletization a step further, consists of loading many smaller bags or cartons into a single large container that can then be loaded directly onto trailers or rail flatcars. Many railroads and truck lines use computerized routing to keep track of freight cars, trailers, and van containers and thereby eliminate delays and lost shipments. Communications advances in telephones, computers, and even satellites have helped to cut transport costs and speed up the movement of products.

New transport procedures and methods and continuing application of technology play a critical role in marketing food. Cargo planes, ships, barges, trucks, and rails all play vital roles in meeting the volume and quality demands of food service operations and consumers.

PROCESSING

Applications of machinery in food manufacturing industries in the early decades of this century led to the emergence of large regional processors in many food lines. In part, the rapid growth of food manufacturing industries was due to a transfer of the many processing operations formerly performed in the household and food service operations to the new food industries. The canning industry, for example, grew remarkably.

Following World War II, a very different influence, that of rising consumer incomes, had a profound effect on the structure of processing industries. The demand for convenience food products—partially prepared, mixed, frozen, and ready-to-eat—offered broadened horizons to food manufacturers. New product development, experimentation, and promotional activities required expanded research facilities and encouraged the emergence of conglomerates. Conglomerates were advantageous for many regional processors who found that the costs of central laboratories and promotional facilities could be spread across different processing activities. Significant economies were obtained by the merger of regional distribution systems into a national system. Regional processing firms that did not merge with the postwar food conglomerates experienced difficulty selling their products in competition with national firms. Many of their products became available for private-label programs of emerging food chains.

Many of the major food manufacturers are parts of large industrial firms that deal in many industries other than food. Because of this factor, the level of concentration in any particular industry is reduced somewhat. Although this is true in some product areas, various important industries have become more concentrated through horizontal integration of activities. The highest levels of concentration are found in cereal, wet corn milling, flour, cookie, cracker, beet sugar, and cane sugar refining. In most food processing industries, plants operated by multiunit firms account for most of the output and for more than three-fourths of the value added to farm food products by processors. Although the number of plants has decreased drastically, the volume of products handled by the firms has increased.

Along with the increasing size of plants and firms, food processing companies have vertically integrated into a wide range of activities other than processing. The integration of farming with processing activities has been small in total, but is quite significant for some individual commodities, pa ticularly broiler chickens, turkeys, sugar beets, and vegetables for processing. Contract production by processors is much more commonly used as a means of integration rather than ownership of production facilities.

Some processing firms have integrated with food service and restaurant businesses and with retail product oulets. In the dairy industry, for example, some fluid milk processors have opened retail dairy or convenience food stores. Ice cream manufacturers frequently have their own retail ice cream stores or restaurants featuring their products. Some firms that specialize in canned food processing have diversified into products designed for use in food service operations as well as the further processing and preparation of meals in central commissaries for the institutional market. Firms in the business of preparing ready-to-serve foods and meals are often referred to as food converters or fabricators.

The relative ease with which large industrial firms can change from one industry to another causes instability in the level of concentration in any one industry. This makes it difficult both to measure and to interpret the degree of concentration in food manufacturing as well as to reduce its impact on competition in many instances.

WHOLESALING

Wholesaling is the link in the marketing system for distribution of food from the producer and/or processor to the retailer. The activities involved in the wholesaling process are principally those of assembling foods from many sources and distributing them to retailers, hotel and restaurant operators, and institutions.

With the extensive number of available products and the variety of items stocked in relatively small amounts in food service operations, managers could not possibly search out and deal with the producer and processor sources of all the required food products. Conversely, processors could not, in many instances, profitably service the limited quantities needed by food service units. The job of the food wholesaler is that of setting up an effective and efficient system of assembling the various products in reasonable quantities from the various processors and then selling them in smaller quantities to users. Figure 21, next page, illustrates the structure of the wholesale-retail-mass-feeding food distribution system and shows how the food wholesaler, who buys and assembles the needed products, is the key figure in the distribution process. Some processors can perform the functions themselves through their sales offices or branch warehouses. The fact that manufacturers' sales agents specialize in a limited product line means that they can concentrate their expertise and sales effort on fewer products. These agents do not take title, bill, or set prices for the goods sold.

Another method used by some processors for distributing their limited

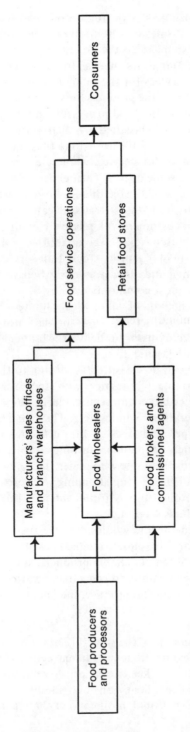

FIGURE 21. Example of the Structure of a Food Distribution System.

line or volume of products is through food brokers and commissioned agents who act as their sales representatives. This group of intermediaries in the distribution system assists the processors by keeping them informed of trade conditions and users' needs. In turn, the broker's sales staff provides goods and services for the retail and food service trade without taking actual possession of the products for sale. Brokers and commissioned agents receive a fee from the food processors in return for their services.

Food wholesalers are classified by their position in the marketing system and on the basis of the functions they perform. One category includes full-function, or full-service, wholesalers, who perform all of the marketing functions to some degree. Their expertise in knowing the market, buying goods, and knowing the techniques for merchandising items to the best advantage are their strongest traits. Because food wholesalers must be able to supply their customers with relatively small quantities at frequent intervals, they must purchase in large quantities and store the food and other goods in the form of inventory stock. Full-service wholesalers extend credit to the customer and deliver goods when ordered. This type of wholesaler is the one most commonly used by food service operations.

In contrast to this method of selling are the limited-function wholesalers, who carry a limited product line, may or may not extend credit, and establish order-size requirements for delivery. Manufacturers' sales branches are usually under this classification.

Wholesalers also can be classified according to the types of products they handle. For example, wholesalers who stock a wide variety of goods so that the food service buyer can secure a large percentage of the needed items are called general-line wholesalers. There has been a trend toward expansion of the types and lines of products and services handled by institutional wholesalers so that mass feeding establishments can purchase virtually all their needs from one wholesaler. This new concept in the food service industry is called one-stop shopping. A more complete discussion of this trend to consolidation is found later in this chapter under the Selecting Food Products section.

In contrast to general-line wholesalers are specialty wholesalers who handle only one line or a few closely related lines of products. For example, they can specialize only in perishable products, such as fresh produce, or can include some frozen fruits and vegetables or other products as well. In total numbers and economic importance, specialty wholesalers are declining.

PRICE TRENDS

Many of the developments in the structure of food processing and manufacturing firms have led to efficiencies in marketing through economies of scale that have tended to keep food prices relatively stable. However, increased worldwide dependency on food supplies, changed government policies, revised international monetary exchange rates, and unstable economic conditions based largely on rising energy costs have caused instability in food prices. Shortages and tight supplies of basic commodities and world demand for U.S. food products have produced unexpected severe fluctuations in prices for certain food products and a general upward trend in the level of all food prices.

Because the costs of marketing food products make up the greater share of food prices, the structure of the marketing system has an important impact on prices paid by consumers. Labor costs make up almost one-half of the marketing costs, followed by packaging and transportation costs. In the food service sector of the marketing system, which makes up about one-fourth of the total marketing bill, the labor cost component is higher than in any other category of marketing firms. Although prices for raw agricultural products fluctuate as supply conditions and demands for the commodities change, marketing costs have shown steady increases over the years as a result of the growth in volume of food marketed, increased marketing services, and the cost of performing these services. Increased marketing services involve the use of more highly prepared forms of food and result in more food being consumed in away-from-home eating places. In the short run, consumer prices may actually rise while the prices paid to producers decline.

Inflation in the general economy, as reflected in the Wholesale Price Index, affects the costs of all inputs into food production and marketing. Therefore, if inflationary trends continue, it is unlikely that prospects for reducing marketing costs will improve. Because profit margins are not usually high in most food marketing industries, reduction of marketing costs requires increased productivity, control of waste or materials, or reduction of services performed. These strategies for price control are applicable in all food marketing firms, including food service operations.

REGULATION

The efforts throughout history to control the quality and safety of the food supply made major advances with the advent of extensive urbanization. Food laws go hand in hand with urbanization because most people do not cultivate or slaughter their own food products. However, the fact that today's foods go through many hands—growers, manufacturers, distributors—increases the possibility of mishandling, fraudulent practices, or misrepresentation. Advances in science and technology also have contributed to the need for food regulation. Although the use of chemicals in food production and processing has increased crop yields, improved shelf life and product quality, and created new products, their use also has created problems. To ensure against overuse or misuse of chemicals, government controls have been established.

Food laws protect both the consumer and the food industry. Responsible growers, processors, and distributors are protected against the unfair

competition of the irresponsible. Food laws have several purposes:
- To ensure real food value
- To maintain integrity of foods
- To protect quality and quantity of all basic foods
- To protect the health of the buyer
- To promote honesty
- To provide informative and accurate labeling

The first pure food law in the United States was the Pure Food and Drug Act of 1906. This act made significant progress in decreasing misbranding and adulteration of foods. However, the act became outdated with advancing technology and was replaced by the more comprehensive Food, Drug, and Cosmetic Act of 1938. This act, amended several times since 1938, does the following:

- Prohibits the shipment of misbranded food products in interstate commerce
- Prohibits the shipment of adulterated (containing any harmful substances) foods in interstate commerce
- Gives the Food and Drug Administration (FDA) authority to regulate the use of food additives
- Gives the FDA authority to establish standards of identity, fill of container for food products, and minimum quality

Standards of identity describe the nature and character of a food product and specify the kinds and amounts of ingredients that go into it. This standard tells what the product is and how it is made and sets limits on certain ingredients, such as moisture content, fat content, and so forth. The FDA has established standards of identity for a wide range of food products, with the exception of meat and poultry products. The U.S. Department of Agriculture sets standards for meat and poultry products.

Standards of fill regulate the quantity of food in the container by telling the packer the amount of food that must be in the container to avoid deceiving the buyer. In general, standards of fill require packages to contain the maximum quantity of food that can be sealed in the container and processed without damage to the food. Standards of fill have been established for most canned fruits and vegetables, tomato products, and shellfish.

Standards of quality also have been established by the FDA for a number of canned fruits and vegetables to supplement the standards of identity by limiting and describing the number and kinds of defects permitted. These standards of quality are minimum standards. Products that do not meet the standard must be labeled substandard if they are to be sold. However, very few, if any, are available on the market. All of the FDA standards are mandatory in nature; that is, food manufacturers, packers, and processors are required by law to comply with them.

The Fair Packaging and Labeling Act of 1966 supplements the Food,

Drug, and Cosmetic Act and sets up requirements for complete information in labeling and for nondeceptive packaging. Under these laws, the following kinds of information are required on labels:

- Common or usual names of all ingredients, listed in descending order of predominance by weight
- Name and address of manufacturer, packer, or distributor
- Statement of quantity of contents in weight, measure, or numerical count
- Name of the artificial flavorings, colorings, or chemical preservatives

Descriptive information such as brand names, recipes, or number of servings may be voluntarily added by processors. Although nutritional information is not usually on the labels of food packed in institutional-sized containers, it can be requested and obtained from the packer or processor.

Meat, poultry, and other animal products are regulated by the U.S. Department of Agriculture's Food Safety and Quality Service (FSQS), by authority of the 1906 Meat Inspection Act, the Wholesale Meat Act of 1967, and the Poultry Products Inspection Act of 1959 and 1968. The purpose of these laws is to control the sanitary conditions of slaughter and processing facilities, to ensure that animals and birds were healthy and free from harmful disease before slaughter, and to set standards of identity that specify the kinds and proportions of ingredients in meat and poultry products.

Labeling of the products also is controlled by the USDA regulations. The regulations require inspection of all meat, poultry, and egg products moving in interstate commerce by federal inspectors or by state inspectors if the firms involved do business only within the state. A round inspection stamp, on the product itself or on its package, means that the requirements have been met and that the product is wholesome and truthfully labeled.

Although no federal law requires grade standards, such measures of quality are provided by the U.S. Department of Agriculture on a voluntary use basis. The number of grades varies with the particular products and indicates the eating quality, other characteristics of appearance, uniformity, and size, or the absence of defects of a food. Although manufacturers are not required to grade products, if a grade shield appears on the product or if a grade name is used, the product must have been actually graded by federal inspectors. Grade standards have been developed for more than 300 farm products and are revised periodically to reflect changes in production, use, and marketing practices. Whenever a producer or processor wants a product graded, a fee must be paid for the service.

MANAGEMENT DECISIONS

Procurement of food involves much more than simply ordering food. It consists of the entire decision-making process, which includes determining quality and quantity standards for the institution; specifying and ordering foods that meet the standards; and receiving, storing, and controlling of inventory of these products. Effective procurement requires that buyers have a great deal of information and knowledge in order to make the best decisions.

MENU PLANNING

The planned menu is the actual starting point in the procurement process because it states the operation's food needs for a specific period. Some of the points to be considered when planning menus to meet the food department's service objectives include:

- *Food budget.* By estimating the cost of food items as each menu is planned, cost can be kept in line with the budget. Before food is purchased, the estimated costs should be checked against current food prices. The foods purchased should make the best possible nutritional contribution for the money spent.
- *Availability of food items.* Food items appearing on the menu should be available to the user in the desired form and quality. Seasonality of various products affects quality and price. The choice among fresh, canned, or frozen items varies, depending on the season. Weather conditions affect the movement of food supplies through market channels and may necessitate changes of planned menu items, particularly fresh fruits and vegetables. Adverse weather can create short supplies and increased prices.
- *Labor budget.* The number and skill of employees and the cost of their labor should be considered in relation to the cost of purchasing certain food items in a partially or fully prepared state. If the number of labor hours cannot be reduced, the higher cost of convenience foods may not fit within the total budget.
- *Equipment and space.* Availability of both equipment and space for preparation and storage of food directly affects menu planning. If a facility is adequately supplied with preparation equipment, menus should make maximum use of what is available. In order to provide menu variety, different forms of food products should be purchased if the kitchen is not adequately equipped. The type and amount of storage space affect both the type and amount of foods purchased. When ample storage space is available, many managers maintain large inventories, believing that they have saved money by large-quantity buying. However, the cost may be greater than the rate of return on money invested in other ways. The desired inventory amount will vary among food service departments; the size of the institution, inventory policies, available space, and location of suppliers greatly affect quantities. Carrying more inventory than

needed can result in loss of food quality as well as poor use of funds.

PURCHASING PROCESSES

Purchasing is one of the functions of the procurement system. Purchasing can be defined as obtaining the quantity and quality of materials required, where and when they are needed, at a price within the operating budget. The purchasing system and procedures used to achieve this objective will vary from one institution to another.

Systems

Centralized purchasing of all materials and supplies by one department is a recognized system in health care institutions, although the degree of centralization can vary from one to another. A purchasing department may perform only the ordering function, whereas the individual departments or groups of departments within the institution perform the receiving and storage functions.

Another system gaining acceptance is to have a materials management department responsible for performing all procurement functions, including the entire process of ordering to the final disbursement of goods to the user department. This system of purchasing has several advantages. Staff time for meeting with sales representatives, placing orders, receiving goods, and doing paperwork is greatly reduced. Central storage provides greater inventory control and security and releases storage space within the food service department for other uses. Quality of products purchased is often improved because central purchasing requires well-written, precise specifications that are clearly understood by vendors, the purchasing department, and the food service department. Personnel with purchasing expertise are usually more aware of market trends, are better able to negotiate with vendors, and are able to follow through on the completion of transactions. To be successful, centralized purchasing systems require open channels of communication and cooperation among the purchaser, vendor, and user of the food products.

For several institutions with similar needs in a community, group purchasing has become an accepted way to control costs through greater efficiency in buying. One of the needs, as well as one of the difficulties in group purchasing, is that participating food service departments must agree on the specifications for each item to be purchased. The potential savings of group purchasing can be nullified if members of the group have wide variations in specifications or continue to purchase many items independently. Purchasing power is greater with several institutions participating because the volume of purchases is larger.

When group purchasing systems are not available in a community or if institutional policy dictates that departments purchase individually, the food service manager will find that a considerably greater amount of time will need to be spent on the buying function. In addition, responsibility for storage and inventory control will rest within the food service department.

Methods

The two general methods of buying are formal competitive bid purchasing and informal buying. Competitive bid purchasing is a formal process using a signed agreement between the vendor and the purchaser and bound by a legal contract. Food service personnel develop a written specification for each product and an estimate of the quantity needed for the bid period. A written notice of requirements, called a bid request, is made available to vendors, inviting them to submit prices based on the quality and quantity needed. The bid request includes instructions about the method of bidding, delivery, and frequency of payment; when bids are due; what is the basis for awarding contracts; and any other information deemed necessary for the buyer and the seller. Figure 22, next page, is an example of a bid request. Firm, fixed prices for the specified period are desirable, but when product prices fluctuate frequently or are steadily rising, vendors may be unable or unwilling to quote firm prices for an extended period. Bid requests that state a maximum amount required, as well as a minimum quantity to be purchased from the successful bidder, allow some flexibility for both buyer and vendor when prices of the product needed are likely to fluctuate considerably. Although price is a major consideration in awarding the contract, the buyer should carefully consider product quality and the ability of the vendor to meet the time specifications of the contract. In addition, the reputation, previous performance, and vendor's compliance with specifications and laws are important. All bidders, successful or unsuccessful, should be informed of the award.

Informal buying is done through verbal and written communication between buyer and vendor by telephone sales representatives. Price quotations should be obtained from two or more suppliers. Call sheets, or quotation sheets as the ones should in figure 23, page 200, are useful. A quotation sheet has spaces for the name and description of food items, amount of food needed, and prices quoted by various suppliers. After careful analysis of price quotes, vendor service, and dependability of quality, a vendor should be selected. Orders are generally placed with the supplier who gave the lowest quotation. Although small institutions may purchase most of their foods in this fashion, larger ones may purchase only perishable fresh products or foods in limited quantity by this method. A disadvantage of informal buying is the amount of time required to check and compare prices, visit with sales representatives, and place orders.

Problems also can result from verbal commitments to buy. Some of these problems, however, can be avoided by providing vendors with a list of accurate product specifications as a communication aid.

Regardless of the purchasing method used, order quantities should be large enough to make it economically worthwhile for vendors. The advantages of price comparison and product choice are lost if small orders are split among several vendors because of price. Delivery schedule requests should be considered carefully; steadily increasing transportation costs will affect food costs if deliveries are requested more often than necessary. In general, economic delivery of food can be scheduled as follows:

- Meat, poultry, fish delivered once a week or less, depending on a chilled or frozen state of delivery
- Fresh produce delivered once or twice a week, depending on storage space available and quantities needed

---

BID REQUEST

Bids will be received until ___(date)___ for ___(indicate type of)___ delivery on the date indicated.

Issued by: *Name of Purchaser* Address: *Street*
Institution *City, State*

Date issued: ___(date bid issued)___ Date to be *(5-10 days after bid* delivered: *is awarded)*

Increases in quantity up to 20 percent will be binding at the discretion of the buyer. All items are to be officially certified by the U.S. Department of Agriculture for acceptance no earlier than two days before delivery; costs of such service to be borne by the supplier.

Item No.	Description	Quantity	Unit	Unit Price	Amount
1	Chickens, fresh chilled fryers, 2½ to 3 lb., ready-to-cook, U.S. Grade A	500	lb.		
2	Chickens, fresh chilled hens, 4 to 5 lb., ready-to-cook, U.S. Grade A	100	lb.		
3	Turkeys, frozen young toms, 20 to 22 lb., ready-to-cook, U.S. Grade A	100	lb.		
4	Eggs, fresh, large, U.S. Grade A, 30 doz. cases	150	doz.		
5	Eggs, frozen, whole, inspected, 6 4-lb. cartons per case	60	lb.		

Vendor _____

FIGURE 22. Example of a Bid Request.

QUOTATION SHEET

Type of Product: Fresh Produce   Day: Monday   Date: 2/10   Approved by: DL

Quantity	Unit	Description and Specification	Suppliers and Quotations Per Unit			
			Smith	Brown		
1	50# bag	Carrots	11.40	13.85		
1	40# bag	Bananas, #4	12.00	13.40		

QUOTATION SHEET

Type of Product: Canned Goods   Day: Wednesday   Date: 4/6   Approved by: DL

Quantity	Unit	Description and Specification	Suppliers and Quotations Per Unit			
			S & H	B & G		
6	case	Applesauce, regular #10	10.09	10.83		
6	case	Peas, early June, #10 can.	11.39	13.46		

FIGURE 23. Examples of Quotation Sheets.

- Canned goods and staples delivered weekly, bimonthly, monthly, or quarterly, depending on storage space, quantities needed, and price quotes for specific volume
- Milk, milk products, bread, baked goods delivered daily or every other day, although suppliers should be consulted because many dairies and bakeries have reduced the number of deliveries
- Butter, eggs, cheese delivered weekly
- Frozen foods delivered weekly, bimonthly, monthly, or quarterly, depending on storage space, usage rate, and price quotes for quantities needed

One-stop shopping, or limited supplier purchasing, is another system used by many small health care facilities. One vendor supplies the buyer with most of the food and supplies needed. The efficiency of food purchasing is improved by eliminating the time-consuming processes of placing bids and getting price quotations. A substantial reduction in warehousing costs is possible if deliveries are frequent. Lower net costs of products can result because the supplier knows relatively far in advance that certain food services are going to be needing specific products and can buy accordingly.

Many one-stop vendors provide other services to their customers, such as assistance with menu planning and inventory control. There can be some disadvantages, including the loss of back-up suppliers, if the main vendor fails to deliver goods. Also, the quality of foods available may not be of the type wanted or needed. For larger food service departments, the number of firms able to supply one-stop services may be limited, but the number of suppliers providing this service is definitely increasing. The effectiveness of this purchasing method is directly related to the efficiency and credibility of the supplier. However, many food service departments have found this method to be very satisfactory.

Guidelines

The following 10 purchasing guidelines are suggested:

1. A specification for each food item should be developed. A specification is a clear, concise, yet complete description of the exact food item wanted. Specifications should be realistic and not include details that cannot be verified or tested or that would make the product too costly because they are not available from processors. Up-to-date product information is essential if specifications are to be useful. Government and industry specifications can provide a starting point to assist food service departments in developing their own. Specifications are an essential communication tool between buyer and seller. A buyer's needs must be expressed in precise terms to give all vendors a common basis for price quotations and bids. For some products, specifications can be quite brief; others will require greater detail. The specific information needed varies with each type of food but all specifications should include at least the following information: name of product, grade or quality designation, size of container or package on which price will be based, and number of purchase units.

2. A copy of the specifications developed by the food service department should be available to and used by the purchasing agent. Many food service departments find it convenient to provide a complete set of their specifications to vendors with whom they routinely do business. The time required to get a price quote on a product is decreased if the vendor has a set of specifications classified by commodity group and number on file.

3. Food quality and yield in relation to price should be compared. A food of higher quality and higher unit price may yield more serving portions of better quality, at a lower cost per serving, than the same food of lower quality and price. Frequent studies of the net yield in serving portions and of cost per serving of various brands

make it possible to base buying decisions on cost per serving rather than on purchase unit price.

4. Only the types, quality, and quantities required for the planned menu should be purchased. However, if a special buy is available and the quality is acceptable, a surplus of the product may be purchased if storage space and conditions permit. For example, prices on the past year's pack of fruit or vegetable items may be quite reasonable just before the new pack reaches the market.

5. Foods should be purchased by weight or size and count per container. Minimum weights acceptable for purchase units should be stated.

6. Food should be purchased from vendors who maintain high levels of sanitation and quality control in accordance with regulations and recommended practices of food handling and storage.

7. Price quotations should be obtained by using the formal bid or informal methods described earlier.

8. Written purchase and receiving records for all foods and supplies ordered and received should be kept on file.

9. All purchases should be inspected upon delivery. If it is necessary to reject an item, it should be done at the time of delivery unless there is a prior agreement whereby the vendor will give credit for any defective products or gross errors. Delivery sheets or invoices should not be initiated or signed until the quality and quantity of foods delivered have been checked against the purchase order.

10. A purchase and delivery schedule should be established. To do this, the storage life of various foods, location of vendor in relation to the food service department, delivery costs, storage space, inventory policies, and the food needs specified by the menu should be considered.

Vendors

Sound business practices and well-stated purchasing policies are the basis for good purchasing. Careful planning and an accurate statement of food needs are the starting point in building good relations with vendors. Fairness and honesty are essential when communicating with them. Product needs should be specified, and complete information about availability and prices should be obtained. The person responsible for purchasing should set up an appointment schedule with sales representatives and adhere to it. One vendor's prices and information should not be discussed with another vendor. Accepting gifts, favors, coupons, or other promotional favors can create a position of obligation to a vendor that can adversely affect the manager's freedom to act in the future. Every manager should be aware of and follow the ethical policies of the institution.

Whenever products or services provided by a vendor are unsatisfactory, the problem should be dealt with promptly through procedures approved by the institution. To maintain fairness, the vendor should be allowed to remedy problems in a businesslike manner. Accurate and complete records of problems should be kept in case a need to justify a discontinuation of purchases from any vendor develops. Special services that ordinarily may not be available from vendors should not be requested.

Selection and Quantities

The planned menu tells the food buyer what kinds of food are needed, but only careful planning will ensure sufficient food for the anticipated number of meals, with a minimum of leftovers. The quantities of food needed can be calculated by following the steps listed below:

1. The number of serving portions required for each item on the menu should be forecast as accurately as possible. If a selective menu is used, the forecast can be based on accurate records of selections previously made when the same food item combinations were served, plus any additional portions anticipated.
2. A standard portion size for each food item should be determined. This should correspond to the portion size stated on the standardized recipes used in the food service department. Standardized recipes also should state the amount of each ingredient to be purchased for the stated yield.
3. The quantities of food required to prepare the number of serving portions needed should be determined.
4. The amount of food on hand in refrigerated, frozen, and dry storage areas should be checked and the amount of food on hand from the quantity needed for the planned menus subtracted. A list of the supplies that must be purchased and those that will be requisitioned from the storeroom should be made.

. Records

When purchasing is centralized, the food service department usually completes a purchase requisition form such as the one shown in figure 24, next page, to inform the purchasing agent of the quantity and quality of specific foods that need to be purchased by that department. The purchase requisition should contain the complete specification, purchase unit, total quantity of each item, and data needed. In addition, a vendor and price may be suggested. However, the purchasing agent is responsible for obtaining bids, if that is the policy, or getting the best possible prices and terms. This system will work well if the food service department head and the purchasing agent pool their knowledge and communicate freely.

Administrative policy will usually require that all purchase requisitions be approved by a designated person in the food service department before being sent to purchasing. The purchase requisition should be prepared in multiple copies, the number of which is based on the organization's policies. One copy should be kept on file in the food service department for future reference.

Whether purchasing is done by a purchasing department or by the food service department, a purchase order should always be used to inform the vendor of specific requirements. A purchase order is a legal document authorizing a supplier to deliver merchandise in accordance with the terms stated. Purchase order forms, such as that shown in figure 25, next page, are standardized by the institution and are used by all departments.

The information contained on these forms includes the name and address of the supplier; a complete specification for each item, except when the vendor already has the specification (in which case the specification number can be used along with a brief description); total quantity of each item ordered; price per unit quoted by the vendor; total price for the amount ordered; terms of delivery; and method of payment. The number of copies of the purchase order needed will vary with the institution, but because it is the record of merchandise ordered and the form used to check receipt of deliveries, all departments dealing with the merchandise or with payments will need a copy.

PURCHASE REQUISITION

To: Purchasing Office   Requisition No.: _____

Date: _____   Purchase Order No.: _____

From: _____   Date Required: _____

Unit	Total Quantity	Description	Suggested Vendor	Unit Cost	Total Cost

Requested by _____ Approved by _____ Date Ordered _____

FIGURE 24. Example of a Purchase Requisition.

PURCHASE ORDER

Purchase Order No.: _____

Please refer to the above
number on all invoices

To: _____   Date: _____
_____   Requisition No.: _____
_____   Dept.: _____
Date Required: _____

Ship to: F.O.B.   Via: Terms:

Unit	Total Quantity	Description	Price Per Unit	Total Cost

Approved by _____

FIGURE 25. Example of a Purchase Order Form.

Food
Selection

MEAT

Meat, the most costly component and also one of the major sources of protein in the daily menu, requires careful selection. Because there is a wide range of quality in many meats, the quality needed should be based on the intended use. The USDA Meat Quality Grades cover the entire range of quality factors and can help a manager make wise decisions in meat purchasing. Meat grades are based on the following:

- Conformation or general form or shape of a carcass, and the ratio of meat to bone and total weight
- Maturity of the animal, determined by skeletal characteristics, color of the lean meat, and fat
- Marbling or the amount of fat distributed through the muscle
- Color, firmness, and texture of the lean muscle
- Amount of external fat

When the carcass is graded, the external surface of the meat is marked with a shield indicating the federal grade, as shown in figure 26, next page. Because grading is not required by law, the food service buyer must state the USDA grade of meat desired in the specification if graded meat is to be purchased.

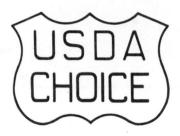

FIGURE 26. Federal Grade Stamp for Meat.

BEEF GRADES

USDA Prime. Beef of Prime grade provides the ultimate in tenderness, juiciness, and flavor because of the abundant marbling and the amount of external fat as compared with meat in lower grades. However, the price per pound for all USDA Prime cuts is usually too costly for most health institutions to use except for special occasions. The supply of this quality beef is also limited in quantity.

USDA Choice. Beef of Choice grade is of high quality but has less fat than Prime grade. More Choice-grade beef is produced than any other grade and is preferred by most consumers and institutions because it is tender and flavorful. Rib and loin cuts are tender and can be cooked by dry heat methods. Other cuts, such as those from the round or chuck, are also tender and have a well-developed flavor when prepared by moist-heat methods.

USDA Good. Cuts of Good grade have less marbling within the muscle and less outer fat cover. The meat is relatively tender, but because of less marbling it lacks some of the juiciness and flavor associated with higher grades. Rib and loin roasts and steaks prepared by dry heat can yield fairly satisfactory products, but other cuts are best prepared by moist heat.

USDA Commercial. Beef of Commercial grade is produced only from mature animals and lacks the tenderness of the higher grades. Institutions find it economical to use this grade for ground beef and stew meat, which becomes tender and full flavored when cooked slowly with moist heat.

There are three other USDA grades for beef. These are Utility, Cutter, and Canner, which are usually not sold as fresh beef but are used in processed meat products.

In addition to the quality grades for beef, there are also yield grades, which are guides to the amount or cutability of usable meat in a carcass. High-cutability carcasses combine a minimum of fat covering with very thick muscling and yield a high proportion of lean meat. The USDA yield grades are numbered 1 to 5, with 1 having the highest cutability. All beef that is quality graded is also yield graded.

LAMB GRADES

The USDA grades for lamb are USDA Prime, USDA Choice, USDA Good, USDA Utility, and USDA Cull. Standards for these grades are similar to those for beef. Choice or Good is the grade selection usually specified for institutional use.

VEAL GRADES

USDA Prime. A veal carcass of Prime grade is superior in quality and has thick muscling and firm, fine-textured flesh. The cut surface of the flesh is velvety to sight and touch. Bones are small in relation to size and weight of the carcass.

USDA Choice. A veal carcass possessing the minimum qualification for this grade is moderately blocky and compact, with fairly thick fleshing. The flesh is firm, fine-textured, and may be moist to sight and touch. All bones are moderately small in proportion to the size and weight of the carcass.

USDA Good. A veal carcass of Good grade is blocky and compact, with thin fleshing and no evidence of plumpness. The flesh is moderately soft and, in a cut surface, moist to sight and touch. All bones are large in proportion to the size of the carcass.

USDA Standard. A veal carcass of Standard grade is not thickly fleshed and has a higher proportion of bone to meat. Moist-heat methods of cooking are needed to ensure juiciness and development of flavor.

Other Grades. The two other grades of veal are Utility and Cull, which are rarely used in food service departments.

PORK GRADES

Pork is produced from young animals and is less variable in quality than beef. USDA grades reflect only two levels of quality: acceptable or unacceptable. The USDA grades for pork are numbered from 1 to 4 for acceptable-quality animals. Unacceptable quality for fresh meat, or pork that is watery and soft, is graded U.S. Utility. The grades for pork are similar to yield grades for beef, but the grades for pork reflect the differences in carcass yield for the four major cuts rather than the differences in eating quality. Most pork marketed today is either No. 1 or No. 2.

MARKET FORMS

Meat can be purchased by food service departments in several market styles: by the half or quarter carcass, in wholesale or primal cuts, or in oven-ready or portion-control cuts. Carcass and primal cuts seldom are used in today's food service departments because of the amount of chilled storage space, cutting equipment, and skilled labor needed to prepare them for use. There is the additional problem of disposing of bones and other waste plus the difficulty of utilizing all the different meat cuts effectively within the menu cycle. In fact, carcasses or primal cuts are not even available from many institutional meat purveyors. These suppliers purchase only the wholesale cuts they use most frequently and break them down into the oven-ready and portion-control cuts used by their food service customers.

There are many advantages for using oven-ready and portion-control meats. Roasts can be purchased in uniform sizes, weights, and trim, thus giving the manager greater control over portion yields and per serving costs. Specification of serving size for individual portion cuts offers maximum control of production quantity and quality, with little or no waste. Greater customer satisfaction can be achieved because each person receives the same size portion.

SPECIFICATIONS

All meat products should be purchased by specifications that are based on a sound knowledge of the factors that influence preparation needs. Recognition of meat cuts and quality is essential. The National Association of Meat Purveyors has prepared the *Meat Buyer's Guide* for use by the meat industry and food buyers. This illustrated manual is coordinated with the Institutional Meat Purchase Specifications (IMPS), which have been developed by the U.S. Department of Agriculture. Copies of the following IMPS general reqirements for meat and meat products are available from the U.S. Government Printing Office.

IMPS for Fresh Beef, No. 100
IMPS for Fresh Lamb and Mutton, No. 200
IMPS for Fresh Veal and Calf, No. 300
IMPS for Fresh Pork, No. 400
IMPS for Cured, Cured and Smoked, and Fully Cooked Pork Products, No. 500
IMPS for Cured, Dried, and Smoked Beef Products, No. 600
IMPS for Edible By-products, No. 700
IMPS for Sausage Products, No. 800
IMPS for Portion-Cut Meat Products, No. 1000

However, the *Meat Buyer's Guide* may be a more useful reference because of the color illustrations and the precise descriptions of all cuts.

Health care facilities making relatively small purchases of meat may not find it practical either to use the lengthy specifications found in IMPS or to make use of the Meat Acceptance Service offered by the U.S. Department of Agriculture. The Meat Acceptance Service is based on IMPS. When a purchaser makes use of this service, the supplier has a USDA meat grader examine the product requested to certify that meat and meat products comply with IMPS. This method of meat purchasing assures the buyer of a wholesome product, grade, trim, weight, and other options requested. The service is provided on a fee-per-hour basis.

If meat items are not going to be used within three to five days after delivery (within one day for ground beef), they should be purchased in the frozen state for best quality. The blast-freezing processes used by meat purveyors provide the best conditions for quality retention. The frequent practice of freezing meat in the food service department usually results in quality deterioration because of the slow rate of freezing. Most food service departments have freezers that are capable only of holding meat in the frozen state, not of freezing meat rapidly.

Regardless of the amount of meat that is purchased at any one time, the information that should be communicated to the vendor through written specifications include the following:

- Name of cut (see figures 27 through 30, pages 212-215, for names of many of the food service or retail cuts and the references previously cited)
- Requirements for boning, rolling, and tying, if applicable
- USDA grade or other quality designation
- Weight of cut or individual portion (state tolerances allowed)
- IMPS number when using these specifications
- Chilled or frozen state of delivery
- Packaging or number of units per shipping container

Examples of specifications following these rules are:

Beef, inside round roast, USDA Choice, 8 to 10 lb., IMPS No. 168, chilled, 32-to-40-lb. polylined boxes preferred

Beef, ground (special) bulk, USDA Commercial or Utility, 18-22 percent maximum fat content, IMPS No. 137, frozen, 10-lb. bag

Beef liver, portion cut, Selection No. 1, 4-oz. portion, IMPS No. 703, frozen, 10-to-15-lb. polylined boxes preferred

Bacon, sliced, layout pack, skinless, cured and smoked, Selection No. 1, 8-to-12-lb. bellies, 18-22 slices per lb., IMPS No. 539, chilled, 10-to-15-lb. polylined boxes preferred

SEAFOOD

The species and prices of fresh fish and shellfish products available vary with geographic location and season of the year. Because of the wide availability and ease of using frozen fishery products, these are usually purchased by the food service department. Most species are available in the frozen form throughout the year. The increasing popularity of fish has taxed the supply and caused an increase in the price of many of the most popular species. As a result, there are many less familiar (underutilized) fish being marketed in fresh and frozen forms. Many of these are satisfactory

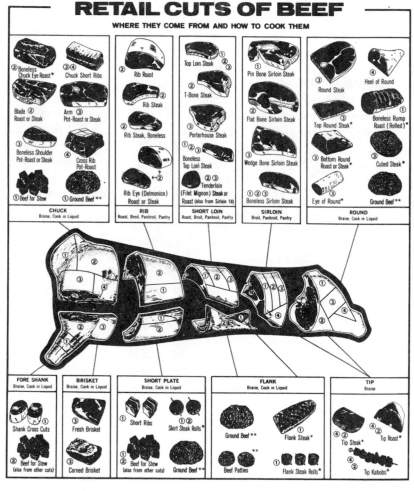

Source: National Livestock and Meat Board

FIGURE 27. Food Service Cuts of Beef.

*May be roasted, broiled, panbroiled, or panfried from high-quality beef.

**May be roasted (baked), broiled, panbroiled, or panfried.

RETAIL CUTS OF PORK

WHERE THEY COME FROM AND HOW TO COOK THEM

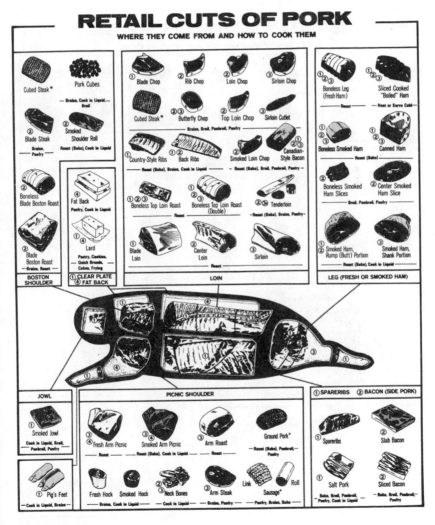

Source: National Livestock and Meat Board

FIGURE 28. Food Service Cuts of Pork.

*May be made from Boston shoulder, picnic shoulder, loin, or leg.

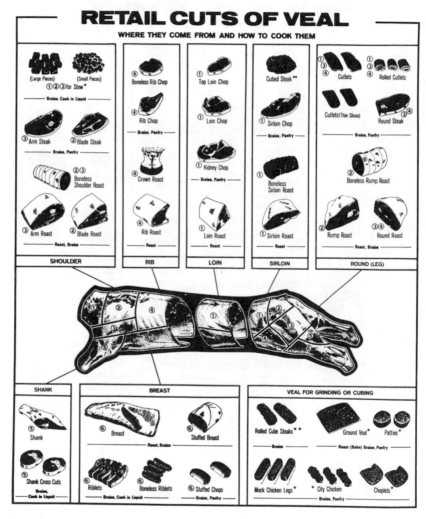

Source: National Livestock and Meat Board

FIGURE 29. Food Service Cuts of Veal.

*Veal for stew or grinding may be made from any cut.

**Cube steaks may be made from any thick solid piece of boneless veal.

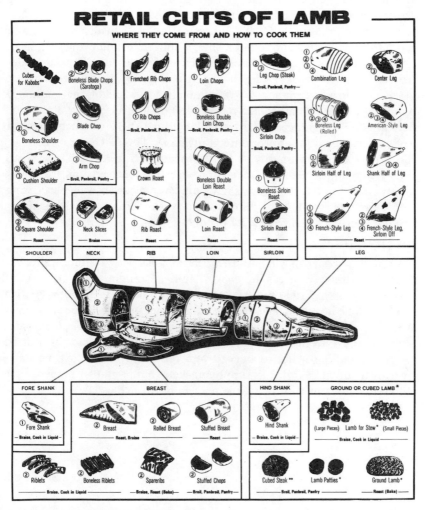

Source: National Livestock and Meat Board

FIGURE 30. Food Service Cuts of Lamb.

*Lamb for stew or grinding may be made from any cut.

**Kabobs or cube steaks may be made from any thick solid piece of boneless lamb.

to use, more economical, and should be considered for purchase.

Inspection for sanitary conditions and wholesomeness, which is required for meat, poultry, and egg products, is not as widely applied to seafood. The Seafood Quality and Inspection Division of the National Marine Fisheries Service, U.S. Department of Commerce, conducts a voluntary seafood inspection program on a fee-for-service basis for processors and other interested parties. Contract plant inspection means that the processing plant, equipment, and food-handling personnel have met required sanitation standards. In addition, a federal inspector has statistically sampled and examined the product and found it safe, wholesome, and properly labled.

Seafood packed under federal inspection will bear the Packed Under Federal Inspection mark (PUFI), as shown in figure 31, below, or statement on the label. Product grading, which is voluntary, is an additional guarantee to the consumer that the product meets a certain level of quality. Presently, there are 23 U.S. grade standards available for fishery products. Graded products may bear the appropriate grade mark: USDC Grade A, B, or C. This service is used primarily by large processors and rarely by the small fishery companies. However, the food service buyer can find excellent-quality fresh and frozen products from uninspected sources by purchasing from a reputable vendor with known sanitary standards and by recognizing the characteristics of high-quality products.

FRESH FISH

High-quality fresh fish will have firm, elastic flesh with a smooth, slippery slime and shiny surface. The eyes should be bulging and clear. Gills should be pink to bright red, and there should be no fishy odor. As fish ages, the slime increases in viscosity and becomes grainy; the odor changes from that of a seaweed to a fishy or ammonialike odor. The flesh becomes softer. Because fresh fish deteriorates quite rapidly, great care must be taken in handling it during harvest and processing. This task becomes more difficult when trying to supply markets that are far from the source of harvest. For this reason, a large percentage of fish is frozen.

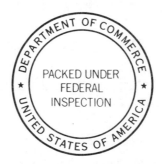

FIGURE 31. Federal Inspection Stamp for Fish.

FROZEN FISH

High-quality frozen fish will be properly processed, packaged, and stored under conditions such that surfaces show no sign of freezer burn and packages are free from drip or ice. The fish should have little or no odor. Frozen fish will remain in good condition for relatively long periods if handled properly. Periodically, the ratio of fish to breading should be determined to be sure of the best buy.

SHELLFISH

Shellfish are marketed live, cooked whole in the shell, headless, or shucked. The meat can be purchased fresh or frozen, cooked or raw, plain or breaded, or canned. Shellfish purchased live in the shell must be kept alive until cooked. Buyers of fresh shellfish should be well acquainted with the source of supply and should check to make sure that the products have been harvested from uncontaminated waters. Because much shellfish is marketed frozen, the quality characteristics before purchasing should be the same as described for other frozen fish.

MARKET FORMS

Fresh and **frozen** fish are available in several forms, including:
Whole and drawn—Only the scales and entrails are removed.
Whole and dressed—Scales, entrails, and usually the head, tail, and fins are removed.
Steaks—Cross-section slices are cut from large dressed fish, usually 5/8-inch to 3/4-inch thick.
Fillets—Sides of fish are cut lengthwise away from the bone. Fillets are practically boneless and come with or without skin.
Portions and sticks—Large, solid, frozen blocks of boneless fish are machine cut. Pieces are dipped in batter or breading and may or may not be partially cooked. Fish purchased precooked means that only the batter or breading is cooked; the fish is raw. Fillets are available in many shapes and sizes and are ready to cook as purchased.

Currently, there are many other seafood products processed and sold in a convenience form, either frozen or in a **freeze-dried** state. Frozen fish fillets or portions may be packed with stuffing, sauces, or nuts. Shrimp and crab are available freeze-dried, which helps to reduce labor time. Both products can be stored for long periods because they are cooked, cleaned, frozen, freeze-dried, and canned. Reconstitution in water takes little time, flavor and color are good, and cost may be less than the fresh product at certain times during the year.

SPECIFICATIONS FOR FISH AND SHELLFISH

When developing specifications for fresh or frozen fish and shellfish, the

following information should be included:
- Species of fish or shellfish
- USDC inspection mark or grade, if applicable
- Market form or portion shape and size
- Raw or precooked, plain or breaded
- Chilled or frozen
- Pounds per package
- Packages per case

Some sample specifications include:

Cod, breaded, 4-oz. portions, U.S. Grade A, 10/6 lb. boxes per case

Cod fillets, skinless, 4-oz. portions, U.S. Grade A, 10/5 lb. boxes per case

Pollock, breaded, 2-oz. precooked portions, minced white meat, packed under federal inspection (PUFI), USDC, 6/5 lb. boxes per case

Shrimp, round, breaded, 30/35 count, U.S. Grade A, 6/4 lb. boxes per case

CANNED FISH

Many kinds of **canned** fish products are available, such as salmon, tuna, mackerel, crab, shrimp, sardines, clams, and so forth. Of these, only salmon and tuna are available in several species and styles.

On the Pacific Coast, salmon is usually sold by species name because of differences in color, texture, and flavor. Chinook or king salmon ranges in color from white to deep salmon color and is the highest quality and highest priced. Very little of these species of salmon is canned because most is sold fresh or smoked. Sockeye is the reddest of all varieties, is of high quality, and is also high priced. Silver, medium red, or coho salmon is usually a rich orange color, slightly touched with red, and widely used for canned salmon. Pink or humpback salmon is lighter in color, but of excellent flavor and good for use in many combination recipes. Chum or keta salmon is light colored and somewhat lacking in flavor.

Tuna canned in the United States is produced from four species of the mackerel family: albacore, yellowfin, bluefin, and skipjack. Albacore has the lightest meat and is the only tuna that may be labeled white meat. The other species are labeled light meat.

Both salmon and tuna are available in oil, water, or brine pack. Four styles of pack are available: fancy or solid pack, which must contain 82 percent solid pieces; chunk style, in which 50 percent of the weight must be pieces one-half inch or larger in diameter; flakes, in which 50 percent or more of the pieces are less than one-half inch in diameter; and grated. When developing specifications for canned fish, the species and variety, packing medium, style of pack, size of can, and cans per case should be

stated. Some sample specifications are:
Tuna, solid pack, light meat, oil pack, 6/64 oz. per case
Tuna, solid pack, light meat, water pack, 24/6-1/2 oz. per case
Salmon, pink, packed under federal inspection (PUFI), 6/64 oz. per case

POULTRY

Poultry products are listed extensively in food service menus because of their great versatility in both general and modified diets. The availability of poultry is rarely a problem because the production and processing techniques used today provide a consistent supply of the desired kind, quality, and quantity of poultry at almost any season. Prices will fluctuate according to market conditions and prices of red meats, but, in general, most poultry products are more reasonable in price than other meat items.

SPECIFICATIONS

The wide variety of poultry products and market forms makes it essential for the food buyer to keep abreast of the marketplace and to have well-written specifications for all poultry items. Adequate descriptions of poultry items include the following information:

1. Kind: Refers to the species, such as chicken, turkey, duck, capon, goose, Rock Cornish game hen, quail, and so forth.
2. Class: Refers to the physical characteristics related to age and sex as follows:

   Chicken:
   Broiler-fryer—A young chicken of either sex, 8 to 12 weeks old, weighing 2-1/2 to 4 lb., ready to cook.
   Roaster—Young chicken of either sex, 3 to 5 months old, weighing 4 to 6 lb. or more, ready to cook.
   Capon—Surgically desexed male chicken, about 8 months old, weighing 5 to 8 lb., ready to cook.
   Hen or stewing chicken—Mature female chicken, more than 10 months old, weighing over 4 lb., ready to cook.
   Rock Cornish game hen—5 to 7 weeks old, weighing less than 2 lb., ready to cook.

   Turkey:
   Fryer-roaster—Less than 16 weeks old, weighing 3 to 7 lb., ready to cook.
   Young hen or young tom—16 to 24 weeks old; and may be called simply young turkey because the sex affects weight range more than eating quality; hens usually weigh 8 to 16 lb. and toms 16 lb. and over; ready to cook; cooked yield higher for heavier birds, as illustrated in table 17, above.
   Yearling or mature turkeys—over 12 months old of heavy weight.

TABLE 17. PERCENTAGE OF COOKED YIELD FOR ALL MEAT AND BREAST MEAT OF READY-TO-COOK TURKEYS

Type of Turkey	Raw Weight, lb.	All Meat, %	Breast Only, %
Hen	6-8	47.1	18.6
	10-12	50.5	19.0
	14-16	53.3	20.0
	17-19	54.3	22.3
Toms	13-15	49.7	17.3
	17-19	53.1	21.0
	21-23	55.4	21.7
	25-29	57.0	23.0

Reproduced with permission of the Department of Poultry Science, University of Wisconsin-Madison.

3. Grade: Refers to the degree of excellence of the product and is determined by factors such as conformation, fleshing, fat covering, and freedom from various types of defects such as cuts, tears, broken bones, discoloration, and so forth. USDA grades for ready-to-cook poultry are A, B, or C. Almost all chicken or turkey marketed fresh-chilled or frozen is Grade A; Grades B and C are used for processed forms. All poultry must be inspected for wholesomeness. Inspection and grade marks are shown in figures 32 and 33, next page. Birds that have a wing, tail, or drumstick missing, resulting from damage that occurs during processing but not affecting eating quality, are labeled *Parts Missing*.

4. Style: Indicates if the bird is to be cut or left whole. When ready-to-cook poultry is purchased, preference for parts, quarters, 8-piece cut, 9-piece cut, breasts, legs, thighs, boneless, and so forth should be indicated.

5. State of delivery: Indicates whether the poultry should be fresh-chilled, frozen, or precooked and frozen.

6. Weight or size: Indicates weight range allowable for individual birds and/or ounces per portion for convenience forms. Tables 17, above, and 18 and 19, pages 222 and 223, provide helpful information for use in determining which form or size poultry can be the better buy from a cost or yield standpoint.

7. Delivery unit: Refers to weight or number per delivery box or package.

MARKET FORMS

The many different market forms of poultry that are available to the food service buyer are becoming increasingly popular because they save time in preparation and labor and eliminate waste. Turkey rolls are available in

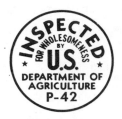

FIGURE 32. Official USDA Poultry Inspection Mark.

many variations: all white meat, all dark meat, or both in specified proportions by weight. Light and dark may be mixed together throughout
the roll or be distinct in sections of it. They are most frequently precooked
and ready to heat and serve, but sometimes are available raw.

Turkey roasts of boneless white, dark, or mixed meat are available in
a range of weights. They are raw, usually preseasoned, and ready to cook
from the frozen state. Frozen, precooked, diced white or dark meat of
chicken or turkey, separate or mixed, is an ideal item for many food
service recipes. Precooked fried chicken products, breaded or battered,
are available in a wide range of portion sizes and styles. Preformed,
precooked turkey or chicken patties are among the many newer products
in a market that changes rapidly.

All poultry products should be handled carefully after delivery and
should be stored under the refrigerated or frozen conditions appropriate
and recommended for the specific item. Of course, all precooked or
uncooked frozen products should be thawed under refrigeration or reheated
without thawing.

Some sample specifications for poultry are:

Chicken, U.S. Grade A, 2-1/2-to-3-lb. broiler, quartered, fresh,
chilled, or frozen as specified

Chicken, boned, cooked, ready to use, minimum 91 percent meat,
maximum 6 percent broth and 3 percent fat, natural proportion of
light and dark meat, seasoning to be salt only, 6/30 oz. rolls per
case, prepared under continuous USDA inspection

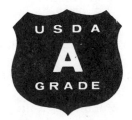

FIGURE 33. Official USDA Poultry Grade Mark.

TABLE 18. COMPARATIVE COSTS OF CHICKEN PARTS

If the price per pound of whole fryers, ready to cook, is—	Chicken parts are an equally good buy if the price per pound is—					
	Breast half Without rib	With rib	Thigh	Thigh and drumstick	Drumstick	Wing
$ .31	$ .42	$ .41	$ .35	$ .33	$ .32	$ .25
.33	.45	.44	.37	.35	.34	.27
.35	.48	.46	.39	.38	.36	.28
.37	.50	.49	.41	.40	.38	.30
.39	.53	.52	.43	.42	.40	.31
.41	.56	.54	.46	.44	.42	.33
.43	.59	.57	.48	.46	.44	.35
.45	.61	.59	.50	.48	.46	.36
.47	.64	.62	.52	.50	.48	.38
.49	.67	.65	.55	.53	.50	.39
.51	.70	.67	.57	.55	.53	.41
.53	.72	.70	.59	.57	.55	.43
.55	.75	.73	.61	.59	.57	.44
.57	.78	.75	.63	.61	.59	.46
.59	.80	.78	.66	.63	.61	.48
.61	.83	.81	.68	.66	.63	.49
.63	.86	.83	.70	.68	.65	.51
.65	.89	.86	.72	.70	.67	.52
.67	.91	.89	.75	.72	.69	.54
.69	.94	.91	.77	.74	.71	.56
.71	.97	.94	.79	.76	.73	.57
.73	1.00	.97	.81	.78	.75	.59
.75	1.02	.99	.84	.81	.77	.60
.77	1.05	1.02	.86	.83	.79	.62
.79	1.08	1.04	.88	.85	.81	.64
.81	1.10	1.07	.90	.87	.83	.65
.83	1.13	1.10	.92	.89	.85	.67
.85	1.16	1.12	.95	.91	.88	.69
.87	1.19	1.15	.97	.93	.90	.70
.89	1.21	1.18	.99	.96	.92	.72

Prices are given per pound at which ready-to-cook whole chicken and chicken parts provide equal amounts of cooked chicken meat for the money, based on yields of cooked chicken meat with skin (only ½ skin on wings and backs included), from frying chickens, ready to cook, that weighed about 2¾ pounds.

Chicken, diced, 1/2-inch cubes, white, dark, or mixed meat, precooked, frozen, 3/10 lb. polybags per case

Chicken, precooked, fryer battered, frozen, 9-piece cut, quartered, or individual parts, 9 lb. per case

Turkey, young hen, U.S. Grade A, whole, fresh or frozen, 12 to 14 lb.

Turkey, young tom, U.S. Grade A, whole, fresh or frozen, 20 to 26 lb.

Turkey breast, U.S. Grade A, boneless, frozen, uncooked, natural skin cover, 4/8 to 10 lb. per case

Turkey roll, natural proportions white and dark meat, precooked, frozen, 4-1/2-to-5-inch diameter, 4/10 lb. rolls per case

Turkey, diced, 1/2-inch cubes, white, dark, or mixed meat, pre-

TABLE 19. COMPARATIVE COSTS OF TURKEY PARTS

If the price per pound of whole turkey ready to cook is—	Turkey parts and products are an equally good buy if the price per pound is—										
	Breast, quarter	Leg, quarter	Breast, whole or half	Drum-stick	Thigh	Wing	Turkey roasts		Boned turkey, canned	Turkey with gravy,[c] canned or frozen	Gravy with turkey,[d] canned or frozen
							Ready to cook[a]	Cooked[b]			
$ .51	$ .57	$ .55	$ .65	$ .52	$ .62	$ .47	$ .89	$1.17	$1.15	$ .45	$ .19
.53	.60	.57	.68	.54	.65	.49	.93	1.22	1.19	.46	.20
.55	.62	.59	.70	.56	.67	.51	.96	1.26	1.24	.48	.21
.57	.64	.61	.73	.58	.70	.53	1.00	1.31	1.28	.50	.21
.59	.66	.63	.75	.60	.72	.55	1.03	1.36	1.33	.52	.22
.61	.69	.66	.78	.63	.75	.56	1.07	1.40	1.37	.53	.23
.63	.71	.68	.80	.65	.77	.58	1.10	1.45	1.42	.55	.24
.65	.73	.70	.83	.67	.80	.60	1.14	1.50	1.46	.57	.24
.67	.75	.72	.85	.69	.82	.62	1.17	1.54	1.51	.59	.25
.69	.78	.74	.88	.71	.85	.64	1.21	1.59	1.55	.60	.26
.71	.80	.76	.91	.73	.87	.66	1.24	1.63	1.60	.62	.27
.73	.82	.78	.93	.75	.89	.68	1.28	1.68	1.64	.64	.27
.75	.84	.81	.96	.77	.92	.69	1.31	1.72	1.69	.66	.28
.77	.87	.83	.98	.79	.94	.71	1.35	1.77	1.73	.67	.29
.79	.89	.85	1.01	.81	.97	.73	1.38	1.82	1.78	.69	.30
.81	.91	.87	1.03	.83	.99	.75	1.42	1.86	1.82	.71	.30
.83	.93	.89	1.06	.85	1.02	.77	1.45	1.91	1.87	.73	.31
.85	.96	.91	1.08	.87	1.04	.79	1.49	1.96	1.91	.74	.32
.87	.98	.94	1.11	.89	1.07	.80	1.52	2.00	1.96	.76	.33
.89	1.00	.96	1.13	.91	1.09	.82	1.56	2.05	2.00	.78	.33
.91	1.02	.98	1.16	.93	1.11	.84	1.59	2.09	2.05	.80	.34
.93	1.05	1.00	1.19	.95	1.14	.86	1.63	2.14	2.09	.81	.35
.95	1.07	1.02	1.21	.97	1.15	.88	1.66	2.18	2.14	.83	.36
.97	1.09	1.04	1.24	.99	1.19	.90	1.70	2.23	2.18	.85	.36
.99	1.11	1.06	1.26	1.01	1.21	.92	1.73	2.28	2.23	.87	.37

Prices are given per pound at which ready-to-cook whole turkey and turkey parts and turkey products provide equal amounts of cooked turkey meat for the money, based on yields of cooked turkey meat, excluding skin, medium to large birds.

[a]Roast, as purchased, includes 15 percent skin or fat.
[b]Roast, as purchased, has no more than one-fourth-inch skin and fat on any part of surface.
[c]Assumes 35 percent cooked boned turkey, minimum required for product labeled Turkey with Gravy.
[d]Assumes 15 percent cooked boned turkey, minimum required for product labeled Gravy with Turkey.

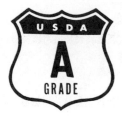

FIGURE 34. Official USDA Shell Egg Grade Mark.

cooked, frozen, 3/10 lb. polybags per case
Turkey ham, precooked, frozen, 2/7 to 8 lb. per case
Turkey franks, chilled 10 per lb., 10 lb. per case

SHELL EGGS

The application of science and engineering has made egg production a highly automated business, yielding a superior-quality fresh egg for the food service and retail markets. Careful feeding and rigid sanitary control of flocks, rapid cooling of eggs, and prompt shipment to market all help to maintain top quality. This technology and the federal regulations for shell eggs, as stated in the Egg Products Inspection Act of 1972, prevent the distribution or use of undergrade eggs, such as leakers, checks, and dirties, in consumer channels.

GRADES

The U.S. Department of Agriculture provides a voluntary grading service for shell eggs. Eggs that have been graded under this program can be identified by an official USDA shell egg grade mark, as shown in figure 34, above. The mark indicates that the eggs have been graded for quality under both federal and state supervision.

Grades refer to the interior quality and condition of the egg, as well as to the appearance of the shell. Official consumer grades are U.S. Grade AA, U.S. Grade A, and U.S. Grade B. The higher-quality eggs—AA and A—have a firm, thick white, high yolk, and a delicate flavor. They are ideal for any purpose, but are particularly good for frying and poaching, when appearance is important. Grade A eggs are less expensive than Grade AA and are highly satisfactory for the same purposes as the higher grade. Grade B eggs have thinner whites and somewhat flatter yolks that may break easily; they are less expensive and are suitable for general cooking and baking.

WEIGHT AND SIZE

Shell eggs are also classified according to size, although size has no relation to quality. Large eggs can be of any quality, just as any quality eggs can be of any size.

Official size categories are based on the minimum weight per dozen. Eggs for institutional use are purchased in cases containing 30 dozen. The official size categories and weights per dozen and the minimum weights per case, excluding the weight of the container, are as follows:

U.S. Weights or Classes, size	Minimum Weight per Dozen, oz.	Minimum Weight per 30-Dozen Case, lb.
Jumbo	30	56
Extra large	27	50-1/2
Large	24	45
Medium	21	39-1/2
Small	18	34
Peewee	15	28

The most common sizes are extra large, large, and medium.

The weight of a case of eggs should be checked periodically. An empty carton that contains the filler flats should be weighed to get an approximate weight of the carton. Then, a full case minus the weight of the carton should be weighed and the results checked against the weights stated above.

SIZE AND PRICE

The size and grade of eggs purchased should be considered with regard to the price and intended use. In some areas, shell color can affect the price even though color has no effect on grade, nutritive value, flavor, or cooking performance of the egg.

Egg prices vary by size for the same grade, but the degree of price variation depends on the supply of the various sizes. To determine which size is the most economical, the price per ounce should be compared among the various sizes. To do this, the price per dozen is divided by the weight in ounces for that size egg. For example, if large eggs are 80 cents per dozen, with a minimum weight of 24 ounces for that size, the price per ounce would be 3.3 cents. Medium eggs at 70 cents per dozen, weighing 21 ounces per dozen, would cost 3.3 cents per ounce. In this case, either size would be an equally good buy. However, medium eggs at any price per dozen over 70 cents would cost more per ounce than large eggs at 80 cents and would not be a good buy.

ACCEPTANCE SERVICE

The USDA Poultry and Egg Acceptance Service aids buyers in the purchase of shell eggs. Information can be obtained from the Poultry Division, Consumer and Marketing Service, U.S. Department of Agriculture, Washington, DC 20250, or the nearest regional office of this agency. For a fee, a federal grader will examine each order to verify that specifications are met by the supplier. Because of the costs involved, only institutions purchasing large quantities of eggs at any one time would use this service.

EGG PRODUCTS

Egg products are a convenience item for food service operations and commercial food manufacturers. Whole eggs, yolks, whites, and various blends can be obtained in *liquid, frozen,* and *dried* forms.

The Egg Products Inspection Act of 1970 provides that liquid, frozen, and dried egg products must be inspected under the U.S. Department of Agriculture's continuous mandatory inspection program. This applies to products shipped between states, within a state, or in foreign commerce. The official USDA egg products inspection mark, shown in figure 35, below, means that the products were processed under continuous supervision of a USDA-licensed inspector, that the products were processed in an approved plant with proper facilities, and that the products were pasteurized in accordance with the USDA's requirements and were truthfully and informatively labeled.

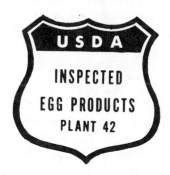

FIGURE 35. Official USDA Egg Products Inspection Mark.

Institutional packs of liquid, frozen, and powdered eggs are available in various sizes. Frozen packs range from 3-pound to 45-pound containers. Many food service operations find the smaller containers, resembling a one-half gallon milk carton, to be the most convenient to use within a short period of time after thawing. They should be stored at 0° F. (-18° C.) or lower and thawed under refrigeration. Dried egg products are also available in many pack sizes, the 5-pound container being the easiest to use. Because dried egg products can be contaminated easily and deteriorate in quality rapidly, they should be stored in the refrigerator in a tightly covered container.

The food service buyer should become familiar with the product variety provided by local vendors and develop specifications in accordance with need and market availability. Table 20, next page, summarizes the manufacturing and inspection specifications for several egg products.

SPECIFICATIONS

Specifications for fresh eggs should include the form, quality designation, size, and unit of purchase. A quality designation such as grade is omitted from egg products because they are not graded. The words *USDA inspected* are used in place of this.

Some sample specifications for eggs and egg products are:

Eggs, fresh, Grade AA, Large, 45-lb. net per 30-doz. case

Eggs, frozen, whole, pasteurized, homogenized, USDA inspected, 6 4-lb. cartons per case

Eggs, dried, whole, 6 3-lb. cans per case

DAIRY PRODUCTS

MILK

Milk is a basic food that patients and residents of any age need every day. It is a source of calcium, protein, and riboflavin and contains many other vitamins and minerals as well.

The key to quality in milk and other dairy products is effective sanitation in production, transport, and processing. For this reason, the regulations concerning the sanitary production of dairy products are very strict. The U.S. Public Health Service's Milk Ordinance and Code is the basis for state and local milk regulations. The Grade A classification for milk and milk products is a designation based on compliance with the sanitation requirements of the applicable laws. Only Grade A pasteurized milk is shipped interstate, and in most states it is the only grade available for purchase and use as a fluid product. The food service buyer should be familiar with the state or local regulatory standards.

The grades of milk are related to the bacterial count. Pasteurization destroys pathogenic organisms and most of the other common bacteria found in milk. Most fluid milk is homogenized, a process that divides the fat globules into tiny particles that remain as a permanent emulsion in milk.

FDA standards for the composition of milk specify the minimum amounts of milk fat and milk solids that are not fat contained in each kind of milk or cream product.

Milk, whole, plain or flavored	8.25 percent milk soilds	3.25 percent milk fat
Milk, lowfat, plain or flavored	8.25 percent milk solids	0.5 to 2.0 percent milk fat
Milk, skim, plain or flavored	8.25 percent milk solids	Less than 0.5 percent milk fat

TABLE 20. MANUFACTURING AND INSPECTION SPECIFICATIONS FOR EGG PRODUCTS.

| Specification | Liquid or frozen | | | Solids | | | | | | |
| | | | | Whites | | Whole | | Yolk | | |
	White	Yolk[a]	Whole	Spray Dried	Pan Dried	Plain	Free[b] Flowing	Plain	Free[b] Flowing	Scram. Egg
Moisture—%	—	—	—	8.0	14.0	5.0	3.0	5.0	3.0	2.5
Total solids—%	11.0	43.0	24.7	—	—	—	—	—	—	—
Crude protein—%	10.0	14.0	12.0	80.0	74.0	45.0	45.0	30.0	30.0	34.3
Total lipids—%	nil	28.0	10.5	<.02	nil	40.0	40.0	56.0	56.0	36.5
pH	8.9±.3	6.2±.1	7.3±.3	7.0±.5	5.5±.5	8.3±.3	8.3±.3	6.4±.3	6.4±.3	
Carbohydrates[c]—%	—	—	—	glu. free	glu. free	SOP	SOP	SOP	SOP	17
Total microbial count—gm	<5,000	<5,000	<5,000	<10,000	<10,000	<10,000	<10,000	<10,000	<10,000	<10,000
Yeast—gm	10 max.	10 max.	10 max.	10 max.	10 max.	10 max.	10 max.	10 max.	10 max.	—
Mold—gm	10 max.	10 max.	10 max.	10 max.	10 max.	10 max.	10 max.	10 max.	10 max.	—
Coliform—gm	10 max.	10 max.	10 max.	10 max.	10 max.	10 max.	10 max.	10 max.	10 max.	—
Salmonellae—gm	Neg.[d]	Neg.	Neg.	Neg.	Neg.	Neg.	Neg.	Neg.	Neg.	Neg.
Granulation	—	—	—	100%[e]	SOP	100%	100%	100%	100%	—
Others[f]	—	—	—	USBS-60	—	USBS-16	USBS-16	USBS-16	USBS-16	—

Source: American Egg Board

[a]Egg yolk contains 17% egg white; natural egg yolk contains about 52% solids.
[b]Free flowing products contain less than 2% sodium silicoaluminate.
[c]Most egg white solids are desugared. Whole egg and yolk products are desugared if specified on purchase (SOP).
[d]Negative by approved testing procedures.
[e]U.S. Bureau of Standards Screen No. 80.
[f]Additives and performance specifications may be specified on purchase.

Milk, cultured	No federal standards
buttermilk	established
Cream, half-and-half	10.5 to 18 percent fat
Cream, light	18 to 30 percent milk fat
Whipping cream, light	30 to 36 percent milk fat
Whipping cream, heavy	Not less than 36 percent
	milk fat

Lowfat milk must be fortified with vitamin A at levels specified by FDA regulations. Fortification with vitamin D is optional. Standards for milk products within certain states may vary from the federal standards.

Cultured milk has a characteristic flavor that is produced by bacterial fermentation. Cultured buttermilk is processed from pasteurized skim milk to which lactic acid bacteria have been added and is partially fermented to produce some coagulation of the milk protein. Small butter granules may be added. Buttermilk produced as a by-product of making butter is almost never available today.

Evaporated milk is prepared by removing about one-half of the water from fresh whole milk. The milk fat content is not less than 7.5 percent, and the milk solid content is not less than 25.5 percent. It must contain 25 international units (IU) vitamin D per ounce; the addition of vitamin A is optional. Evaporated lowfat and skim milks are also available. These are useful in reducing the amount of fat offered in the diet.

Another type of milk used occasionally is *sweetened condensed milk*. This is made from whole milk by removing approximately one-half of the water and adding 40 percent sugar in the form of sucrose, dextrose, and/or corn syrup before evaporation takes place.

Yogurt, which has grown tremendously in popularity, particularly among young people, is available plain or flavored and with variation in fat content. Yogurt can be made from whole milk, lowfat milk with added milk solids, or skim milk with added milk solids. Because of the variation in yogurt composition, the buyer should check local sources for product information and nutrient composition.

Sour cream and *sour half-and-half* are other cultured milk products used by food service operations. Cultured sour cream contains approximately 20 percent milk fat, and cultured half-and-half approximately 12 percent milk fat. Sour half-and-half can be substituted for the richer product in many recipes and is less expensive.

Nonfat *dry milk* is economical for institutional use in cooked or baked products. U.S. standards for grades of nonfat dry milk are U.S. Extra Grade and U.S. Standard Grade. Nonfat dry milk contains not more than 5 percent moisture and not more than 1.5 percent milk fat unless otherwise specified. Instant nonfat dry milk, made by a special process that gives it improved solubility, is the most popular form. However, noninstant nonfat dry milk is available and can be used satisfactorily in baked products when mixed with the dry ingredients. Fortification of nonfat dry milk with vitamins A and D is optional and if desired should be stated in the specification.

Dry buttermilk is another useful product for baking purposes. The grade names for this product are the same as for nonfat dry milk. All dry milk products are made from pasteurized milk.

The federal standards of identity for *ice cream* specify a minimum content of 10 percent milk fat and 20 percent milk solids. The quality of ice cream is related to composition, quality of ingredients, weight per gallon, and the quality and quantity of flavoring materials. Differences in these components influence the price of the various products. Ice cream is available in a wide selection of forms suited to food service use; individually wrapped slices or individual cups are time savers. Novelty items add an interesting change to the menu.

Ice milk, hardened or soft serve, is available in a wide variety of flavors. Ice milk contains a minimum of 2 percent milk fat and 11 percent milk solids. *Fruit sherbets* contain a minimum of one percent milk fat and two percent milk solids. State standards for sherbets and other frozen dessert products can vary in compositional requirements, so buyers must be familiar with state regulations.

SPECIFICATIONS

Written descriptions of exact needs for milk and other dairy products are just as important as for other foods. Additions or deletions from the following sample specifications may be needed to meet any particular situation:

Milk, whole, homogenized, pasteurized, fortified, minimum 3.25 percent milk fat, 1/2-pint carton

Milk, lowfat, homogenized, pasteurized, fortified, minimum 2 percent milk fat, 1/2 gallon carton

Buttermilk, cultured, homogenized, pasteurized, minimum 8.25 percent milk solids, 1-quart carton

Cream, half-and-half, pasteurized, 10.5 to 18 percent milk fat, 1-pint carton

Milk, nonfat, dry, instant, U.S. Extra Grade, 5-lb. bag

Yogurt, lowfat, minimum 8.5 percent nonfat solids, plain flavored, 8-oz. carton

NONDAIRY PRODUCTS

Cream substitutes, dessert toppings, and *imitation milk* are among a group of products developed to simulate dairy products. There are no compositional standards for these products, so the buyer needs to check ingredient lists provided by the manufacturers. Some of the nondairy products, including many of the coffee whiteners, contain no milk or other dairy products and are available in fresh and frozen liquid or powdered forms. Dessert toppings are found in pressurized containers and in powdered or frozen forms. The stability of nondairy toppings and their lower cost have made them extremely popular for food service use.

Imitation milk is available in some states and can have utility value for some modified diets. These products combine fats or oils other than milk fat with food solids, but exclude milk solids. Sodium caseinate is frequently used as the protein source.

Cultured nondairy sour cream is another of the imitation dairy products. Lauric acid oils, including coconut oil, hydrogenated coconut oil, and/or palm kernel oil, are frequently used in this product. The manufacturer should be consulted for specific content.

CHEESE

The varieties of cheese available to consumers provide a tremendous potential for interesting menus and are a challenge to the food service buyer. To buy cheese effectively requires knowledge of the quality and flavor characteristics of each cheese and of the ways they can be used.

Natural cheeses are classified into several groups by degree of hardness: soft, like cottage, ricotta, or cream; semisoft, like brick, Muenster, or mozzarella; hard, like cheddar or Swiss; and very hard, like Parmesan or Romano. Further distinctions are made on the basis of the organism (bacteria or mold) used for ripening and the length of ripening or aging.

Natural cheeses are made from whole, partially defatted, or skim milk, depending on the variety of cheese. Federal standards of identity specifying the processing methods and setting minimum fat and maximum moisture contents have been established for major cheese varieties.

CHEDDAR

This whole milk cheese is perhaps the most popular of all natural cheeses in the United States. It is also called American or American cheddar cheese and can be identified by its shape or style, such as longhorn or daisy. In addition, it is often identified by the locality where it was produced, such as Wisconsin, New York, and so forth. The standards for cheddar cheese specify a minimum of 50 percent milk fat and content and a maximum of 39 percent moisture. The USDA grades for cheddar cheese are AA, A, B, and C and are based on flavor, body, texture, color, and appearance. Various states also may have their own grades.

Flavor terminology is also used to specify the age of the cheese to be purchased. As cheddar cheese increases in age, the flavor becomes sharper. Market flavors available are: fresh or current, medium or mellow, aged or sharp, and very sharp. Aged cheddar melts faster and produces a smoother product than cheese less than three months of age.

When purchasing cheddar cheese, the desired form and size should be specified: 20- 40- or 60-lb. blocks; 12-lb. cylindrical longhorns; 20-lb. cylindrical daisies; 5-to-20-lb. loaves; or any other size or form available from vendors. Presliced forms are also available. In addition, the desired degree of aging and USDA or state grade should be specified.

SWISS

Swiss cheese is produced from pasteurized whole and skim milk and has a lower fat content than cheddar. Standards require a minimum of 43 percent milk fat and not more than 41 percent moisture. The characteristic holes, or eyes, are produced by bacteria during aging, which also develop the most desirable sweet nutty flavor. USDA-graded Swiss cheese is available. Aging for 3 to 9 months is typical, although the desired aging should be specified.

COTTAGE

Cottage cheese is the soft, uncured curd from pasteurized skim milk. Cream is added to the dry cheese curd to make creamed cottage cheese. Creamed or dry cottage cheese comes in small curd, with particles about 1/8 to 1/4 inch in diameter, and in large curd, with particles up to 3/8 inch in size. When purchasing this product, the curd size should be stated. Cottage cheese is available in many container sizes, from 1 to 30 lb. Because cottage cheese, particularly large curd, has limited shelf life after the container has been opened, the quantities served and the amount of time it takes to use a container should be considered when purchasing.

OTHER NATURAL CHEESES

Because the variety of natural cheese is so extensive, other specific types are not described here in detail. Table 21, next page, gives examples of cheese classifications and describes the characteristics of frequently used cheeses. Federal grades and standards have not been established for most of these varieties, with the exception of mozzarella. However, familiarity with the quality standards of various manufacturers and careful product evaluation will help the food buyer develop the ability to make selections of high-quality cheeses.

PROCESSED

Pasteurized processed cheese is a blend of two or more lots of cheddar cheese, fresh and aged, that are heated to a point at which further ripening is halted. Emulsifying agents are added to give a smooth texture and prevent separation. Because of the heating process, the texture and the flavor of the cheese remain constant after processing. Other cheeses can

TABLE 21. CHARACTERISTICS OF COMMONLY USED CHEESES

Cheese	Characteristics
American (pasteurized process)	Semisoft to soft; light yellow to orange; mild. Made of cow's milk (whole), Cheddar, and/or Colby cheese.
Blue	Semisoft; white with blue-green mold; flavor similar to Roquefort. Made of cow's milk (whole).
Brick	Semisoft; smooth; light yellow to orange; flavor mild but pungent and sweet. Made of cow's milk (whole).
Brie	Soft, edible white crust; flavor resembles Camembert. Made of cow's milk (whole, lowfat, or skim).
Camembert	Soft, almost fluid; mild to pungent flavor. Made of cow's milk (whole).
Cheddar	Hard; smooth; light yellow to orange; mild to sharp. Made of cow's milk (whole).
Cottage	Soft; moist, delicate, large or small curd. Mildly acid flavor. Unripened; usually made of cow's milk (skim). Cream dressing may be added to cottage dry curd.
Cream	Soft; smooth; buttery; mild, slightly acid flavor. Unripened; made of cream and cow's milk (whole).
Edam	Semisoft to hard; rubbery; mild, sometimes salty flavor; cannonball shape. Made of cow's milk (lowfat).
Gorgonzola	Semisoft, less moist than blue; marbled with blue-green mold; spicy flavor. Made of cow's milk (whole) or goat's milk or mixture of these.
Gouda	Hard; flavor like Edam. Made of cow's milk (lowfat).
Gruyère	Hard with tiny gas holes; mild, sweet flavor. Made of cow's milk (whole).
Monterey Jack	Semisoft (whole milk), hard (lowfat or skim milk); smooth; mild to mellow. Made of cow's milk (whole, lowfat, or skim).
Limburger	Soft; strong, robust flavor; highly aromatic. Made of cow's milk (whole or lowfat).
Muenster	Semisoft; flavor between brick and Limburger. Made of cow's milk (whole).
Neufchatel	Soft; creamy; white; mild flavor. Unripened or ripened 3-4 weeks. Made of cow's milk (whole or skim), or a mixture of milk and cream.
Parmesan	Very hard (grating) granular texture. Made of cow's milk (lowfat).
Provolone	Hard, stringy texture; bland acid to sharp, usually smoked flavor; pear, sausage, or salami shaped. Made of cow's milk (whole).
Roquefort	Semisoft; white with blue-green mold; sharp, piquant flavor. Made of sheep's milk.
Stilton	Semisoft; white with blue-green mold; spicy but milder than Roquefort flavor. Made of cow's milk (whole with added cream).
Swiss	Hard with gas holes; mild, nutlike, sweet flavor. Made of cow's milk (lowfat).

Adapted from *Newer Knowledge of Cheese*, Chicago: National Dairy Council, 1980.

be used in making processed cheese. The varieties will be noted on the label.

Pasteurized processed cheese is similar to natural cheese, except that it has a lower fat content, higher moisture content, and added whey or milk solids. Additional ingredients, such as sausage, vegetables, or nuts, are sometimes added. The cheese flavor is usually less pronounced in processed cheese than in natural cheese, but processed cheese melts more readily during cooking.

Pasteurized processed cheese spread has a still lower fat and higher moisture content than the other products described above. It is soft and can be spread with a knife. A stabilizer is usually added to prevent separation of the ingredients. None of the processed cheese products are federally graded. The food buyer should become acquainted with the large variety of natural and processed cheeses available.

IMITATION

The Filled Cheese Act of June 6, 1896, imposed a tax on cheese and licensed its manufacture and sale under special labeling and packaging procedures. Various states also imposed other restrictions that inhibited or discouraged the *development* of filled-cheese products. The Filled Cheese Act was repealed in October 1974. As a result, filled-cheese foods are now subject solely to the provisions of the Federal Food, Drug, and Cosmetic Act and the Fair Packaging and Labeling Act and move freely in interstate commerce as nonstandardized foods, but their sale can be prohibited in some states.

Presently there are two types of imitation cheese available to consumers: skim milk plus vegetable fat, and calcium or sodium caseinate plus vegetable fat. Most of these products have the body, texture, and appearance of regular cheese, although some people think that the flavor is different. Cheese substitutes are also functionally equivalent to their natural cheese counterparts. Various convenient package sizes are available for food service use.

SPECIFICATIONS

Sample specifications for cheese include the following:
> Cheese, American, processed, medium blend, pasteurized, 6/5 lb. blocks
> Cheese, cheddar, natural, U.S. Grade A, medium aged, 6/5 lb. blocks
> Cheese, mozzarella, part skim, low moisture, 6/5 lb. blocks
> Cheese, cottage, creamed, minimum 4 percent milk fat by weight, maximum 80 percent moisture, small curd, 5-lb. container

FRESH FRUITS AND VEGETABLES

A significant amount of information is needed to purchase fresh or processed fruits and vegetables. As with other food products, it is important to select the form (fresh, canned, or frozen), style, and quality best suited to the planned use on the menu.

GRADES

The USDA's Agricultural Marketing Service has developed quality grade standards for fruit and vegetable products. Grading of fresh, frozen, and canned fruits and vegetables is voluntary; that is, any grower, processor, or buyer who wants the product graded requests and pays for the grading service. When the products have been graded by a USDA inspector, they can be labeled with the U.S. grade name. If a product is labeled with one of the official grade names, such as Fancy, but without the prefix *U.S.*, that product still must meet the USDA's standard for the grade, whether or not it has actually been inspected.

Grades for each product cover the entire range of quality, so there are more grades for some products than for others. The grade names for all products are not uniform, but progress is being made to standardize them. The terms *U.S. Fancy*, *U.S. No. 1*, *U.S. No. 2*, and *U.S. No. 3*, which are the grade names used in establishing or revising standards for fresh fruits and vegetables, were effective July 1, 1976.

Although most fresh fruits and vegetables are sold at wholesale on the basis of U.S. grades, not many are marked with the grade when resold. The typical range of grades for fresh fruits and vegetables include U.S. Fancy, U.S. No. 1, and U.S. No. 2. For some products, there are grades above and below this span, which is the basis for the new policy of reclassifying grade names.

The grades for canned and frozen fruits and vegetables are U.S. Grade A (Fancy), U.S. Grade B (Choice for fruits and Extra Standard for vegetables), and U.S. Grade C (Standard). Grade A fruits and vegetables are the most tender, succulent, and uniform in size, shape, and color. Grade B is very good quality, but may be slightly less uniform in size and color and there may be a few blemishes. Grade C products are fairly good quality, just as wholesome and nutritious as the higher grades, and may be the best buy for use in combination recipes when the appearance is not important.

Most processors and distributors have their own quality control programs and quality designations, whether or not they use USDA's grading service, and pack more than one grade of product. Food buyers should be aware of the various quality designations used by companies in their areas.

NET WEIGHTS

A statement of net quantity is required by federal and various state laws to appear on the label of canned fruits and vegetables. However, none of these laws specifies what the labeled weight or volume should be for these products. The fill, which affects the net weight or volume, varies with each product, but is required to be as full as practical, usually about 90 percent.

PRODUCT USES

The intended use of a product will determine which product style to buy. The product style will affect the cost of fruit and vegetables. Canned whole fruits and vegetables usually cost more than cut styles, but should be used when appearance is important. Short cuts, dices, and pieces of vegetables are the least expensive and are good for use in soup and stews. Less perfect fruits can be chosen for cooked desserts and mixed salads when appearance is not so important.

When purchasing fresh fruit and vegetable products, the quality, variety, and size of product needed should be considered. On some fresh items, the labor and waste in trimming and preparation should be considered. For example, fresh broccoli will require some pre-preparation time and there will be some loss in trimming stems and cutting the bunches into uniform serving sizes. Apples that are purchased for eating out-of-hand will be a different variety and size than those purchased for cooking purposes.

CONTAINERS

The container size selected can affect the cost and quality of the food as well as the ease of handling. Larger container sizes can provide a lower per serving cost if the quantity of food they contain can be used while the food is at peak quality. If purchased in too large a unit, some food may have to be discarded because of staleness or spoilage, which results in an increase in food costs.

The No. 10 can, packed six per case, is the most common packing container for canned fruits and vegetables. However, for items used in smaller quantities, the No. 303, or 2-1/2-oz., cans, packed 24 per case, may be a better purchase size.

Frozen vegetables are most commonly found in 2- or 2-1/2-lb. packages and are packed 12 per case. However, some are available in 20-, 30-, or even 50-lb. packages.

The initials IQF in relation to frozen fruits and vegetables mean individually quick frozen. The pieces of the product are frozen separately, then loose packed so that the right amount of product can be measured without having to thaw the complete package. IQF fruits and vegetables are usually packed in 20-lb. polybags or in larger quantities.

In order to retain color and flavor, many fruits are packed with sugar. Because fruit-sugar ratios vary, purveyors should be consulted for specific information.

Fresh fruits and vegetables are usually purchased by weight, but in some cases the count per shipping container also should be specified. A wide variety of sizes of cartons, boxes, and other shipping containers are used for fresh produce, depending on the type of product and the area where the product is produced. A list of common container sizes for fresh fruits and vegetables is available from the United Fresh Fruit and Vegetable Association (see references).

SPECIFICATIONS

Specifications for fresh, frozen, and canned fruits and vegetables should include the following:

- Name of product
- Style or type of product (whole, cut, trimmed, and so forth)
- USDA grade, brand, or other quality designation
- Size of container
- Quantity or weight per shipping unit
- Other pertinent factors, depending on product (packing medium, syrup density, variety, stage of maturity, drained weight, and so forth)

Specifications for fruit and vegetable products should be developed according to the quality and type of product needed in a particular operation. Following are some sample specifications for fruit and vegetable products.

Bananas, fresh, No. 1, green tip, 6-8 inches, 40-lb. carton

Fruit cocktail, canned, U.S. Grade A (Fancy), heavy syrup, min. dr. wt. 72 oz., 6/#10 per case

Blueberries, frozen, whole, U.S. Grade A, IQF, 20-lb. box

Cabbage, fresh, green, U.S. No. 1, 1-1/2-to-2-lb. heads, 50-lb. mesh sack

Corn, canned, yellow, whole kernel, U.S. Grade A (Fancy), liquid pack, min. dr. wt. 70 oz., 6/#10 per case

Broccoli, frozen cuts, U.S. Grade A, 12/2 lb. per case

DEHYDRATED FRUITS AND VEGETABLES

Dehydrated fruits and vegetables have been available to consumers for years. At present, more and more products, particularly potatoes, are being used in food service operations. There are two major types of dehydrated foods available. Regular moisture-dried foods contain 18 to 20 percent of the original moisture of the food. Apples, apricots, raisins, dates, peaches, and prunes are available in this form. Low-moisture dehydrated foods contain only 2.5 to 5 percent moisture and are less perishable. Onions, parsley, green peppers, potatoes, garlic, and many other vegetables are sold in this form.

Two methods of preservation are used for drying foods. Fruits are dried in the sun in warm, dry areas of the country. New technology allows foods to be dried by vacuum dehydration. Foods are placed in enclosed chambers, and dry, warm, inert gas under vacuum conditions is used to extract moisture.

Federal standards of quality exist for most all dried and low-moisture fruits. These standards are U.S. Grade A, U.S. Grade B, and U.S. Grade C. No standards are available for low-moisture vegetables except dried legumes, including beans, peas, and lentils. Nearly all peas and lentils and about one-third of all beans are officially inspected before or after processing, even though retail packages seldom carry the federal or state grade stamp.

USDA grades are generally based on shape, size, color, and foreign material. State grades are based on quality factors similar to those for federal grades. The lower grades usually contain more foreign matter and more kernels of uneven size and off-color. The higher grades are U.S. No. 1 for dry, whole, or split peas, lentils, and black-eye peas (which are actually beans). USDA No. 1 Choice Handpicked or simply Handpicked is for great northern, pinto, and pea beans. U.S. Extra No. 1 is for lima beans, large and small.

When purchasing dehydrated fruits and vegetables, a buyer should specify a clean product that has been prepared and packed under sanitary conditions. The product should have a bright characteristic color and good aroma. Specifications for dehydrated potatoes should include the style: flakes, granules, sliced, or diced. In addition, for instant mashed potato products, which may have dried milk and/or vitamin C added, this information should be specified. Other important considerations are the quality and yield of instant dehydrated potatoes. The pounds of reconstitution stated on the label should be checked by sampling. Cooking is recommended to check quality. Some specifications for dehydrated foods follow:

Potatoes, sliced (cross-sliced 1/8-inch-thick chip), dehydrated, max. 7 percent moisture, 4/5 lb. bags per case
Potatoes, instant, granules, without milk, Fancy, 6/10 per case
Beans, dry, navy, U.S. Grade No. 1, 25-lb. bag
Peas, dry, split, green, U.S. Grade No. 1, 25-lb. bag
Raisins, processed, Thompson Seedless, natural, U.S. Grade A, small, 30-lb. box

FATS AND OILS

Food service operations require several kinds of shortening and oil products designed for specific purposes. Manufacturers offer products for baking, frying, and general-cooking purposes.

Lard is rendered fat from hogs. Quality varies according to the color, texture, and flavor of the product. The shortening power and textural characteristics of lard are well suited for use in pastry. However, lard is not a satisfactory product for frying because the smoking point is lower than vegetable oils. Hydrogenated lard is available with improved quality and a higher smoking point than pure leaf lard. Blends of lard and tallow are marketed, as well as blends of meat fat and vegetable shortenings. These products are suited to most general-cooking purposes. There are also *hydrogenated meat fat shortenings*, particularly designed for stability in deep-fat frying.

Hydrogenated vegetable shortenings can be used for many purposes in food production. The process of hydrogenization changes vegetable oils from liquid to a creamy, plastic texture at room temperature. *All purpose* vegetable shortening is used in baking, grilling, and other cooking operations. *High-ratio* vegetable shortenings have added emulsifiers, usually monoglycerides or diglycerides, which increase the shortening power. The high-ratio shortenings are desirable for bakery products, but break down more rapidly during deep-fat frying than other types of shortening.

Vegetable oils for general or specialized uses include those from a single source and blends of several different vegetable oils. The vegetable oils most widely used include corn oil, cottonseed oil, soybean oil, and peanut oil. Safflower, sunflower, and sesame seed oils are more unsaturated than the other common oils and therefore are being incorporated in many new products on the market. Most vegetable oils are deodorized, bleached, and clarified for use in foods, but any one or more of these processes may be omitted for specialized oils. The quality of vegetable oils can deteriorate from exposure to air, light, and moisture. Oils also can become cloudy in appearance when placed in cold temperatures if they have not been winterized, a processing treatment that keeps oils clear at refrigerator temperatures. *Cooking oils* are not processed in this way and become solid at low temperatures.

Specially designed shortenings and oils are recommended for good performance in deep-fat frying. High smoke points are needed to help prevent fat breakdown. For purchasing products for deep-fat frying, baking, and for general-purpose cooking, detailed information on ingredients and performance should be obtained from the manufacturer. Specifications for these products may be similar to the following:

Oil, mixed (cottonseed, soybean, and corn), 5-gallon container

Shortening, all vegetable high-ratio hydrogenated, 50-lb. container

Shortening, all vegetable, all-purpose (smoking point 435°F. [223°C.]), hydrogenated, 50-lb. container

Shortening, liquid, all vegetable with stabilizer (smoking point 440°F. [227°C.]) 3/10 qt., 6/5 qt., or 6/1 gal. containers per case

BUTTER

Butter has been defined, by an act of Congress, to contain not less than 80 percent milk fat and may or may not have salt and coloring added. The U.S. grades for butter are based on flavor, body or texture, salt, and color. The grades, arrived at through a numerical point system, are U.S. Grade AA (93 score), U.S. Grade A (92 score), and U.S. Grade B (90 score). In addition, many states have established grades for butter. Purchase units for butter include pound prints, chips, patties or reddies, and cubes. Local suppliers can offer information about availability of forms that meet specific needs. The quality desired, style (prints, chips, and so forth), number of chips per pound, and total weight of container should be included when writing a specification for butter.

MARGARINE

Margarine is manufactured under federal standards of identity and must contain 80 percent fat, which may be of approved animal or vegetable origin. The kinds of fats used in the manufacture of margarine must be listed on the label. If animal fat is used, the margarine must be manufactured under government inspection. Other ingredients include milk, salt, flavoring, color, emulsifiers, and preservatives. Fortification of margarine with 15,000 IU of vitamin A per pound is mandatory; vitamin D fortification is optional. Margarine for cooking purposes can be purchased in pounds. For table use, chips, patties, and reddies are available in different sizes. Many states have laws requiring food service operators to inform customers when margarine is used as a table spread. Information in the written specifications is similar to that for butter.

GRAIN AND CEREALS

FLOUR

Several types of flour, made from different kinds of wheat, are available for specific uses. Flours are classified by density (hard, semihard, or soft), color, protein strength, and use. *Bread* or *hard flours* contain higher protein content than other types of flour. These proteins help form gluten, the strong elastic structure needed in yeast-leavened doughs. *All-purpose* flours can be blends of hard-wheat flours or soft-wheat flours or both. Although all-purpose flours are suited to many purposes, they are not as satisfactory as bread flour if high-volume breads are desired. However, all-purpose flour can be used for almost any other baked product with excellent results. All-purpose flour is available bleached or unbleached. *Self-rising* all-purpose flour is also available; this flour contains baking powder, baking soda, and salt.

Pastry and *cake flours* are usually milled from soft wheats and are used mainly in pies, cakes, and other desserts. These flours have a lower protein and higher starch content than other flours. In purchasing any of these white flour products, buyers should specify that the flour be enriched with thiamin, riboflavin, niacin, and iron. Fifty- and 100-pound bags are the most convenient size for food service use.

Whole wheat or *graham flour* is made from the entire wheat kernel with only the outer bran layer removed. Because the wheat germ, which is high in fat, is left in whole wheat flour, it will become stale or rancid if not stored properly.

Rye flour is made from rye grain and contains the proteins needed for gluten formation, but not in the same proportion as in wheat. For that reason, some wheat flour is used in rye bread recipes.

Soy flour with varying amounts of fat removed is high in protein. Incorporation of some soy flour in bakery products improves the protein content, moistness, and tenderness.

Specifications for flours commonly include a percent protein and ash content. The following examples illustrate suggested specifications for some wheat flours:

Flour, wheat, white, all-purpose enriched, .46 percent max. ash, 9 percent min. protein on 14 percent moisture basis, 50-lb. bag

Flour, wheat, bread, enriched, .46 percent max. ash, 9 percent min. protein on 14 percent moisture basis, 50-lb. bag

Flour, whole wheat or graham, 1.9 percent max. ash, 11 percent min. protein on 14 percent moisture basis, 25-lb. bag

PASTA

Enriched macaroni products are made from wheat. A basic ingredient in high-quality macaroni products is obtained from a hard, amber durum wheat. The wheat is milled into a golden-toned, coarse product called semolina; into granulars that contain more flour; or into flour itself. Water is added to a mixture of durum meals or flour, semolina, and farina to make a dough that is forced through dies to make the many shapes of tubular macaroni products or cordlike spaghetti. Because enrichment of these products with thiamin, riboflavin, niacin, and iron is not mandatory, the buyer needs to specify that the product be enriched when purchasing. Macaroni products can be made with other kinds of wheat flours, so durum wheat should be specified for high quality.

Noodle products are similar in composition to macaroni, except they must contain liquid eggs, frozen eggs, dried eggs, egg yolks, dried yolks, or any combination of these at a minimum level of 5.5 percent. Enrichment is optional and, if desired, should be stated in the specification. The product name and purchase unit also should be included. The following are examples of pasta specifications:

Macaroni, shell, durum, enriched, small, 10-lb. box
Egg noodles, durum, enriched, broad, 10-lb. box
Spaghetti, durum, enriched, long, 10-lb. box

CORNMEAL

Cornmeal is made from white or yellow corn and is available in either coarse or fine grinds. Enrichment with B-vitamins and iron is common but not mandatory. Calcium is an optional enrichment ingredient. Regular cornmeal contains most of the corn kernel and has a fat content over 3.5 percent. Degermed cornmeal has a fat content under 2.25 percent. Self-rising cornmeal, with added baking soda, baking powder, and salt, also can be purchased. Common purchase units are 5-lb. or 25-lb. bags. The size that best suits an institution's needs should be selected. If only small amounts are used at any one time, smaller bags are easier to handle.

RICE

Rice can be classified as short, medium, or long grain. Each has different cooking characteristics. For example, short-grain rice tends to be stickier after cooking and is suitable for use in recipes where it is needed as an extender and binder. Medium and long-grain rice will remain separate and more distinct in form after cooking.

Rice is available in several forms: regular milled white; parboiled, or converted, white; precooked white; and brown or husked.

Regular milled white rice has the outer hull removed and is polished. Because this processing removes the major amounts of B-vitamins and some of the minerals, enrichment is desirable and should be specified when purchasing.

Parboiled or converted rice is regular white rice treated to retain the B-vitamins by either parboiling or subjecting the rice to steam pressure before hulling. After cooking, the grains tend to be more separate and plump and have better holding qualities than regular white rice. Precooked rice is milled, cooked, and dehydrated; it is usually enriched.

Brown, or husked, rice has only the rough outer husk removed, and thus has a higher calorie, protein, and mineral content than enriched white rice. The firmer texture and characteristic nutty flavor has helped increase the popularity of brown rice. It is well suited to many kinds of recipes and is a staple for vegetarian fare. Purchase information needed is similar to that for other kinds of rice.

Wild rice is not actually a rice but is a seed of a grasslike plant. Because it is a costly product, it is usually purchased as a mixture that includes white or brown rice and may be preseasoned. Relatively small quantities of wild rice produce large cooked yields because wild rice continues to absorb water throughout the cooking process.

BREAKFAST CEREALS

Many kinds of hot cooked cereals are found on the menus in health care facilities. These include oatmeal (rolled oats), farina, grits, cream of wheat, cream of rice, rolled wheat, and others. Regular, quick-cooking, and instant forms are available for many of these products. Except for the whole-wheat products, enrichment should be specified.

Ready-to-eat breakfast cereals add great variety to breakfast alternatives. Individual boxes and ready-to-serve individual bowl packs are available for the most popular varieties. If the clientele is unable to handle individual boxes, bulk retail packages should be considered; these are less expensive but require more labor time. Presweetened cereals cost more per ounce than unsweetened cereals.

The following are sample specifications for several grain and cereal products:

Cornmeal, yellow, enriched, coarse, 25-lb. bag
Farina, enriched, regular, 6/5-lb. packages per case
Cereal, whole wheat meal, malted, 6/5-lb. packages per case
Rice, milled, long grain, enriched, U.S. Grade No. 1, 25-lb. bag

OTHER STAPLES

A great many other food items are basic staples in any food service operation, but purchasing decisions for these are less difficult to make than those decisions previously discussed. For example, many kinds of prepared bread and bakery products are available. Developing specifications requires knowledge of local market offerings and terminology. For breads, specifications should include size or weight of loaf, number of slices, and enrichment. Although federal laws require enrichment of some bread products traded interstate, some states do not require enrichment of breads produced and sold within the state. Frozen bread and roll doughs have become very popular because they provide fresh-baked characteristics with greatly reduced labor and equipment requirements. Quality characteristics of products from various vendors as well as cost should be evaluated before purchase decisions are made.

The consistent quality and laborsaving advantages of baking mixes make them mainstays in many food service operations. Cake mixes, pudding mixes, quick bread mixes, and other dessert mixes are just a few that can add variety to the menu yet reduce labor time. When purchasing, a food buyer should compare product quality and yield from various brands and calculate cost per serving.

In setting up specifications for other miscellaneous items, such as spices, condiments, sweeteners, and beverages, the various brands available should be considered and the quality of each evaluated. Prices for various package sizes should be compared, and the food service buyer should keep up to date with price trends. Package sizes, particularly for spices, should be considered. Some may be used in much larger quantities than others and should be purchased in one pound or larger units; others used only occasionally should be purchased in the smaller retail market packages to retain better quality until used. Where they have been established, federal standards and grades should be used. There are federal grades for honey, maple syrup, nuts, olives, pickles, and catsup. Federal standards of identity are also available for many products.

The following specifications for some staple foods may be useful in developing others:

Walnuts, U.S. No. 1, small pieces, latest season crop, 6/5 lb. boxes per case

Olives, green, queen, giant, U.S. Grade A or Fancy, 6/#10 per case

Pickles, dill, thin, crosscut, fresh pack, U.S. Grade A or Fancy, 6/#10 per case

Honey, light amber, U.S. Grade A, extracted, 6/5 lb. per case

INVENTORY CONTROL, RECEIVING, AND STORAGE

Determining inventory levels, proper receiving, storage, and issue of goods are critical processes in controlling food service costs and maintaining quality of food. All these activities can be centralized in the materials management department or can be the responsibility of the food service department head. Wherever they take place, the tasks of checking food and supplies for quantity and quality plus distribution to the point of use must be performed according to the organization's policies and sound business practices.

INVENTORY

Inventory is money. In other words, money is converted into goods in the form of food, supplies, and equipment. Management must be aware of the value of these goods and the costs involved in controlling the size of the inventory and the security of these goods once they are on hand. How should a buyer plan what and how much stock to keep? Obviously, the answer goes back to that all-important management tool, the menu. The quantities of food needed are projected from menu item frequency and product popularity based on past usage. Inventory levels are established and monitored and adjustments are made periodically to correct overage or shortage problems.

The methods used by some managers to determine inventory levels are known as the par stock or the mini-max system. The par stock system requires that a certain quantity level be established for each item that must be kept on hand to meet the needs of the planned menu and any unusual circumstances that may occur. Orders are placed at a regularly fixed interval for a specific period. Each time the ordering date comes around, enough stock is purchased to replenish the supply to the predetermined amount. The usage rate of each item must be carefully planned and coordinated with the period between order dates.

The mini-max system involves establishing both a minimum and a maximum amount of stock to have on hand. Goods are ordered whenever the minimum is reached and only in the quantity needed to attain the maximum level. With this system, the amount of each food ordered will be the same each time, but the time it is purchased will vary. Again, the usage rate of each item must be carefully scrutinized so that the determined minimum and maximum levels are feasible.

Figure 36, next page, illustrates both these systems of controlling the quantities of food in inventory. Either will be helpful in preventing overstocking and avoiding shortages of foods used frequently.

CONTROL

Equally significant to inventory management is control of goods kept in dry and low-temperature storage areas and the issue of these to the user department. Formalized methods of issuing stock usually are used only for those goods obtained from the dry storage area. Many facilities have two or more types of storage areas for dry goods, one for bulk supplies and the other for daily supplies. The main storage area is kept locked, and goods are issued by a stock clerk upon receipt of a stores requisition sheet, such as that shown in figure 37, page 247. When this system is used, daily or weekly supplies needed are determined in relation to the menu and a requisition is written. Supplies are delivered and stored in an area within the kitchen and may or may not be locked; a locked storeroom affords better control.

However, in small operations, where a storeroom clerk is not available to issue foods and keep records, other alternatives can be considered. One person could be designated to issue foods and keep the record during a specific time of day. Or, a sign-out sheet can be placed in the storeroom and foods removed can be noted by the person taking them.

A third alternative is to have each person responsible for food production keep a list of the kinds and amounts of foods used. At the end of each day, these lists are given to the manager, who records them on the inventory record. The last two methods provide the least amount of security and control.

Perpetual Inventory

The process of recording all purchases and food issues is called keeping a perpetual inventory. This is a continuous record of the quantity on hand

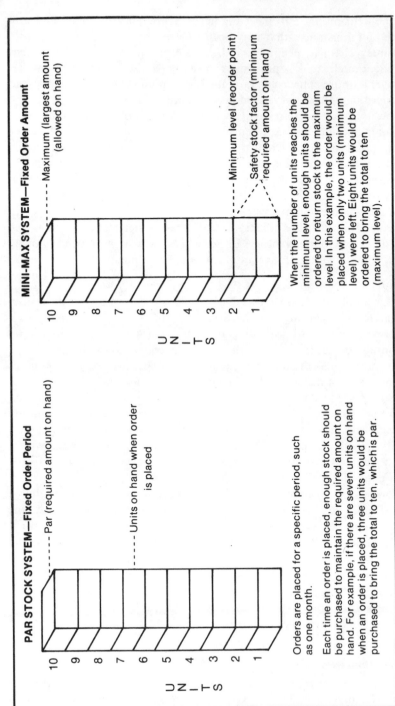

PAR STOCK SYSTEM—Fixed Order Period

- - - - Par (required amount on hand)

- - - - Units on hand when order is placed

Orders are placed for a specific period, such as one month.

Each time an order is placed, enough stock should be purchased to maintain the required amount on hand. For example, if there are seven units on hand when an order is placed, three units would be purchased to bring the total to ten, which is par.

MINI-MAX SYSTEM—Fixed Order Amount

- - - - Maximum (largest amount (allowed on hand)

- - - - Minimum level (reorder point)

- - - - Safety stock factor (minimum required amount on hand)

When the number of units reaches the minimum level, enough units should be ordered to return stock to the maximum level. In this example, the order would be placed when only two units (minimum level) were left. Eight units would be ordered to bring the total to ten (maximum level).

Note: The number of units (1 to 10) above are for purposes of example only. Numbers of units that represent par, maximum, and minimum will vary according to the requirements of each food service department.

FIGURE 36. Comparison of Inventory Systems.

STORES REQUISITION						
			_____ Hospital			
Day to be used _____			Day issued _____			
Ordered by _____			Issued by _____			
Stock no.	Total quantity	Order unit	Item description	Issued to	Price per unit	Total cost

FIGURE 37. Stores Requisition Sheet.

at any given time, as well as the value of food and supplies. Perpetual inventory records provide the manager with up-to-date information on product usage and give direction for further purchases.

For accurate accounting of all food and supplies, a perpetual inventory record only is not sufficient. This inventory should be verified monthly by taking a physical inventory of goods on hand and adjusting the inventory accordingly.

Perishable foods delivered directly to the kitchen are not usually kept on the perpetual inventory, because they are considered to be consumed shortly after receipt. These supplies may require only a monthly consumption record, compiled from purchase records.

Maintaining a perpetual inventory system is time-consuming. Therefore, small institutions may not have the personnel or need for such detailed records. For them, particularly if limited amounts of supplies are kept on hand, a physical inventory and a record of purchases would be sufficient.

Forms or cards for perpetual inventory systems are available from suppliers, who can assist in selecting a system that best meets the specific needs of an institution. Although details will vary, the information recorded always includes the quantity on hand, quantity received, quantity issued, and unit cost for each food and supply item. Larger, more sophisticated food service operations are converting their manual inventory systems to computerized systems for greater control.

Physical Inventory

Periodic physical counts of all stock are necessary even when a perpetual inventory is maintained. Even with the best of systems and personnel, errors can be made in recording transactions, foods can spoil, and pilferage can occur. In small operations where the labor involved in keeping a perpetual inventory is impractical, physical inventories can be made monthly to determine the cost of foods used during the month.

Taking a physical inventory is simplified when the storeroom is organized by food categories and the foods within each category are stored alphabetically. A form for recording goods on hand should be developed to correspond to the storeroom organization. Each item on the inventory form should be listed on a separate line; if more than one package size of an item is stocked, it should still be listed separately. The form should include space for the product description, unit size, quantity on hand, unit cost, and total value of the amount on hand.

By using a physical inventory, the cost of food used can be calculated in the following manner:

Cost of beginning inventory
+Cost of foods purchased
_____

=Cost of food on hand
-Cost of ending inventory
_____

=Cost of food used

A sample physical inventory record is shown in figure 38, page 250. Inventory records are essential not only for calculating costs but also for managing purchases and making the best use of available money. With increased emphasis on cost containment, management must be aware, at all times, of what is taking place in the food service department and make every effort possible to control costs.

RECEIVING

Effective procurement requires adequate receiving procedures to ensure that food and supplies delivered match the quality and quantity of items ordered. Economic advantages gained by competitive bidding based on well-written specifications can easily be lost by poor receiving practices. If poor-quality products or incorrect amounts are accepted, it can mean a financial loss to the food service department. This can be prevented by setting up sound receiving procedures and properly training the person responsible for the task.

Receiving procedures vary among institutions, but some basic rules apply to all. The responsibility of checking quantities should be assigned to receiving or storeroom personnel. In very small organizations, this may be one of several tasks assigned to kitchen personnel. Inspection for quality should be the responsibility of a person who has previously determined the specifications, or of someone who at least is qualified to judge products.

The person responsible for receiving should:

1. Be prepared for deliveries. Delivery dates and approximate times should be known so that space and equipment are available for receipt of the items. Because most deliveries are on a regular schedule, this is relatively easy to accomplish.
2. Check the merchandise immediately. On arrival, all items should be checked, preferably in the presence of the delivery person. Perishable items should be checked first. The count, weight, quality, and condition of the merchandise should match the purchase order or quotation sheet before delivery is accepted. Cases or cartons that appear damaged should be opened and the quality of fresh produce at top and bottom of each container should be checked. The internal temperature of all frozen foods should be at 0°F. (-18°C.); if the temperature exceeds 0°F., they should be rejected. If this type of check is impossible, visual inspection of packages will often show if the product has been subjected to undesirable high temperatures. Wet or dripping packages should not be accepted.
3. Date or tag all chilled, frozen, and nonperishable foods as they are received, so that they can be used on a first-in first-out basis. These foods should be stored immediately.
4. Sign the delivery slip from the vendor only after these steps have been taken. Unordered or rejected merchandise should be returned at this time.
5. Fill out the required receiving report. Institutions with a centralized receiving department usually require a written report for all merchandise received.
6. Transfer nonperishable foods and supplies to storage in appropriate areas as soon as possible.

Methods

Two receiving methods are in general use by food service operations:

1. Invoice receiving. This frequently used method involves having the receiving clerk check the items delivered against the purchase order or telephone order and note any discrepancies. This method makes it easy for the clerk to check quantity and quality against the specifications and order the proper amounts. It is quick and economical but somewhat unreliable if the person fails to make the comparison

Quantity on hand	Order unit	Article	Description	Unit cost	Total
	#10	Apples	Sliced, 6/#10/case		
	#10	Apples	Dehydrated, low moisture, 6/#10/case		
	#10	Apple rings	6/#10/case		
	#10	Applesauce	6/#10/case		
	#10	Apricots	Unpeeled halves, 6/#10/case		
	#10	Blueberries	Water pack, 6/#10/case		
	#10	Cherries	RSP, water pack, 6/#10/case		
	gal.	Cherries	Maraschino halves, 4/1 gal./ case		
	#10	Cranberry sauce	6/#10/case		
	lb.	Dates	Pieces, 25-lb. box		
	#10	Fruit cocktail	6/#10/case		
	#10	Fruits for salads	6/#10/case		
	#3	Grapefruit sections	Whole, 12/#3		

PHYSICAL INVENTORY

Date _____ Taken by _____ Beginning Inventory $ _____

#3	Grapefruit-orange sections	Whole, 12/#3 cyl/46 oz./case		
#10	Mincemeat	Solid pack, 6/#10/case		
#10	Mandarin oranges	6/#10/case		
#10	Peaches	Halves, 6/#10/case		
#10	Peaches	Sliced, 6/#10/case		
#10	Pears	Halves, 6/#10/case		
#10	Pineapple	Crushed, 6/#10/case		
#10	Pineapple	Sliced, 6/#10/case		
#10	Pineapple	Tidbits, 6/#10/case		
#10	Plums	Purple, 6/#10/case		
#10	Prunes	6/#10/case		
lb.	Raisins	Dried, seedless, 24/16 oz./case		
#10	Rhubarb	6/#10/case		

FIGURE 38. Physical Inventory Record.

and simply uses the delivery invoice.

2. Blind receiving. The receiving clerk uses an invoice or purchase order that has the Quantity Ordered column blanked out. The person must record the quantity received for each item. This method requires that the clerk actually check each item because the amount ordered is unknown. The purveyor's invoice should not be available to the receiving clerk. This method takes more time than invoice receiving because it requires that the clerk prepare a complete record of all merchandise delivered, but it is more reliable.

Records

Maintaining records of all merchandise delivered is as important as inspecting for quality and quantity. The method and forms used may be simple or complex. However, the fact remains that some record must be kept so all persons involved with the purchase, use, and payment of goods are informed of what was received. One or more of the following records may be used, depending on whether receiving is centralized or takes place within the food service department.

1. A merchandise receipt, such as that shown in figure 39, below, may be required for each shipment received. This type of form is completed by the receiving clerk in central stores and duplicate copies are sent to appropriate persons in purchasing, food service, accounting, and

MERCHANDISE RECEIPT		
Date_____		
No._____		
Received from:_____		
Purchase Order No._____		
Quantity	**Description**	**Distribution**
Merchandise received and inspected by:_____		

FIGURE 39. Merchandise Receipt.

so forth to inform them of the goods received. Notation of items ordered but not delivered, or those returned, may be included on this form or a separate form, called a credit memo, that is used for this purpose. The merchandise receipt and credit memo should be signed by the person responsible for receipt of goods and attached to the invoice or sent separately, as stated in the policy manual.

2. A daily receiving record similar to that shown in figure 40, below, may be required, along with a merchandise receipt, or may be the only form used to record incoming goods. Either or both records can be used to verify receipt of items and are a source of information for payment of goods by the accounting department and/or for updating the inventory records.

RECEIVING RECORD									
Date 8/1									
Quantity	Unit	Description of Item	Name of Vendor	Quantity Verified by:	Unit Price	Total Cost	Distribution		
							To Kitchen	To Store-room	
10	cases	Peas, Early June #10	S&H	77	11.39	113.90		✓	

FIGURE 40. Daily Receiving Record.

STORAGE

Dry and low-temperature storage facilities should be accessible to both receiving and food preparation areas to reduce transport time and corresponding labor costs. It is desirable to locate these facilities on the same floor as the kitchen. When this is impossible because of building constraints, ample space should be allocated in the kitchen area for one or more days' supply of foods.

Dry Storage

The amount of space required depends on many factors, such as the types and amounts of foods needed to meet menu demands, frequency of deliveries, and policies regarding inventories and monetary investments.

The storage areas should be constructed so that they are free from dampness, easy to clean, and easy to keep free of rodents and insects. Walls and ceilings should be of nonporous, easily cleaned materials. If windows are provided, they should be screened and equipped with an opaque security sash to protect foods from direct sunlight and located to avoid interference with shelving. Floors should be constructed of quarry tile, terrazzo, or concrete that has been sealed to make an easily cleanable surface. All floors should be slip resistant. The ceiling should be free from water and heating pipes. Storerooms should be well lighted so that supplies in all parts of the room can be seen easily and to contribute to better housekeeping. Approximately two to three watts per square foot of floor area and light fixtures centered over each aisle will provide adequate light.

Dry storage rooms should be well ventilated and temperature controlled to reduce the rate of deterioration of food. A temperature range of 50 to 70°F. (10 to 21°C.) is recommended for this area. A thermometer placed in an easy-to-read location is essential. Ventilation should be provided by fans or other mechanical means.

A single entrance facilitates control of deliveries and food issues. Access to the storeroom should be limited to those persons responsible for storage and issue of goods. Secure locks should be installed on doors and keys should be carefully safeguarded. A door width of 42 inches is recommended for ease in transporting goods in and out of the area.

Miscellaneous supplies and broken case lots can best be stored on adjustable metal shelves at least 2 inches from the walls. Shelves 16 inches deep will hold two rows of No. 10 cans or three rows of No. 2 or 2-1/2 cans. Clearance of 12 to 16 inches between upper shelves and 18 to 36 inches between lower shelves is desirable. Sectional slatted platforms (pallets) or wheeled metal platforms provide the best storage for bags and for case lots of canned products. All shelving should be 6 to 12 inches above the floor, in accordance with local health department requirements. Aisles between shelves and platforms should be wide enough for the use of mobile equipment.

Metal or plastic containers with tight-fitting covers should be used for storing cereals, cereal products, flour, sugar, dried foods, and broken lots of bulk foods. They can be placed on dollies for ease of movement from one place to another. All containers should be legibly and accurately labeled.

Poisonous materials used for cleaning and sanitation purposes should be clearly labeled and kept in a locked area away from the food supplies. Empty food containers must not be used for storage of broken lots of these materials. Likewise, empty containers from sanitation supplies must not be used for foods. Food should be stored only in food grade containers.

A worktable should be provided near the entrance of the storeroom for unpacking supplies, putting up small orders of bulk products, and assembling orders. Large and small scoops should be provided for each food container in use, such as bins for flour, sugar, cereal, and so forth. Scales should be available for weighing both small and large quantities of food. Mobile equipment is necessary for delivering supplies to the various work areas. Usually, several types are needed such as platform dollies and shelf trucks. Hand washing facilities are essential and should be located near the storeroom.

The floor, walls, ceiling, lights, shelves, and equipment in the storeroom should be kept clean. A cleaning schedule should be developed and someone assigned to this task. Routine inspections should be made and any violations of sanitation standards corrected immediately.

Refuse containers should be provided and emptied at least daily. Leaking or bulging cans and spoiled foods should be disposed of promptly. The storeroom should be treated regularly for the control of rodents and insects. Further information for safe and sanitary preservation of food and supplies in dry storage areas is available from city or state health departments.

Stock should be systematically arranged and inventory records should follow the same system to save time when stock is issued or inventoried. New stock should be placed in back of items of the same food so that older stock will be issued first. Each item should be marked or stamped with the date of delivery and unit cost as it is placed on the shelf. The cost can thus be noted on the inventory sheets as the actual count is taken in the physical inventory, permitting a rapid computation of the cash value of the inventory on hand. Price marking is an effective way of familiarizing kitchen employees with the cost of foods.

Quantity lots of bagged items, such as flour and sugar, should be cross-stacked on slatted platforms or racks raised to the proper height above the floor to permit air circulation. Bulk cereal, dried vegetables, and dry milk should be refrigerated if the storeroom temperature cannot be maintained below 70°F. (21°C.). When cases of canned foods are stacked, the labels should be exposed for easy identification. Cartons of foods packed in glass jars should be kept closed because light tends to change the color and flavor of some foods. Dried fruits can be stored satisfactorily for a limited time in the original boxes if the temperature in the storeroom can be kept below 70°F. (21°C.) and humidity below 55 percent. If refrigerated space is available, prevention of mold growth could be inhibited by using the lower temperature.

Bananas should be kept in the dry storage area or at a temperature of 60 to 70°F. (15 to 21°C.). To prevent bruising, they should be left in the delivery box. Because a temperature of 55°F. (13°C.) or below darkens the flesh of bananas, they should not be refrigerated. Unripe fruits and vegetables should be put into dry storage until they reach a good quality edible stage. Unripe melons, peaches, pears, pineapples, plums, avocados, and tomatoes will ripen at 65 to 80°F. (18 to 27°C.); colder temperatures can cause injury to these products and they will not ripen.

Potatoes should be stored away from light, if possible, in a dry, well-ventilated room at a temperature of 40 to 60°F. (4 to 15°C.). If peeled potatoes are purchased, they should be stored under refrigeration for the number of days suggested by the processor. Sweet potatotes and winter squash keep best in a well-ventilated room at a temperature of 50 to 60°F. (10 to 15°C.). Sweet potatoes will spoil more quickly under refrigeration than in dry storage. Onions keep best in dry storage at a temperature of 40 to 60°F. (4 to 15°C.). It is important to remember not to overbuy, because even under the most ideal conditions food quality can deteriorate.

Low-Temperature Storage

Perishable foods should be held under refrigeration or in frozen storage immediately upon delivery and kept under these conditions until ready to use in order to preserve their nutritive value and appealing quality. The type and amount of low-temperature storage space required will vary with menu and purchasing policies. Some food service operations are fortunate to have separate refrigerated units for meats and poultry, fish and shellfish, dairy products, and vegetables and fruits, and separate freezers for ice cream and other frozen foods because the ideal temperatures for each of these commodity groups vary. However, satisfactory storage of these products can be maintained with fewer units kept at the temperatures stated below.

Fruits and vegetables (except those requiring dry storage)—40 to 45°F. (4 to 7°C.)

Dairy products, eggs, meat, fish, poultry, and shellfish—32 to 40°F. (0 to 4°C.)

Frozen foods— -10° to 0°F. (-23 to -16°C.)

In large institutions, walk-in refrigerators and freezers are common; in smaller operations, the trend is away from walk-ins and toward reach-ins because the available storage space is used more efficiently, less floor space is required, and cleaning is much easier. Regardless of the type available, location is the key for saving labor and avoiding unproductive work. Walk-in refrigerator doors should be flush with the floor so that movable racks or shelves can be wheeled in and out of them easily. Both types should be close to the work area where foods will be used. Employees should be trained to obtain all supplies needed at one time to eliminate constant opening of doors, which increases the use of energy.

All refrigerators and freezers should be provided with one or more thermometers, such as a remote-reading thermometer, a recording thermometer, or a bulb thermometer. The remote-reading thermometer is placed outside the refrigerator and permits reading the temperature without

TABLE 22. RECOMMENDED STORAGE TEMPERATURES AND TIMES

FOOD	REFRIGERATOR STORAGE 32-40°F. (0-4°C.)	FREEZER STORAGE 0°F. (-18°C.) or below	DRY STORAGE 50-70°F. (10-21°C.)
MEAT Roasts, Steaks, Chops	3-5 days	Beef and lamb: 9-12 months Pork: 6-9 months Veal: 4-6 months Sausage, ham, and slab bacon: 1-3 months Beef liver: 3-4 months Pork liver: 1-2 months	No ↑
Ground meat, Stew meat	1-2 days	6-8 months	
Ham, not canned	1-3 weeks	1-3 months	
Hams, canned	1 year	Not recommended	
POULTRY Chicken, Turkey, and so forth	2-3 days	Chicken, 6-8 months Turkey, 4-5 months Giblets, 2-3 months	
FISH or SHELLFISH	30-32°F. (-1-0°C.) on ice, 2-3 days	3-6 months	
EGGS Shell Frozen	1-2 weeks 1-2 days after thawing	Not recommended 9 months	
Dried	6 months	Not recommended	
FRUITS & VEGETABLES Fresh Frozen Canned Dried	5-7 days — — Preferred	Not recommended 10-12 months Not recommended Not recommended	↓ No 12 months 2 weeks
CEREAL PRODUCTS Regular cornmeal, whole wheat flour	Required over 60 days	Not recommended	2 months
Degermed cornmeal, all-purpose and bread flour, rice, and so forth	Preferred	Not recommended	Satisfactory

opening the door. The recording thermometer is also mounted outside of the refrigerator and has the added feature of continuously recording the temperatures of walk-in low-temperature storage. One can see at a glance the fluctuations in temperature that have occurred. The bulb type is probably the most common one used if the refrigerator or freezer does not have a thermometer built into the door. The warmest area of the unit should be determined and the thermometer placed there. Regardless of the type of thermometer used, someone should be assigned to check the temperatures in all units at least once a day.

Humidity also is important for maintaining food quality. Perishable foods contain a great deal of moisture. Evaporation will be greater when the air in the refrigerator is dry. Evaporation causes foods to wilt, discolor, and lose weight. Food held at low humidity will shrink considerably and will require extra trimming. Although a humidity level as low as 65 percent is suggested for some products, a range between 80 and 95 percent is recommended for most foods.

Good air circulation should be provided throughout the refrigerators and freezers at all times. All foods stored in them should be placed in a manner such that air can circulate to all sides of the pan, box, or crate. For sanitary reasons, foods should not be stored on the floor. All foods should be covered. Most foods should be left in their original containers; this is mandatory for frozen foods, particularly to reduce the possibility of freezer burn and drying out of foods. Fresh produce should be examined for ripeness and spoilage before storing. These products may be transferred to specially designed plastic containers after inspection. Paper wrappings on fruit should be left on to help keep them clean and prevent spoilage and moisture loss.

Recommended food storage temperatures and times are shown in table 22, page 257.

Quality Assurance in Food Production

Producing high-quality food that meets the objectives of the food service department and satisfies consumer expectations is essential in health care facilities. Nutritious foods that are properly prepared, flavorful, and attractive are vital for restoring and/or maintaining the general health of patients or residents Microbiological safety is also a concern throughout the food production process.

The food service manager is responsible for knowing food quality standards, implementing these standards, and developing procedures to control and ensure that the quality and quantity of food needed are provided. Unless the manager and all employees have a clear understanding of the standards and are constantly striving to attain them, quality food will not be produced consistently.

The purpose of this chapter is to introduce the management techniques and production methods used to ensure quality in quantity food preparation.

ASPECTS OF FOOD QUALITY

What is high-quality food? Perhaps no question is more difficult to answer, because quality standards are usually very personal, developed through life experiences, and differ among geographic areas, age groups, ethnic groups, and economic levels. The challenge to food service managers is to select quality standards acceptable to the clientele being served yet consistent with those identified through scientific study and research. Often, it is necessary to arrive at a compromise among the variations in standards to secure consumer satisfaction. Most people, however, agree that the key aspects of food quality are the sensory, nutritional, and microbiological characteristics of food products.

SENSORY ASPECTS

A substantial proportion of the population selects food not for its nutritional qualities, but for its sensory qualities. Color is the primary factor affecting the sense of sight, although food shapes also have some effect. If menu items are to have the most attractive appearance, food production personnel must fully understand what happens to the colors in foods when various cooking and holding procedures are used. For example, a menu that depends heavily on the distinct green of broccoli spears for attractiveness will certainly be less appealing if the broccoli is overcooked to a brownish-olive color. The basic principle for managing food color changes in preparation is to maintain the natural color of the food product as much as possible or to enhance it through a cooking process.

Food flavor is a combination of sensations and is perceived differently by each person. If a food stimulates a pleasant response by the senses of taste, smell, feel, sight, and hearing, it is acceptable. Because of individual likes and dislikes as well as variable perceptions, an acceptable flavor is very hard to define in precise terms.

Taste is perhaps the most important component of flavor perception because it is often the most intense. The four fundamental taste sensations are sweet, sour, salty, and bitter. Many food tastes are a blending of these.

Aroma is important in flavor perception because it excites and stimulates the flow of gastric juices that make a person eager to eat. Unpleasant food odors have an opposite effect on food acceptance. Individuals who have an impairment of smell lose a significant degree of flavor perception.

The feel, or texture, of foods also plays a large part in determining whether an individual thinks a food has good flavor. The characteristics of crispness, mushiness, graininess, smoothness, stickiness, and dryness are some of the food textures that affect acceptance.

Temperature is another aspect of food feel that influences flavor perception. For example, hot roast lamb may excite favorable responses, but loses much of its appeal when served lukewarm or cold.

Sight plays a surprisingly large role in the acceptance of food flavors. Certain foods have an expected appearance, and if a food does not look the way it should, the flavor will probably be unacceptable. This phenomenon can be illustrated by simply tinting applesauce samples with small amounts of red, green, and blue food coloring. even though the applesauce is identical in each sample, most people will rate the flavor of the green and blue samples as bad, because of the unexpected and unnatural appearance of the products.

Even the sense of hearing affects perceptions of flavor. The sizzling of a steak on a platter heightens anticipation of delicious flavor, just as the crunch of crisp salad ingredients increases flavor acceptance.

NUTRITIONAL ASPECTS

Conservation of nutrients in food is of prime importance in health care facilities. Fresh foods are often regarded as representing perfection in terms of nutritive value and processed foods as nutritionally inferior. This is often an inaccurate view, particularly if fresh foods have been improperly stored and held too long in storage. Some vitamins, especially vitamin C in fresh vegetables, can severely degrade in improper storage. The rate of vitamin loss is affected by temperature and extent of peeling or cutting. In general, fruit and meat held at temperatures above freezing are less susceptible to vitamin loss than are vegetables.

Nutritive losses occur during food preparation. Some nutrients can be lost through oxidation when cut food surfaces are exposed to air. The water-soluble vitamins and minerals can be lost when fruits or vegetables are soaked or cooked in large amounts of water. Careless preparation or extended preparation periods also decrease the nutrient value of many foods. Overcooking and high cooking temperatures can destroy significant amounts of heat-sensitive nutrients. In general, preparation procedures that retain peak sensory qualities of foods also are effective in conserving nutrients. However, more research is needed concerning nutrient loss that takes place during quantity food production.

MICROBIOLOGICAL ASPECTS

The healthful quality and safety of finished food products depend on wholesome food ingredients that are processed with care and critically evaluated at each stage of production. In quantity food preparation, there is always a potential danger of microbial contamination and growth if sanitation practices are not carefully followed. Controls are needed to ensure that ingredients, packaging, and other supplies brought into the food service operation are sanitarily acceptable for use. Pest control, cleanliness, and temperature regulation are necessary in storage areas to decrease risk of contamination or spoilage.

In the preparation stages, equipment sanitation, employee personal hygiene, and work habits are critical to food safety. Care must be taken to avoid possible contamination of prepared foods by raw food ingredients and work surfaces. This is particularly important when prepared foods are held prior to cooking, as in many conventional food production systems, or after cooking in cook/chill and cook/freeze systems. Bacterial control is more difficult during the chilling processes because it requires several hours to lower the temperature of masses of hot food to the 40 to 45⁰F. (4 to 7⁰C.) range, at which bacterial growth is slowed.

Food distribution systems must be carefully monitored to ensure that safe temperature and time relationships exist. Perishable foods must be kept above 140°F. (60°C.) or below 45°F. (7°C.) at all times during holding. Local sanitation codes may require stricter rules for temperature control. In such cases, local regulations should be followed.

MANAGEMENT TECHNIQUES FOR QUALITY CONTROL

It is possible for every food service operation to buy the same ingredients and use the same recipes, equipment, and similar labor skills, yet produce food items that vary greatly in quality. The difference is largely the result of the care and attention the manager gives to quality control throughout all aspects of food production.

PLANNED MENU

Food quality control starts with menu planning, during which the nutritional potential of each meal is carefully considered and balanced to meet the needs of patients. Menus that lack essential nutrients can be corrected at this point. Similarly, esthetic control begins in menu planning. Color combinations, shapes, flavors, and temperature contrasts must be planned into each menu. Because quality problems can occur when employee skills are overtaxed or insufficient preparation time is allowed, a carefully planned menu recognizes the limitations of skills, time, and equipment that can affect food quality.

PROCUREMENT

Quality assurance is not simply an occasional sampling of food products to see if they meet expectations; it is a complete system that encompasses all stages from purchasing to service. Although the menu determines what kinds of food are needed, complete purchase specifications for each item designate the quality, form, style, and other characteristics desired. Careful checking of all items at delivery ensures that the desired quality and quantity of necessary foods are actually received. Control of storage conditions protects the quality of foods until they enter the preparation stages.

FORECASTING

Although a forecast of quantities needed must precede purchase of food, a more refined production forecast for each meal should be developed. Accurate forecasting can have a positive effect on overall food quality.

Overproduction results in excess food, which must be stored and offered at a later time, with potential quality loss. Conversely, underproduction can result in substitution of menu items with other products. Replacements may be lower in quality because of insufficient time to prepare them. Food costs may increase if substitutions are made very often, because convenience items are usually relied upon. Because these foods have labor costs already added to the cost of ingredients, the cost per portion can be higher.

Forecasting systems used in health care facilities vary among institutions. Selection of procedures for determining production quantities is directly related to the type of facility, costs of overproduction and underproduction, and the degree of accuracy desired. The costs associated with the effort needed to produce accurate forecasts should be considered.

In many health care facilities, an informed estimate is the most commonly used forecasting method. In a long-term care facility where there is little turnover in residents or staff, an experienced manager can, with little difficulty, accurately project the needed production requirements for a nonselective menu. This method is less accurate when a selective menu is used and in short-term care facilities where occupancy fluctuates daily. In such situations, a tally system is used. Patient selections are recorded for each meal one day or one meal in advance. From this tally, the total production quantity is calculated. Most of the problems involved in this method are related to fluctuation in patient count and the inability to predict what menu choices will be made by the new patient.

Overproduction and underproduction in cook/chill systems can become a real problem because food production takes place far in advance of the time an accurate census is available. Even in conventional production systems, many items must be prepared a day or more in advance with similar risks. The tally system is time-consuming and may be expensive, because of the clerical personnel needed to produce accurate production data.

Statistical methods for generating food production orders have been reported in research journals. Most of these methods require long-term records of total patient census, tray census, and menu item selections. A consultant can be used to develop a mathematical formula that uses these data to more accurately predict menu item demand.

When facilities have computer access, programs for computer-assisted forecasting can be developed. However, an extensive data base is needed to generate a reliable computer forecast. Even when such sophisticated methods are used, routine evaluation of their accuracy is needed. For example, any change in the menu will affect the forecast's accuracy.

STANDARDIZED RECIPES

The standardized recipe is one of the most effective management tools available for controlling quality, quantity, and cost. A standardized recipe is one in which the amounts and proportions of ingredients, as well as the method of combining ingredients, will consistently produce a high-quality product and yield a given number of portions. Any substitutions for specified ingredients or changes in procedures can affect the quality and yield of the product. When standardized recipes are used, changes in personnel do not affect food quality because all ingredients and preparation details are precisely stated in the recipe. Purchasing is simplified because exact quantities and forms of food have been established when the recipe is tested. Job satisfaction is increased because employees can be assured of a quality product if they follow directions carefully. In addition, new employees can be trained much more rapidly.

Although standardized recipes are available from many sources, each food service department should reevaluate and test all recipes used to ensure that quantities produced, portion sizes, and overall quality meet the needs of clientele and are suited to the available equipment.

Each food service department must determine portion sizes for each category of foods served. In setting portion sizes, the type of clientele, the nutritional needs, the type of menu served, and the food budget should be considered. When reviewing new recipes, food service managers should compare the stated portion size with the established portion sizes for their institutions. In most situations, clientele evaluations are very helpful in judging acceptance of portion sizes and overall quality of food products.

Before standardizing any recipe, each of the following should be analyzed.

1. *Proportion of ingredients.* Each recipe should be read thoroughly, particularly if it has not yet been tried, because it may prove to be inappropriate or the numbers of different ingredients used or the complexity of the procedures may make it impractical. The proportion of ingredients should be analyzed in relation to each other. For example, in a cake recipe, the sugar, flour, and shortening ratios should be appropriate for the product. However, the exact ratio between flour and fluids will vary according to the kind of flour used. Also, if hydrogenated shortening or margarine is used instead of butter or lard, a greater amount will be needed to achieve the same degree of shortening power. Finally, the new recipe should be compared with other tested recipes for a similar product.

2. *Amount of ingredients.* The ingredient quantities should be listed in both weights and measures on the recipe. Because it is usually more accurate to weigh ingredients, measures should be converted to the appropriate weight. Small amounts of spices and seasonings can be measured rather than weighed.

3. *Form of ingredients.* The form of the ingredients should be described on the recipe. Descriptive terms placed before the name of the

ingredient designate the kind and form of food as purchased or the cooking or heating required before the food is used, such as *canned* tomatoes, *fresh chopped* spinach, *cooked* chicken, and *hard-cooked* eggs. Descriptive terms placed after the ingredient name indicate the preparation necessary to make the form of the ingredient different from the form as purchased or cooked, such as onions, *chopped*; canned diced carrots, *drained*; and apples, *pared, sliced.* If waste is likely to occur in the initial preparation steps for some ingredients, the quantity should be listed as *edible portion* (EP) rather than as *as purchased* (AP). The purchase amount should be recorded in a separate section on the recipe card.

4. *Order of ingredients.* Ingredients should be listed in the order in which they will be combined. For example, ingredients for the fruit mixture in an upside-down cake should be listed first because that part of the recipe is prepared and placed in the pan before the batter is prepared. Any ingredients that need pretreatment before combining should be listed first or specially marked indicating advance preparation needed.

5. *Procedures.* If possible, the procedures should be simplified or some of the preparation steps eliminated in order to save time, equipment, and warewashing. For example, in a kitchen equipped with steam-jacketed kettles, the easiest way to prepare a cooked pudding is to place measured cold milk in the kettle, combine all dry ingredients, blend them into milk with a wire whip, and then heat the entire mixture. The procedure for combining ingredients should be stated clearly. Specific terms, such as blend, whip, cream, or fold, tell the cook exactly what to do. Mixing speeds and times, as well as type of beater to use, should be stated on recipes that will be prepared in the mixer. When the batch size is increased or decreased, mixing times may have to be adjusted accordingly. If a chilling time is required before the entire recipe can be completed, the time should be stated.

6. *Recipe format.* There are a variety of ways in which standardized recipes may be written. Standard formats for all recipes should be developed so that it is easier for personnel to use them. A sample format is shown in figure 41, next page. Spaces for recording calculations of portion cost and for other batch sizes also can be included. Recipes can be filed according to types of items in a standard recipe box, a file drawer, or notebook. Duplicate copies should be kept in a master file. Transparent plastic envelopes or laminated cards can be used to protect recipes in the kitchen.

7. *Batch size adjustment.* A tested recipe that yields a high-quality product may need to be altered in batch size for ease of handling or to suit the capacity of equipment available. For example, if a 30-quart mixer bowl is the largest size available, the batch size should not

Recipe: *Pizza Casserole*

Portions 96
Pans 3
Pan size 12 x 20 x 2½

Cooking temperature 350°F. (177°C.)
Cooking time 20-25 minutes
Portion size 8 x 4
Portion utensil Spatula

Total recipe cost _____
Cost per portion _____
Date calculated _____

INGREDIENTS	AMOUNT	PROCEDURE
Ground beef Pork sausage, bulk	3 lb. 3 lb.	1. Sauté ground beef and sausage until cooked. 2. Drain excess fat
Spaghetti, thin Salt Cooking oil	4 lb. + 8 oz. 4 tbs. 2 tbs.	3. Cook spaghetti in boiling salted water in steam-jacketed kettle. Add 2 tbs. oil to water to prevent boiling over. 4. Drain. 5. Put in pans.
Canned tomato sauce	1 #10 can	6. Pour equal amounts of sauce over spaghetti. 7. Sprinkle cooked meat over sauce.
Oregano, crushed Sweet basil, crushed Mozzarella cheese, grated Onions, chopped Green peppers, chopped Mushrooms, drained Ripe olives, sliced	3 tbs. 3 tbs. 9 lb. 1½ c. 1½ c. 3 1-lb. cans 3 c.	8. Sprinkle oregano and basil over meat. 9. Sprinkle cheese over oregano and basil. 10. Top with chopped onions, green peppers, mushrooms, and ripe olives. 11. Bake.

FIGURE 41. Example of a Recipe Format.

exceed this amount. To adjust the total recipe yield, the number of servings needed must first be determined. That number should then be divided by the number of servings stated on the original recipe to arrive at a factor for adjusting the ingredient quantities.

To increase the batch size, the amount of each ingredient should be multiplied by the factor and rounded off to the nearest convenient weight or measure. To decrease the batch size, the amount of each ingredient on the original recipe should be divided by the factor to arrive at the appropriate quantity for the reduced recipe. *Proportions of ingredients should not be changed when recipes are increased or decreased*, although mixing or cooking times may change in some cases. Decimal equivalents and rules for rounding weights and volume measures of ingredients in recipes are listed in tables 23, 24, and 25, pages 267, 268, and 269.

8. *Other details.* The recipe should specify the type and size of pans to be used, the amount to be placed in each pan, and pretreatment of the pans. To get an accurate yield of uniform portions, the weight or

TABLE 23. DECIMAL EQUIVALENTS FOR DIFFERENT UNITS, IN PARTS OF 1 LB., 1 CUP, OR 1 GALLON

Number of Units, oz., tbs., or cups[a]	Decimal Equivalent of 1 Lb., 1 Cup, or 1 Gallon					
	+0 Unit	+1/4 Unit	+1/3 Unit	+1/2 Unit	+2/3 Unit	+3/4 Unit
0	—	0.016	0.021	0.031	0.042	0.047
1	0.062	.078	.083	.094	.104	.109
2	.125	.141	.146	.156	.167	.172
3	.188	.203	.208	.219	.229	.234
4	.250	.266	.271	.281	.292	.297
5	.312	.328	.333	.344	.354	.359
6	.375	.391	.396	.406	.417	.422
7	.438	.453	.458	.469	.479	.484
8	.500	.516	.521	.531	.542	.547
9	.562	.578	.583	.594	.604	.609
10	.625	.641	.646	.656	.667	.672
11	.688	.703	.708	.719	.729	.734
12	.750	.766	.771	.781	.792	.797
13	.812	.828	.833	.844	.854	.859
14	.875	.891	.896	.906	.917	.922
15	.938	.953	.958	.969	.979	.984

Source: USDA Guides for Writing and Evaluating Quantity Recipes for Type A School Lunches, September 1969.

[a] The units are read at the side and top of the table. If the units are ounces, the decimal equivalents given in the body of the table are parts of 1 pound. If the units are tablespoons, the decimal equivalents are parts of 1 cup. If the units are cups, the decimal equivalents are parts of 1 gallon. Example 1: To convert 10½ ounces to the corresponding decimal equivalent of a pound, find 10 in the first column and follow this line across to the column headed ½, which shows that 0.656 ounces corresponds to 10½ ounces. Example 2: To convert the decimal 0.531 pound to ounces, find 0.531 in the body of the table. Then, in the first column find the number that is on the same horizontal line, which is 8. Next, add the number from the heading of the column in which 0.531 was found, which is ½. Thus, 0.531 pound corresponds to 8½ ounces.

TABLE 24. RULES FOR ROUNDING WEIGHTS AND VOLUME MEASURES OF INGREDIENTS IN RECIPES

If the Total Amount of an Ingredient Is:	Adjust as Follows[a]	Example
Weights[b]		
Less than 2 oz.	Volume measure only unless weight is ¼, ½, ¾ oz., and so forth	⅞ oz. of salt would be shown only as 2 tbs.
From 2 to 10 oz.	Nearest ¼ oz.	Round 2⅓ oz. to 2¼ oz.
More than 10 oz. but less than 2 lb. 8 oz.	Nearest ½ oz.	Round 1 lb. 5⅜ oz. to 1 lb. 5½ oz.
2 lb. 8 oz. to 5 lb.	Nearest full oz.	Round 3 lb. 6⅝ oz. to 3 lb. 7 oz.
More than 5 lb.	Nearest ¼ lb.	Round 5 lb. 9½ oz. to 5 lb. 8 oz.
Volume Measures[b]		
Less than 2 tbs.	Nearest ¼ tsp.	Round 1⅔ tsp. to 1¾ tsp.
2 tbs. to ½ cup	Nearest tsp.	Round 3 tbs. ⅓ tsp. to 3 tbs.
More than ½ cup but less than ¾ cup	Nearest tbs.	Round ½ cup 1⅓ tbs. to ½ cup 1 tbs.
More than ¾ cup but less than 2 cups	Nearest 2 tbs.	Round 1 cup 2¾ tbs. to 1 cup 2 tbs.
2 cups to 2 qt.	Nearest ¼ cup	Round 1 qt. 3 cups 11⅓ tbs. to 1 qt. 3¾ cups.
More than 2 qt. but less than 4 qt.	Nearest ½ cup	Round 3 qt. 9 tbs. to 3 qt. ½ cup.
1 gal. to 2 gal.	Nearest full cup	Round 1 gal. 1 qt. 3¼ cups to 1 gal. 1¾ qt.
More than 2 gal.	Nearest full qt.	Round 2 gal. 1 qt. ½ cup to 2¼ gal.

Source: *USDA Guides for Writing and Evaluating Quantity Recipes for Type A School Lunches*, September 1969.

[a] When a weight or volume measure is at the midpoint, round up.

[b] The weights and volume measures have been grouped so that the percentage error in rounding does not exceed the error normally introduced in handling food ingredients.

volume of mixture for each pan must be stated and followed. It is helpful to note the total weight or volume of the batch as well. Cooking times and temperatures should be double-checked. Those on the original recipe may not be suited to the type of equipment available. For example, baking temperatures and times for standard ovens may have to be reduced for convection ovens. Portioning instructions should be stated, as well as any instructions for cooling or holding prior to portioning. Portioning tools may be stated on certain recipes. Garnishes also may be listed.

TABLE 25. RULES FOR ROUNDING AMOUNTS TO PURCHASE
FOR A MARKETING GUIDE

If the Total Amount of an Ingredient Is:	Adjust as Follows[a]	Example
Weights[b]		
Between 2 to 10 oz.	Up to next ¼ oz.	Round 6⅛ oz. to 6¼ oz.
More than 10 oz. but less than 2 lb. 8 oz.	Up to next ½ oz.	Round 1 lb. 3¾ oz. to 1 lb. 4 oz.
Between 2 lb. 8 oz. and 5 lb.	Up to next 1 oz.	Round 4 lb. 7¼ oz. to 4 lb. 8 oz.
More than 5 lb.	Up to next even 2 oz. Use only amounts of 2 oz., 4 oz., 6 oz., 8 oz., 10 oz., 12 oz., 14 oz., or full pounds.	Round 8 lb. 8¾ oz. to 8 lb. 10 oz.
Cans, packages, loaves[b]		
No. 10 can	Up to next ⅛, ¼, ⅓, ½, ⅔, ¾, or 1 can.	Round 0.60 can to ⅔ can.
No. 3 cyl	Up to next ¼, ⅓, ½, ⅔, ¾, or 1 can.	Round 0.40 can to ½ can.
Package	Up to next ¼, ½, ¾, or 1 pkg.	Round 0.80 pkg. to 1 pkg.
Loaf of bread	Up to next ¼, ½, ¾, or 1 loaf.	Round 0.57 loaf to ¾ loaf.

Source: *USDA Guides for Writing and Evaluating Quantity Recipes for Type A School Lunches*, September 1969.
[a]When a weight or volume measure is at the midpoint, round up.
[b]The weights and volume measures have been grouped so that the percentage error in rounding does not exceed the error normally introduced in handling food ingredients.

New recipes should be prepared exactly as the procedures state. It is often tempting to begin modifying ingredients, quantities of ingredients, or preparation steps before discovering what kind of product would have been produced. Measurements should be checked for accuracy. If the original recipe does not list weights as well as measures, quantities should be weighed as the recipe is prepared and the actual yield carefully noted to determine whether it is the same as the stated yield. The finished product should be evaluated for eye appeal, quality, and acceptance. However, products acceptable to employees or management may get a less favorable reaction from patients or residents. Therefore, in most operations, clientele evaluations are very helpful in determining acceptance.

If careful evaluation indicates that changes are needed in the recipe, they should be made and carefully noted on the recipe. It is very important to have the cooks' cooperation, because they may find it hard not to assert their individuality by adding ingredients and not reporting the changes.

After the new recipe has been judged acceptable, it can be set up on the standard recipe format in the appropriate batch size.

INGREDIENT CONTROL

Traditionally, each person responsible for food preparation performed all tasks from collecting and weighing ingredients to portioning of the final product. Because of the need for greater control over quality and costs, pre-preparation of recipe ingredients has been centralized in ingredient areas or ingredient rooms. Centralized ingredient control frees skilled cooks from repetitive tasks that do not require their levels of skill. Food quality can be controlled because the possibility of production personnel altering ingredients or batch size can be eliminated. In some operations, only dry ingredients are weighed or measured. In others, all pre-preparation necessary to accurately weigh recipe ingredients is performed in the central location. This system achieves the greatest degree of control, but requires more personnel time and equipment.

In the ingredient area, quantities of ingredients as stated on the standardized recipes are weighed, measured, and collected for each menu item. The person weighing ingredients needs a production forecast that indicates the batch size needed for each recipe. A labeling system for premeasured ingredients is required, listing the recipe name, ingredient name, and quantity. The ingredients are delivered to the kitchen at the time the cooks need to begin combining the items.

Physical layout of the ingredient center can take many forms. Ideally, an area within the storeroom itself can be equipped to handle this function if space is available. Otherwise, a location close to the storeroom and refrigerators can be used. Regardless of the physical layout, the equipment needed includes large and small scales, measures, a sink, storage bins, large and small containers for measured ingredients, trays or baskets, and carts. Even without a separate ingredient area, some of the advantages can still be realized. During slow periods in the workday, employees can be assigned to weigh ingredients for the next day's production.

Accurate measurement is important for consistent results with standardized recipes. Measuring tools and scales must be easily accessible in all work areas when centralized ingredient control is not used. It is quicker and more accurate to weigh ingredients when the right kinds of scales are provided. Standard measuring spoons and measuring cups for both dry and liquid ingredients are needed. The purchase of heavy-grade metal measures is well worth the added cost, because denting and distortion are not likely to occur. In each work center, measuring equipment should be stored for easy access by employees.

EQUIPMENT

High-quality food cannot be prepared efficiently without the proper equipment. Although the basic ideas of cooking foods in heated air, steam, or liquids have not changed in several hundred years, cooking equipment certainly has. Major cooking equipment used in many food service kitchens today includes steam-jacketed kettles in several sizes, compartment steamers, high-pressure steamers, tilting braising pans, and convection ovens in addition to or instead of the more conventional ranges, cook-tops, and deck ovens. Labor time is saved by electric food cutters, shredders, grinders, and mixers. Vertical cutter-mixers can chop, shred, or mix large quantities of ingredients in a matter of seconds.

No matter how a kitchen is equipped, all equipment must be maintained properly and operated correctly to produce quality food. Thermostats on heating equipment and temperature controls on refrigerators and freezers must be accurate. With constantly increasing utility costs, employees in most food service operations need retraining for energy conservation. Key areas for control of energy costs are in the use of ovens, ranges, and fryers and in the use of refrigeration.

Small equipment for mixing and portioning is as essential as the major equipment. Whips, ladles, knives, spoons of several types, scoops, and scrapers are needed in almost every work center. Standardized pans are required if recipes are to yield the correct number of portions of the desired size. The basic pan size used in most standardized recipes is the 12-by-20-inch pan, available in 2-to-8-inch depths. Half-, quarter-, and third-sized pans accommodate smaller quantities of recipes. For baking, the 18-by-26-inch pan is most common. Use of the correct pan size for every recipe is critical in achieving the desired end product quality.

In conventional food service systems, hot-holding equipment is needed. This equipment must be designed to hold food at microbiologically safe temperatures and protect esthetic qualities of foods at the same time. In addition, careful control of production schedules will lessen holding problems.

PRODUCTION SCHEDULING

Daily schedules for food production can be valuable management tools for controlling the use of labor while ensuring the quality of the food. A daily work schedule assigns specific tasks to each employee. The work load is balanced according to the job duties and the specific skills of employees, and a time sequence for all production activities is established. In a conventional food production system, production timing is perhaps the greatest benefit of a daily production schedule. It can ensure that foods will not be cooked too far in advance of service, yet can allow adequate time for preparation.

For each item to be prepared, daily food production schedules should state the name of the item, name of employee assigned, time that preparation should be started and completed, and specific details regarding ingredients, portion control, and so forth. In smaller operations, one production schedule for the entire kitchen staff will be sufficient. Larger operations with several employees in each specialized unit may require separate schedules for each work group. More detailed schedules will be needed for less-experienced employees than for those who are extremely familiar with the recipes, equipment, and job duties. When job duties are not highly specialized, work schedules can eliminate confusion about which tasks are to be performed by each employee.

Daily food production schedules should be developed when menus are planned. Simultaneous planning of the work load and the menu can avoid imbalance from day to day and allow adequate time for prepreparation of foods for service at a later time. When setting up the schedule, the equipment being used for each food item should be considered so that necessary equipment will be available when needed. All cleaning duties, as well as meal and break times for employees, should be included in the work schedule.

QUALITY ASSURANCE PROGRAM

A systematic program of quality assurance requires integration of the management techniques described in this section. In addition, it involves measurement of quality factors after food production and before service. Sampling of food products, temperature measurement, and sensory appraisal of product characteristics allows comparison of observed quality with the standard established for each item. Through evaluation and analysis, management can identify what is wrong, how often, and why, and then corrective action can be taken to eliminate or reduce the quality deficiencies.

The success of a quality assurance program depends on the awareness and commitment of all employees, particularly managers, to the production of high-quality food. Quality control activities should be incorporated in regular job routines and duties for each position.

The following is an example of criteria that can be used for inspecting quality in food preparation and service:

Food appearance:
- Satisfactory and appropriate color for each item
- Pleasant variety of food color combinations
- Attractive garnishes
- Variety in shape and size of food items
- Adequate portion size for the person being served

Food taste:
- Pleasant flavor combinations
- Characteristic taste of each item
- Adequate seasoning
- No undesirable or off-flavors
- Pleasing aroma

- Proper temperature

Food texture:
- Proper texture for each item; not overcooked or undercooked
- Variety of textures
- Suitable moisture content
- Not tough and/or stringy
- Suitable for clientele being served

Food safety:
- Proper hot serving temperatures:

Liquids	185° F. (85° C.)
Cereals	175° F. (79° C.)
Soups	180° F. (82° C.)
Meats	150° F. (65° C.)
Eggs	145° F. (63° C.)*
Vegetables	160° F. (71° C.)

- Proper cold serving temperatures:

Liquids	35° F. (2° C.)
Foods	50° F. (10° C.)†

- Foods are prepared and portioned using utensils or disposable gloves to avoid contamination by employee's hands
- Clean spoons or forks used for tasting food products instead of preparation utensils
- Special care used in handling clean dishes and silver to prevent contamination
- Unused raw ingredients or cooked leftover foods refrigerated promptly and used within 24-48 hours, frozen immediately, or discarded
- Single-use utensils and containers not reused
- Employees' clothing and personal hygiene meet established standards

Tray appearance:
- Adequate tray size, overcrowding avoided
- Specified setup used
- Each item correctly placed on tray and arranged for eating convenience
- Dishes and/or flatware in good condition
- Food neatly served
- Separate dishes for foods that contain liquid
- Neat overall appearance, no spills

Tray accuracy:
- All food items specified on menu present on tray
- Food on tray is allowed on patient diet
- Utensils needed are provided on tray, no unnecessary items

Some states require higher minimum holding temperatures for any hot food.
†Some states require lower maximum holding temperatures for cold foods.

PATIENT QUESTIONNAIRE

We are interested in your comments about meal service in the hospital and appreciate your cooperation in completing this questionnaire. Please keep the completed form with your menu. We will pick it up later. Thank you.

Date: _____

1. Name _____ Room no. _____

2. Length of stay _____

3. Are you on a modified diet? Yes _____ No _____ Name of diet _____

   If you are on a modified diet, has it been explained to you by a dietitian?

   Yes _____ No _____

4. For each topic listed below, check (✓) the box that describes your opinion of that aspect of food service. Please make any additional comments you wish.

	Good	Fair	Poor	Comments
Menu Variety				
Tray Appearance				
Portion Sizes				
Food Flavor				
Hot-Food Temperature				
Cold-Food Temperature				
Overall Food Quality				

5. Have you received all the items marked on your menu? Yes _____ No _____

   If not, what and how often was it omitted? _____

   _____

6. Comments: _____

   _____

FIGURE 42. Food Service Department Patient Questionnaire.

The ultimate test of quality control system in a food service operation is the acceptance or rejection of foods by the patient or cafeteria customer. Plate waste should be routinely noted as trays are returned. Management should try to find out why plate waste occurs, particularly if patterns of waste are noted for certain items or on certain diets. Visiting with patients or residents in the dining room and on patient floors and with cafeteria customers helps to obtain this information. Many short-term care facilities use simple evaluation forms, such as that shown in figure 42, opposite page, for patients to fill out following their stay. In long-term care institutions, periodic evaluations are helpful in getting overall appraisal of food acceptance. Negative comments should be followed up to determine whether they are valid, and any changes warranted to improve the situation should then be made. Avoiding plate waste and food rejection is increasingly important today to reduce food cost as well as to satisfy consumers.

Food
Production
Processes

MEAT

Proper cooking procedures improve the flavor, tenderness, color, and palatability of meat. Management and personnel responsible for cooking meat should understand the basic composition of meat, because this influences choice of cooking method and the ultimate flavor and tenderness of the cooked product.

Meat is a complete protein, approximately 75 percent water and 25 percent solids. Although meat contains all the essential amino acids needed by the human body, it also supplies iron, phosphorus, potassium, sodium, and magnesium in varying amounts. Meat, particularly some of the organ meats, are liberal sources of B-vitamins.

The muscle fibers of meat are the basic structural units of lean tissue. Connective protein tissue surrounds the muscle fibers, binding them in bundles that, in turn, are bound into larger bundles. Two kinds of connective tissues are found in all meat: collagen and elastin. During the cooking process, collagen gelatinizes in the presence of moisture and becomes softer, making the meat more tasty and tender. Elastin, a tough yellowish material, is unaffected by heating.

Fat also is found in all meat as an exterior covering and is deposited between muscles and muscle bundles, within cells, and between muscle cells. The breeding, age, and diet of the animal influence the amount of fat, its location, and its nature. The intermingling of fat and muscle, called marbling, increases tenderness, juiciness, and flavor of the cooked meat product as it melts during heating.

Water, which makes up 70 to 75 percent of animal muscle, is lost to a certain extent during the cooking process through dripping and surface evaporation. Control of water loss is essential because water is important to the ultimate juiciness of the cooked meat and as a carrier of flavoring compounds. Juiciness in a cut of meat is controlled to a large extent by the temperature, time, and cooking method used, as well as by the amount of fat in the meat.

Flavor, tenderness, juiciness, and color of cooked meat are major concerns of both consumers and management. In addition to these sensory qualities, the manager must be aware of the total quantity and number of servings obtainable after meat has been cooked. Cooking temperatures, times, and equipment can affect cooking losses. Cooking methods that produce the highest yield of palatable, edible meat must be selected to control the cost of each serving. Cooked yields are reduced by shrinkage caused by excessive evaporation of water from the surface of meat and through drip loss of fat, water, and natural flavoring substances from the tissue.

Control of cooking temperatures and times is critical in minimizing shrinkage of meat during preparation. Research has shown that low temperatures consistently produce higher yields and more evenly cooked products. The other major factor affecting shrinkage is the length of cooking time. As cooking time increases, losses from evaporation increase, with undesirable changes in meat texture, flavor, and carvability.

Several factors affect cooking time. Among these are the size of cut and the uniformity of shape. Usually, the larger the roast, the longer the cooking time required. If the cut of meat is not uniform in shape, one end of the cut can become overcooked before the remainder is done. A large flat roast will cook in a shorter period than one of similar weight that has been rolled and tied.

Cooking time is affected by the composition of the meat itself. Greater amounts of outside fat covering and fat deposits within the meat will decrease cooking time, because fat is a better conductor of heat than the muscle tissue. For meats that are being roasted, cooking times also will be increased with greater oven loads. The degree of doneness affects cooking time because it takes longer to cook meat to the well-done state than to the medium or rare state. Overcooking is a particularly wasteful practice, because it not only causes greater losses in yield but also damages tenderness and palatability.

PREPARATION METHODS

Meat cooking methods are usually designated as dry-heat methods or moist-heat methods. These terms refer to the atmosphere surrounding the meat. The differences are in the rate of heat transfer to the meat and in the temperatures to which the meat surface is exposed. Water vapor, used in moist-heat cooking, is a more efficient heat conductor than air and helps supply heat energy more rapidly to the meat. The temperature to which meat is subjected in moist-heat cooking is no higher than the boiling point of water. In the dry-heat methods, the heat transfer is slower, but the meat surfaces are subjected to much higher temperatures.

Dry Heat

Dry-heat methods cause carmelization, or browning, of the meat surfaces, which makes meat more palatable, but does not provide any additional moisture to soften collagen. For that reason, the dry-heat methods of roasting, panfrying or grilling, and deep-fat frying are usually recommended for meat cuts that are expected to be naturally tender. Muscles that are less exercised, such as rib and loin cuts of beef and pork, and those that come from higher grade animals are usually suitable for dry-heat cooking. Young animals, such as veal and lamb, are also tender, but are often cooked by moist-heat methods to develop flavor and allow a broader variety of entrees.

Because of some changes in beef production as well as in consumer preferences, other exceptions to these recommendations exist. Less tender chuck and round roasts may be cooked by dry heat to the rare and medium-rare states, and then thinly sliced to yield a flavorful, tender finished product. Other methods are used by food service operations to tenderize less tender cuts sufficiently to allow dry-heat cooking. Some of these treatments also can be used by meat processors. Mechanical means to physically break down muscle fibers and connective tissue, such as cubing, dicing, grinding, or chopping, are often used. Marinating less tender cuts in oil and acid mixtures can break down muscle fibers. Tomato juice, vinegar, lemon juice, wine, and sour cream are commonly used marinades. Enzymatic tenderizers, often containing papain, can be applied to meat surfaces, used as a marinade, or injected into the muscle. Surface applications of such tenderizers are most effective on thinner cuts of meat.

Roasting. Meats can be roasted in several different types of ovens—conventional, convection, deck—but the cooking procedure is similar in each. The meat is placed on a rack in an open pan with no moisture added. The radiant heat from the top of a regular oven or the heated moving air of a convection oven help to produce surface browning. It was once common to sear roasts in a very hot oven for 20 to 30 minutes and then reduce the temperature to about 300°F. (149°C.) for the remainder of the cooking time. Searing, or coagulating the surface proteins, was supposed to prevent the loss of juices and nutrients. However, studies have shown that searing does not prevent the loss of juices and nutrients, and that it can increase total cooking losses from the surface. Without searing, a hard outer crust is prevented, making slicing easier. Repeated studies have shown that low, constant temperatures ranging from 25 to 325° F. (-4 to 163° C.) for roasting produces a meat that is juicier, more uniformly cooked, more tender, and with lower cooking losses. The lower temperature is recommended for convection ovens.

A meat thermometer should be used to determine the interior temperature and doneness of meat. The thermometer should be inserted so that the tip is in the center of the largest muscle and not touching bone or imbedded in fat. The internal temperature will continue to rise after the meat has been removed from the oven. Therefore, it should be taken out of the oven slightly before the temperature reaches the desired end point. If roasts are allowed to stand in a warm place for 10 to 15 minutes, the texture will become more firm and will slice more easily on an electric slicer.

Minutes-per-pound tables are, at best, only a guide to help estimate total cooking time. However, as described earlier in this section, many factors influence cooking time. It is essential to use meat thermometers to determine doneness and to keep careful records of the actual cooking times needed to reach that state of doneness for each quality, style, and size of roast prepared.

Table 26, below, lists standard end-point temperatures for roasted

TABLE 26. STANDARD END-POINT TEMPERATURES FOR ROASTED MEAT

Meat	Internal Temperature
Beef	
Rare	130° F. (54° C.)
Medium-rare	140° F. (60° C.)
Medium	150° F. (65° C.)
Medium-well	155° F. (68° C.)
Well-done	160° F. (71° C.)
Veal	170° F. (77° C.)
Lamb	160° F. (71° C.)-180° F. (82° C.)
Pork, fresh	
Well-done	170° F. (77° C.)
Pork, cured	
Ham, ready-to-eat	140° F. (60° C.)
Ham, uncooked	160° F. (71° C.)
Shoulder	170° F. (77° C.)
Turkey	180° F. (82° C.)-185° F. (85° C.)

meats. It is important to note that the internal temperature for well-done pork (170° F. [77° C.]) is lower than that recommended years ago. Research has shown 170° F. (77° C.) to be ideal for flavor, tenderness, and palatability in pork. It is well above the safety point for destruction of possible *Trichina* (140° F. [60° C.]) and produces a greater yield of sliceable meat.

Broiling. Broiling is a dry-heat cooking method in which direct or radiant heat from gas flames, electric units, or charcoal briquettes provides the heat source. This method is most successful for relatively tender cuts between 1 and 2 inches thick. Thinner cuts tend to dry out and thicker cuts are difficult to broil to the more well-done stages. For optimum juiciness and tenderness, meats should be broiled at moderate rather than high temperatures. Cuts should be turned only once during broiling and should not be seasoned until cooking has been completed. Addition of salt tends to draw moisture from the meat surfaces and delays browning. Equipment used for broiling is variable, so broiling times may differ from one unit to another. Timetables for broiling are not particularly useful because thickness of cut, distance from the heat source, and degree of doneness also affect the total cooking time. Frozen cuts can be broiled with consistent results, but should be placed farther from the heat or at a lower temperature to reach uniform doneness. Broiling time will be almost doubled for most steaks. Cuts over 1-1/2 inches thick should be thawed before broiling.

Frying. Heat is conducted from the surface of a grill, braising pan, or skillet to the meat surface. The metal surface may be oiled before very lean cuts are placed on it. Meats that contain fat will generate enough melted fat to prevent sticking. Moderate temperatures should be used to avoid overbrowning and crusting of meat surfaces. Excess fat can be removed as it accumulates and care should be taken to avoid temperatures high enough to cause smoking that will give off-flavors to the meat. Many meat cuts, such as hamburger, steak, liver, cube steaks, ground lamb, lamb chops, ham steaks, Canadian bacon, or other similar thinner cuts, can be completely cooked by this method. Many recipes combine an initial panfrying, sautéing, or grilling with moist-heat finishing. Frying large quantities of many of the cuts mentioned is too time-consuming to be practical. For that reason, oven frying is often substituted. Meat is placed in well-greased, shallow pans with or without additional fat dribbled over the product. Meats may be dredged in seasoned flour or crumbs, and cooked at temperatures ranging from 375 to 400° F. (190 to 204° C.) The pan is uncovered and no liquid is added.

Deep-fat frying. Deep-fat frying is not one of the major methods of cooking meats. It is usually the initial step for browning meats that will be finished by another method. For example, round steaks or pork chops may be browned in deep fat and then finished in the oven. Meats should be coated or breaded before deep-fat frying. The fat temperature should be controlled at 350° F. (177° C.). This temperature is high enough to avoid overabsorption of fat yet low enough to produce a tender product and avoid breakdown of the fat. Meat that is to be deep-fat fried should be free of excessive moisture and loose particles of breading. Moisture will cause the fat to spatter or bubble and will speed up fat breakdown.

When meat is deep-fat fried, uniformly sized pieces should be loaded into the fryer basket and lowered slowly into the hot fat. The fryer should not be overloaded, because this will reduce the fat temperature and increase fat absorption into the meat. This is particularly important when frying frozen meat. The meat should be cooked until the outside is properly browned or until the cut is completely done. The doneness should be checked by cutting into a sample piece from the batch. When removing the meat from the fat, the fryer basket should be lifted and allowed to drain over the fryer kettle. Care should be taken to avoid shaking excess crumbs from the coating into the fat. The meat can be salted after it has been removed from the fryer basket. (Salt speeds up the deterioration of fat.) Additional fat should be added during the cooking process to maintain the correct frying level and extend the life of the fat. The fat should recover to proper cooking temperature before more meat is fried. Frying fat should be filtered at least once daily or more often if the fryer is used extensively or if breaded foods are fried in it.

Moist Heat

Meats cooked by moist-heat methods are surrounded by steam or hot liquid. The external surface of the meat is exposed to temperatures no higher than that of boiling water, unless the meat is cooked under pressure. Moist-heat methods are used to tenderize tougher muscles and cuts that contain larger amounts of the connective tissue collagen. In general, the cooking times for moist-heat methods are considerably longer because the temperatures are lower than in dry-heat cooking. Many cuts that could be cooked by dry heat are cooked in moist heat to add greater variety and appeal to entree selections. For example, certain tender cuts such as pork or veal steaks, chops and cutlets, and beef and pork liver are cooked in this way. Slow cooking develops flavor, tenderizes meat, and reduces personnel handling time.

Braising. Braising is one of the most frequently used moist-heat methods of cooking. Pot roasting, Swissing, and fricasseeing are terms sometimes used instead of braising. Meat cuts are cooked slowly in a covered utensil in a small amount of liquid. The meat may be browned first in a small amount of fat. If it is browned, the cut can first be dredged in seasoned flour to increase browning.

In food service facilities, several different pieces of equipment can be used to braise meat. Steam-jacketed kettles or tilting braising pans are ideal because of the speed in cooking, ease in controlling uniform heating, and ease of handling the cooked meat. Covered, shallow, heavy-duty pans also can be used for braising on the range top or in a 300 to 325° F. (149 to 163° C.) oven.

Stewing. This method of meat preparation involves cooking in a large amount of liquid at temperatures just below the boiling point. Although the method is sometimes called boiling, temperatures between 185 and 200° F. (85 and 93° C.) produce a more flavorful, tender product. Boiling makes meat stringy and difficult to slice and produces more shrinkage. Stewing is suitable for the less tender cuts, such as fresh or corned beef brisket; beef, lamb, or veal cubes that will be incorporated into stews or casseroles; and any meats such as shank or neck that are being used to make soup stock. For additional flavor and color, some meats may be dredged in seasoned flour and browned before stewing. Although stewing can be done in many different types of equipment, it is important to select pots, kettles, or pans that have sufficient capacity to eliminate labor time in transferring the product from one container to another and to reduce warewashing.

Steaming. Meat can be cooked by steam using pressure steamers or by completely wrapping the meat in heavy foil. When using this moist-heat method, less tender cuts can be tenderized, but shrinkage and drip loss may be greater than in other methods. Many food service operations use compartment steamers to reduce the cooking time for meat that will be used in salads, creamed dishes, or sandwiches. However, flavor and color of steamed meats are usually less attractive than meat cooked by other methods. Experiments with heavy foil wrapping for beef roasts have shown that cooking time is increased, and higher cooking losses as well as less tender, juicy cuts of meat result.

USING FROZEN MEAT

Trends indicate that many food service operations are purchasing more types of meat items in a frozen state. Most meats can be cooked from the frozen state with essentially the same yield and quality as when fully or partially thawed. The same cooking procedures and temperatures apply, but additional cooking time and energy are needed to reach the desired degree of doneness. When roasting meat from the frozen state, the cooking time will be increased approximately 1-1/2 times. This additional time and the cost of fuel for the extra roasting must be considered in production scheduling. A meat thermometer should be inserted midway in the cooking process, so that accurate end-point temperatures can be determined.

Some cuts of meat, such as preformed ground meat patties, fabricated veal, or pork cutlets, should not be thawed before cooking. These cuts become too hard to handle, and, if breaded, there is a tendency for the breading to fall off. Browning also may be more uneven when the cuts are thawed before cooking.

When precooked frozen meats are used, manufacturer's instructions for thawing and reheating should be followed accurately to obtain optimum quality and avoid food safety hazards.

PORTIONING AND HOLDING

Portioning. Standard portion sizes for each type of meat served must be determined to ensure food cost control and consumer acceptance. A chart that states individual portion sizes can be developed and made available to personnel responsible for portioning. For roasts and other large cuts of meat, electric slicers are the most efficient way to slice uniform portions. The sliced meat should be weighed for the desired individual portion size, and equal numbers of portions should be placed in each pan. For fully cooked meats, such as hams, turkey rolls, or preroasted beef, the meat should be sliced and put in the pan prior to heating. The manufacturer's instructions for handling should be followed. The pans should be covered to prevent undesirable moisture loss.

Electric slicers must be cleaned very carefully immediately after use and kept in a sanitary condition at all times. If an electric slicer is not available, sharp knives and properly sanitized cutting boards will be necessary. The work area used for portioning cooked meats also should be in a sanitary condition. Knives and boards used in preparing raw meat or poultry products must always be sanitized before using with cooked products.

Holding. Meats must be held at temperatures of 140° F. (60° C.) or higher. Before holding, the meat should be brought to a safe temperature of at least 140° F. (60° C.) or higher as needed for palatability and safety. Most holding equipment is designed to maintain these temperatures and not to reheat cold foods. Ideally, meat and meat-containing items should be held for as short a time as possible, and never for more than two hours. In many situations, however, holding for transport or an extended service period is necessary. Meats cooked by moist heat are more suitable for extended holding, but beef roasts that are cooked to rare and medium-rare stages can be held for a short period of time without becoming overdone. Pork should be brought to a temperature of 170° F. (77° C.) prior to holding.

In many food service operations, staggered production schedules reduce the necessity for extended holding and decrease the probability of quality loss, shrinkage, and lower acceptability. Batch production is almost essential for fried and breaded items because they do not hold well on the steam table.

STORING COOKED MEAT

Regardless of how accurate the forecasting method is, there may be cooked meat items remaining at the end of the service period, as well as meat items that have had to be cooked in advance of the service time. Despite great care in preparation and/or holding, there is always the risk that these foods have been exposed to microbiological hazards. For that reason, cooked meats must be very carefully stored to avoid foodborne illness.

Cooked meat and meat-containing foods must be quickly chilled to temperatures below 45° F. (7° C.) within 2 hours. For some items, cooling will be more rapid if the hot food is placed in a shallow layer in shallow pans and refrigerated immediately. The food should be covered after it has cooled. For dense foods, such as lasagna or other similar entrees, quick-cooling can be accomplished by placing the pan of food on ice or in a sink containing ice and water. Stews, soups, and other semiliquid foods should be treated similarly, with stirring during the initial cooling period. Hot foods should not be placed in deep pots, jars, or pans because the cooling rate will be very slow. Hot stock, gravy, or other products should not be added to a pan that contains leftovers. The risks of doing so are twofold: the entire batch may be warmed to temperatures that can support bacterial growth, and the safe storage life of the newly cooked food will be decreased.

In a cook/chill system, a specially designed quick-chilling refrigerator should be used to bring hot foods down to 45° F. within 4 hours. After chilling, the foods should be stored at 32 to 38° F. (0 to 3° C.) and used within a maximum of 48 hours to avoid safety risks and loss of palatability.

USING LEFTOVER MEAT

Leftovers should always be stored separately, dated, and kept for no longer than 24 to 48 hours. If it is known that the products cannot be used within that period, they should be frozen immediately after service in a refrigerator that has adequate air circulation. Pans of food should not be stacked or refrigerator shelves covered with foil or trays because this can block air flow.

Leftovers should not be combined with fresh products. For example, leftover beef stew should not be added to a new batch of beef stew. However many kinds of leftover meat can be used in casseroles, salads, sandwich fillings, or soups. When devising ways to use leftovers, the additional labor cost that is going to be added to make the item usable should be considered. If considerable labor will be expended in reworking the item, it may be more economical to serve it with fewer changes or to freeze it until it appears again on the menu cycle.

To freeze leftover meats, they should be packaged in moistureproof and vaporproof materials such as freezer wrap, freezer bags, or heavy-duty foil. Plastic or foil containers are suitable for casseroles, stews, or other semiliquid products that can be thawed before reheating by placing in the refrigerator. These products should be reheated to at least 165 to 170° F. (74 to 77° C.). After one reheating, leftovers should be discarded.

POULTRY

Most poultry purchased today is ready to cook in either the fresh-chilled or frozen state. Many forms of precooked poultry are also available to food service facilities. The most widely marketed poultry—broiler-fryer chickens, turkeys, Cornish hens, ducks, and geese—are all young, tender birds. For that reason, broiling, frying, and roasting are the preferred preparation methods. Moist-heat cooking methods offer great menu variety and appeal, and today's poultry does not need long cooking in moisture to yield a tender product.

Poultry must be properly handled during pre-preparation, preparation, cooking, holding, and cooling to prevent contamination that might cause food poisoning. Chilled fresh poultry should be stored at 28 to 32°F. (-2 to 0°C.) for not more than 2 or 3 days. If the poultry must be purchased more than 2 or 3 days prior to service, it is advisable to purchase it in a frozen form.

Poultry should always be thawed in the refrigerator for 1 to 4 days, depending on the size of the bird or packages. Frozen whole turkeys, ducks, or geese can be thawed more rapidly by placing them, in the original wrapper, in cold water. Defrosting at kitchen temperatures or in warm water is hazardous because bacteria on the surface of the poultry have an opportunity to multiply. The body cavity is especially rich in *Salmonella,* which is capable of causing food poisoning. Thawed poultry should be washed inside and out in cold water, drained, and refrigerated, and should be cooked within 24 hours. Prebreaded or battered chicken pieces, either cooked or uncooked, should not be thawed before cooking or reheating. Fully cooked frozen turkey rolls, boneless frozen diced turkey, chicken, and other similar forms may be thawed in the refrigerator before using. Knives and cutting boards used to prepare uncooked poultry should be sanitized before they are used in preparing any other food products.

DRY-HEAT PREPARATION

Roasting. One of the common methods of preparing poultry uses the dry-heat method of oven-roasting. Turkey may be roasted whole, cut in half, or cut in pieces. Although the results will be similar, available oven space and roasting time may make the cut forms more efficient. If the white meat and dark meat parts are panned separately, overcooking of the white meat can be avoided. Because white meat cooks more rapidly, it should be allowed a shorter roasting time. If a turkey is to be roasted whole, it should not be stuffed; roasting should be done during one continuous period. Raw turkeys can be cooked from the frozen state or partially thawed and cooked.

The turkey or chicken should be placed on a rack in a shallow pan and roasted in a 300 to 325°F. (149 to 163°C.) oven. Low oven temperatures ensure higher yields of edible meat, with better flavor and greater succulence. The skin can be brushed with butter, margarine, oil, or shortening. If desired, the body cavity of whole birds may be seasoned with salt, pepper, and herbs. A meat thermometer can be used to determine doneness. In turkeys, the thermometer should be inserted in the thigh muscle adjoining the body cavity or in the thickest portion of the breast. Doneness is indicated when the thermometer registers 180° F. (82° C.). Doneness also is indicated when thigh or breast meat feels soft or when the leg moves readily at the thigh joint; the juice will be clear, with no pink color.

A tent of aluminum foil placed loosely over the breast of a whole turkey will delay browning and excessive drying of the breast meat, but should be removed during the last 30 minutes of roasting. Wrapping in foil or cooking in a covered pan will tend to steam the bird rather than develop the rich browning and true flavor of roasted poultry. Basting may be done as needed during the cooking process.

When roasting ducks or geese, no basting is needed. Fat should be poured off as it accumulates in the roasting pan. A small amount of water can be added to each pan to reduce spattering, but the birds should be roasted uncovered, following the same procedures as with turkey or chicken.

For easier slicing, roasted poultry should stand for 15 to 20 minutes after it has been removed from the oven. This permits the hot juices to be absorbed into the meat so that they flow less freely during slicing. The flesh will be firm and slice with less tearing and crumbling. Boned and rolled fresh turkey is also easily carved.

Oven frying. Fried chicken is always a favorite. An easy way to prepare it in quantity is to oven fry it. Chicken pieces are washed and dried, dredged in seasoned flour, and placed in a single layer on a well-greased sheet or in 12-by-20-inch pans. Additional melted shortening may be poured over it, and the chicken is cooked in a 400° F. (204° C.) oven for 45 to 50 minutes. There are almost unlimited variations on the basic oven-fried chicken recipe. The chicken may be dipped in milk, buttermilk, undiluted cream soup, or margarine before coating. The variety of coatings includes bread crumbs, cornflake crumbs, and cracker crumbs seasoned with herbs, paprika, or Parmesan cheese. Instant potato flakes make a crunchy coating, and commercial coatings can provide further variety for this frequently used menu item.

Deep-fat frying. This method produces a uniform golden color around the chicken pieces, but more attention is required during the frying process. In order to make sure that deep-fried chicken is thoroughly cooked, many food service operations partially fry the chicken until golden and then place it in a 325° F. (163° C.) oven to complete the cooking. The temperature of the fat should be 350 to 365° F. (177 to 185° C.) and the same procedures described for frying meat apply. Deep-fat frying is also ideal for reheating the prebreaded and prebattered cooked chicken pieces used in many food service operations. The poultry processor's instructions for time and temperature should be followed.

Broiling. Tender young chickens can be broiled, provided there is sufficient broiler capacity for the quantity needed. Halves or parts can be brushed with melted fat, seasoned, and placed skin side down on the broiler rack about six inches away from the heat source. The chicken parts should be turned after 10 or 15 minutes and brushed with fat. Total broiling time will be 35 to 50 minutes, depending on the size of the pieces. For calorie-restricted or fat-restricted diets, brushing the chicken pieces with fat should be eliminated.

In extended care facilities, an outdoor chicken barbeque can provide a welcome change from the regular meal routine in summer. Barbeque grills can be improvised from 30- or 50-gallon oil barrels that are cut in half vertically. Charcoal should be placed in the bottom and a rack over the top side of the barrel. Several times during the cooking period, chicken quarters, halves, or pieces can be brushed with oil, a mixture of equal parts of oil and vinegar, or a seasoned barbeque sauce. Seasoned barbeque sauces should not be added until the last 15 or 20 minutes. The chicken pieces should be turned every 10 or 15 minutes during the 45 to 60 minutes required for doneness. To shorten the cooking time, the chicken pieces can be partially cooked in the steamer or oven immediately before barbequeing.

MOIST-HEAT PREPARATION

Several moist-heat methods may be used for cooking older, less-tender poultry or for menu variety. These methods include braising, stewing, simmering, and steaming. These processes can be used for cooking whole or split poultry to be sliced, creamed, or made into soups and stews. The flavor that develops depends on the concentration of the broth. In braising, only enough liquid is used to cover the bottom of the pan; in stewing or simmering, the meat is fully covered with liquid. In all methods, the pan or kettle is covered tightly, and the temperature is kept at approximately 185°F. (85°C.). Cooking time will depend on the age and size of the bird, as well as the quantity in the container. The poultry should be cooked until fork tender. Poultry parts also can be steamed in low- or high-pressure steamers, following manufacturer's suggestions.

If these methods are used to produce cooked boneless meat to be used in other recipes, the poultry should be removed from the cooking liquid as soon as it is done. The pieces should be placed in a single layer on a flat pan and allowed to cool only enough to ensure safe handling. The meat should be quickly deboned by using a fork, tongs, and plastic disposable gloves. The boneless meat should be placed in a shallow layer on a flat pan, refrigerated immediately, and kept refrigerated until used. The broth should be cooled separately by adding ice if it is already concentrated, or by placing the hot broth in a pan in a sink filled with ice water and stirring until cold.

Cooked poultry meat should be stored in the same manner as other meat products, following the recommendations outlined in that section.

FISH AND SHELLFISH

Good fish that is well prepared can compete with the finest meat or poultry. Fish flesh is delicate and contains some connective tissue and variable amounts of fat. Fat content is one of the characteristics that determine the best cooking method for a particular species of fish, although almost any cooking method will produce a tender product. Most finfish and all shellfish are lean, with less than 5 percent fat. This means that they are susceptible to drying, either by exposure to air or by heat. Other considerations are the size, texture, form, and strength of flavor.

Well-done—or the point at which the flesh becomes opaque, flakes easily, and is moist—is always the stopping place when cooking fish. High cooking temperatures or overcooking will yield a hard, dry, pulpy fish that breaks up easily. Table 27, next page, presents the recommended and possible cooking methods for several common species of fresh fish and saltwater fish. Fish should be served as soon as possible after cooking, because holding will make unbreaded products dry and breaded products mushy.

PRE-PREPARATION

Proper handling and storage is necessary to protect the quality of fresh or frozen fish. Ease of handling, product quality, and microbiological safety are all major concerns. Fresh fish and seafood should be stored in the refrigerator at approximately 35 to 40° F. (2 to 4° C.) for only 1 or 2 days.

Frozen unbreaded fish products should be thawed in the refrigerator, allowing 24 to 36 hours for 1-lb. packages and 48 to 72 hours for 5-lb. solid-pack packages or gallon cans. If faster thawing is necessary, containers can be thawed under cold running water. However, this is not a recommended practice, because if fish pieces become waterlogged, soluble flavors will leach out into the water. Breaded products should not be thawed before cooking. They should always be cooked from the frozen state.

PREPARATION

There are some basic principles and procedures to follow when cooking fish and seafood, no matter what recipe is used.

Baking. One of the easiest ways to prepare fish in quantity is to bake fillets, steaks, or unbreaded pieces. Uniformly sized pieces of fish should be placed on a well-oiled pan that is brushed with butter or margarine, and baked in a 350 to 400° F. (177 to 204° C.) oven for the shortest time

TABLE 27. RECOMMENDED COOKING METHODS FOR FISH

PRACTICAL FISH GUIDE

SPECIES OF FISH	FAT or LEAN	BROIL	BAKE	BOIL STEAM POACH	FRY SAUTÉ
Alewife	Fat		Best	Good	
Barracuda	Fat	Good	Best		Fair
Black bass	Lean	Good	Good		Good
Bloaters	Fat				Best
Bluefish	Fat	Good	Best		Fair
Bonito	Fat	Good	Best		Fair
Buffalo fish	Lean	Good	Best		Fair
Bullheads	Lean		Fair	Good	Best
Butterfish	Fat	Good	Fair		Best
Carp	Lean	Good	Best		Fair
Catfish	Lean			Good	Best
Cod	Lean	Best	Good	Fair	
Croaker (hardhead)	Lean	Good	Fair		Best
Drum (redfish)	Lean		Best	Good	
Eels	Fat		Good	Fair	Best
Flounder	Lean	Good	Fair		Best
Fluke	Lean	Good	Fair		Best
Grouper	Lean		Best		
Haddock	Lean	Best	Good	Fair	
Hake	Lean	Fair	Best	Good	
Halibut	Fat	Best	Good	Fair	
Herring lake	Lean	Good	Fair		Best
Herring sea	Fat	Best	Fair		Good
Hog snapper (grunt)	Lean	Good			Best
Jawfish	Lean		Best		
Kingfish	Lean	Best	Good	Fair	
King mackerel	Fat	Best	Good		
Lake trout	Fat	Fair	Best		Good
Ling cod	Lean	Best	Good	Fair	
Mackerel	Fat	Best	Good	Fair	
Mango snapper	Lean	Good			Best
Mullet	Fat	Best	Good		Fair
Muscallounge	Lean	Best	Good		Fair
Perch	Lean	Good	Fair		Best
Pickerel	Lean	Fair	Good		Best
Pike	Lean	Fair	Good		Best

TABLE 27. *Continued*

PRACTICAL FISH GUIDE

SPECIES OF FISH	FAT or LEAN	BROIL	BAKE	BOIL STEAM POACH	FRY SAUTÉ
Pollock	Lean	Fair	Good	Best	
Pompano	Fat	Best	Good		Fair
Porgies (scup)	Fat	Good	Fair		Best
Redfish (channel bass)	Lean	Good	Best		
Red snapper	Lean	Good	Best	Good	
Robalo (snook)	Lean	Good	Best		
Rockfish	Lean		Good	Best	
Rosefish	Lean		Good		Best
Salmon	Fat	Good	Best	Fair	
Sablefish (black cod)	Fat			Good	
Sardines	Fat		Best		
Sea bass	Fat	Best	Fair		Good
Sea trout	Fat	Best	Good		Fair
Shad	Fat	Good	Best		Fair
Shark (grayfish)	Fat		Best	Good	
Sheepshead (fresh water)	Lean		Good	Best	
Sheepshead (salt water)	Lean	Best	Good		Fair
Smelts	Lean	Good	Fair		Best
Snappers	Lean	Good	Best	Fair	
Sole	Lean	Good	Fair		Best
Spanish mackerel	Fat	Best	Good		Fair
Spot	Lean				
Striped bass (rockfish)	Fat		Good	Best	
Sturgeon	Fat	Good	Best	Fair	
Suckers	Lean	Good	Fair		Best
Sunfish (pumpkin seed)	Lean	Good			Best
Swordfish	Fat	Best	Good	Fair	
Tautog (blackfish)	Lean	Best	Good		Fair
Trout	Lean	Good	Fair		Best
Tuna	Fat	Fair	Best	Good	
Walleye (pike perch)	Lean			Best	
Weakfish (sea trout)	Lean	Best	Good		Fair
Whiting (silver hake)	Lean			Best	
Whitefish	Fat	Good	Best		Fair
Yellowtail	Fat		Good	Best	

Note: All shellfish are lean.

that will produce a cooked product. Herbs, lemon juice, paprika, chopped parsley, chives, or seasoned salts can be used to add flavor and appeal to baked fish. In baking breaded precooked pieces of fish, the manufacturer's instructions should be followed.

Broiling. Broiling requires careful watching and thus increases labor time. However, broiled fish adds variety to menus and, if prepared properly, is well accepted by many people. It is best to thaw frozen fish to reduce cooking time. Lean fish should be brushed with melted butter or magarine; fish containing more fat may not need the added oil. The fish should be placed on an oiled broiler pan, with skin (if any) away from the heat source, and broiled 2 to 4 inches away from the heat for 5 to 15 minutes, depending on the thickness of the fillet. The fillets may be brushed with melted butter or margarine as needed to keep them moist.

Panfrying. If small quantities of fish are prepared, panfrying or sautéing may be a suitable method to use. Thawed, dried fish should be dusted with seasoned flour and/or coated with breading and fried in 1/8 inch of hot oil over moderate heat, first on one side and then the other, until each side is browned. If frozen prebreaded fish is being panfried, it should not be thawed before cooking.

Oven frying. A simple procedure requiring the least amount of direct labor time is the oven-frying method. A standard oven should be preheated to 500° F. (260° C.) or a convection oven to 450° F. (232° C.). Thawed fish fillets can be dipped in beaten egg or milk and then in flour or breading. Frozen breaded portions or sticks should not be thawed. The fish should be placed on a well-greased baking pan, and a thin layer of melted shortening should be poured over the fish, using approximately 1 lb. for each 20 lb. of fish. Melted shortening need not be added to precooked breaded portions. The fish should be oven fried until just well-done. The precooked items will reheat rapidly, so the time should be watched carefully.

Deep-fat frying. Deep-fried fish and shellfish, if properly prepared, have good eye appeal, flavor, and texture. To obtain an attractive brown, crispy crust, the oil designed for deep-fat frying should be used at a temperature of 350 to 365° F. (177 to 185° C.). Fish or shellfish should be dipped in batter, milk, or egg and breading, and the excess breading should be shaken off. The pieces should be placed carefully in the fryer without overloading and fried approximately 4 or 5 minutes, depending on thickness, until the coating is golden brown and done. The fish should then be drained and served as soon as possible. If necessary, they can be held for a short period uncovered in proper hot-holding equipment or in open pans under infrared food warmers. For prebreaded products, the manufacturer's instructions should be followed.

Batter ingredients are a critical factor in producing a good deep-fried product that is crisp, not greasy, and maintains the characteristic flavor of the specific fish. Common batter ingredients are flour, egg, baking powder, salt, or other seasoning and a liquid. Although baking powder helps produce a fluffier, lighter batter, it will increase fat absorption. Many batter recipes use a carbonated beverage instead of baking powder to avoid this problem. Egg also increases the tendency for fat absorption, but helps the batter adhere to the product. It may take some experimentation to develop and standardize a suitable batter recipe or to find an acceptable commercial batter mix.

It is also important to keep the frying oil in good condition by filtering, adding oil, and controlling temperature. Oil that has begun to break down will cause the food to overbrown, absorb more fat, and produce strong off-flavors. Too high a temperature, as well as the presence of food particles, moisture, and salt in the oil, will hasten fat breakdown. During periods when the fryer is not in use, the thermostat should be either at 200°F. (93°C.) or turned off.

Steaming, poaching, and simmering. Steaming or poaching is a good way to prepare fish or shellfish without adding any fat or calories. To steam, the fish should be placed on a rack in a shallow pan with liquid on the bottom, covered tightly, and cooked in the oven or on the range top until the fish is done. A low- or high-pressure steamer also may be used, following manufacturer's instructions.

To poach, the fish should be placed in a shallow pan that contains a small amount of seasoned hot liquid such as water, water and lemon juice, or milk. The pan should be covered and the fish should be simmered gently at approximately 185°F. (85°C.) until it flakes easily. The fish portions should retain their shape.

For some recipes, such as chowder or fish stews, fish is cooked at simmering temperatures in a larger amount of liquid, which is used as stock. Shellfish, such as shrimp, lobster, or crab, also should be cooked in large amounts of seasoned water at temperatures between 185 and 200°F. (85 and 93°C.) only long enough to cook through. However, for most institutions, it is more economical and efficient to purchase such fish in a partially prepared form to eliminate the labor involved in shelling and handling.

EGGS

An egg is one of the most versatile and valuable foods available. Served at breakfast, lunch, or dinner, in appetizers, soup, entrees, salads, or desserts, eggs are a good source of many nutrients.

The shell of an egg is composed basically of calcium substances. When an egg is fresh, the shell is covered by a substance called the bloom. This material limits passage of flavors, odors, and bacteria into the egg as well as the evaporation of moisture from the egg itself. As an egg ages or is held under poor storage conditions, the bloom disappears. The unprotected shell can no longer prevent evaporation of internal materials, so the egg shrinks, the air cell enlarges, and the white becomes more watery.

The white of an egg contains mainly protein. The yolk contains fat, protein, and minerals. The color of the yolk may vary from light yellow to deep orange-yellow, depending on the breed and type of feed eaten by the hen. Color is not related to the age or food value of the egg itself. Shell color does not affect nutritional value; it simply depends on the breed of hen.

Eggs are used in many ways either by themselves or in combination with other foods because of their varied properties. They not only add flavor and color to any recipe in which they are used, but are essential in many cooking processes. Eggs can function as thickening, leavening, binding, emulsifying, or clarifying agents.

Egg proteins, like other proteins, coagulate and become firm when heated. This makes it possible for eggs to function as a thickening agent in puddings, custards, and sauces. Protein coagulation is also the reason eggs can act as a binding agent to hold crumbs together for crust formation on breaded foods or to hold meat loaf ingredients together. In some kinds of batters and doughs, coagulation of the egg protein helps make the cell walls and outer crusts rigid as in cakes or cream puffs. Coagulation also allows clarification of broths or similar foods by enclosing particles that are suspended in the liquid.

Egg yolks act as emulsifying agents, because a protein complex that they contain is capable of forming a thin film around tiny droplets of oil to keep them from separating from a water phase in a mixture of oil and water. The best example of this function is in mayonnaise. Egg yolks keep the oil suspended in the mixture and form a stable emulsion.

The fluid property of an egg and the surface activity of its proteins in the white make it capable of forming a thin film around air bubbles when beaten. When egg white foam is heated, it expands the air, stretches the protein film, and then coagulates forming a light, porous structure. Coagulation of protein in egg white by beating is either hindered or aided by additional ingredients. Fat from the yolk or any other source may prevent coagulation. The addition of small amounts of acid such as lemon juice or cream of tartar stabilizes egg white foam. More air can be held within the protein film and drainage is reduced when acid ingredients are added during the soft peak stage of beating. Sugar added to egg white foam increases stability and improves texture but also increases the beating time.

Foaming also is affected by temperature. Egg whites at room temperature will beat faster and attain greater volume than when cold. A fresh high-quality egg will produce a more stable foam because it contains more thick white. Heating foam also helps coagulate the protein, so underbaking can produce a foam product that will drain or become watery. Egg white foam that is overbeaten until it is dry becomes unstable and loses functional abilities. Although egg yolks do not foam as easily, egg yolk foam can be produced and is the basis for sponge cakes.

Coagulation of egg protein is desired when preparing many food items. This can be accomplished by applying heat or by violent agitation (beating or whipping). Temperature needed for egg protein coagulation depends on whether the whole egg or white only is used. Egg yolk protein coagulates at 149 to 158°F. (65 to 70°C.). The white alone coagulates at a lower temperature of 140 to 150°F. (60 to 65°C.). Other ingredients combined with the egg affect the coagulation temperature. Sugar raises the temperature and retards the rate of coagulation. Acids tend to lower the temperature and speed up coagulation (as in egg white foam). Exposure to high temperatures or prolonged low heat toughens the egg protein network. Liquid separates from the solid mass, leaving a tough, dry product. When this takes place, syneresis, or curdling, has occurred.

USING EGG PRODUCTS

The term *egg products* refers to liquid, frozen, dehydrated, and freeze-dried eggs obtained by breaking and processing shell eggs. These products include separated whites and yolks, mixed whole eggs, and blends of the whole egg and yolk. Food service operations using egg products can save in labor time, effort, and storage costs, and less waste occurs than when shell eggs are used.

Chilled or frozen. Chilled or frozen egg products are available in 4- or 5-lb. paper cartons, or in 30-lb. containers for large batch needs. The products are suitable for use in almost any menu item. Handled properly, these products are even safer to use than fresh shell eggs because they are pasteurized at temperatures high enough to destroy any food-poisoning bacteria that might be present.

Added ingredients and special processes help to improve and preserve the performance characteristics of many egg products. Sugar, corn syrup, or salt is frequently added to egg yolks to keep them from toughening. Buffers such as citric acid, monosodium phosphate, or monopotassium phosphate increase the acidity of the products, thus improving textural and performance qualities. Milk or nonfat dry milk is added to the scrambled egg blends, along with salt or other seasonings.

Chilled egg products should be stored at 38°F. (3°C.) or lower. These products have a relatively longer shelf life than thawed frozen eggs, and can usually be held at least 5 days. Manufacturers usually provide recommended storage conditions and times on label information.

Frozen egg products should be stored at 0°F. (18°C.) or lower. They should be thawed in the refrigerator for 2 or 3 days or held under cold running water for quicker thawing. After thawing, they should be refrigerated and used within 3 to 4 days.

Other available convenient frozen egg products include omelets, scrambled eggs, and hard-cooked eggs. These products should always be handled according to the manufacturer's instructions.

Dehydrated. New processes that remove the small amounts of glucose in eggs have permitted the development of improved dried egg products. Glucose removal is necessary for longer shelf life. The products are treated at temperatures high enough to destroy pathogenic organisms.

Dried egg solids are available in several forms: egg white, whole egg, egg yolk, and fortified products. Egg white solids usually have small amounts of whipping aids, such as sodium lauryl sulfate or triethyl citrate, added to reduce whipping time and improve the volume and texture of the foams. Egg yolk solids are used primarily by food manufacturers for their emulsifying properties and are not likely to be used in most food service operations. Whole egg solids, however, are very convenient for use in many recipes. For quick breads, yeast breads, cookies, or cakes, the dry egg solids are blended with the other ingredients, and the water required for reconstituting is added to other liquids in the recipe. For other kinds of recipes, the dried eggs are reconstituted before they are combined with other ingredients. Table 28, below, gives the conversion factors to use in substituting one form of egg for another.

Most quantity recipe files and manufacturer's labels provide information on reconstituting dried whole eggs. However, as a general rule, equal measures of dried egg and water are used. If products are weighed, one part dried whole egg to three parts water should be used.

EGG SUBSTITUTES

Egg substitutes that contain no cholesterol are useful in some modified diets. Individual manufacturers have different formulas, but, in general, the natural egg white is retained and a substitute for the yolk is added. Yolk substitutes contain vegetable or other oils and carotenoids as coloring and nutritional additives. Although manufacturers suggest various uses, egg substitutes do not have all the functional properties of eggs. They perform satisfactorily as scrambled eggs, omelets, and binders in other

TABLE 28. CONVERSION FACTORS FOR SUBSTITUTING EGG PRODUCTS

	Frozen	Shell Egg Equivalent	Dried Egg Solids
Whole	1 lb.	9 eggs	4 oz. + 12 oz. water
Yolk	1 lb.	23 yolks	7¼ oz. + 8¾ oz. water
White	1 lb.	15 whites	2 oz. + 10 oz. water

recipes. The manufacturer's directions should be followed for storage and preparation.

PREPARATION

Eggs served in hospitals and nursing homes may be cooked either inside or outside of the shell. The typical breakfast fare includes soft- or hard-cooked, poached, fried, scrambled, or baked eggs. To add variety, they can be served as omelets or soufflés or be incorporated in other meal components. Whatever the method of preparation, prolonged cooking and high heat are to be avoided.

Some general suggestions that apply to cooking eggs are:

- Only eggs that are free from dirt or cracks should be purchased or used.
- Eggs should be kept refrigerated until preparation time, unless they are being prepared for egg foam. In that case, they should be allowed to stand at room temperature for 30 minutes before use.
- Eggs and egg combinations should be cooked at moderate to low temperatures. High temperatures and prolonged cooking should be avoided.
- Appropriate techniques should be used when beating eggs. For a binding or coating mixture, whole eggs should be beaten slightly with a fork or wire whip. For lightness and volume, they should be beaten thoroughly with an electric mixer until thick and light lemon-colored. For stiffness they should be beaten until peaks form that fold over slightly as the beater is withdrawn.
- Egg whites should be combined carefully with other ingredients by folding rather than stirring, using a wire whip or an electric mixer at low speed.
- Hot liquids should be added to eggs slowly, beating constantly.

Soft- and Hard-Cooked

Eggs can be cooked in the shell to varying degrees of doneness by using any one of several different pieces of equipment. However, time and temperature are the critical factors regardless of the equipment used. Soft- or hard-cooked eggs can be prepared with a compartment steamer, steam-jacketed kettle, or a pan on the range top. Eggs at refrigerator temperatures are more likely to crack when subjected to hot water if the pan method is used. This can be prevented by placing them in warm water for a few minutes before cooking.

Soft-cooked eggs require approximately 3 to 4 minutes in water brought to a boil (212°F. [100°C.]) and then simmered. Small-batch cooking is necessary when serving soft-cooked eggs. Holding for even a short period of time will cause them to be overcooked. Hard-cooked eggs need 15 to 20 minutes when cooked by this method. Excessively high temperatures and prolonged cooking time cause hard-cooked eggs to toughen. A greenish-black ring also forms around the yolk. This results when hydrogen sulfide in the white combines with iron in the yolk to form ferrous sulfide.

Hard-cooked eggs placed in cold water immediately after cooking will be easier to peel. Quick cooling helps prevent formation of the ferrous sulfide ring. Hard-cooked eggs should be thoroughly cooled before mixing with other ingredients, particularly in salads.

A timesaving method for hard-cooked eggs that are to be chopped is to cook them out of the shell in a shallow, greased pan. The pan should be placed uncovered in a steamer for 20 minutes or covered and baked in the oven at medium temperature for approximately 30 to 40 minutes. The egg should then be cooled, removed from the pan with a spatula, and chopped with a French knife or food chopper.

Poached

When poaching eggs, the addition of 1 tablespoon of salt or 2 tablespoons of vinegar to 1 gallon of water will help to reduce spreading of the egg white. Fresh Grade AA or Grade A eggs and simmering water should be used to retain shape. A 4-inch-deep full-size pan filled with approximately 2 inches of water should be used. The eggs should be gently slipped into the water and cooked for 3 to 5 minutes, depending on the firmness desired. In a cafeteria, eggs can be poached in a counter insert pan in the hot-holding counter. Whichever method is used, small batch cooking is advisable.

Fried

Eggs can be fried to lend variety to the menu, particularly for residents in a long-term care facility. However, more labor time may be needed to produce good-quality fried eggs than eggs prepared by other methods. Careful handling during the preparation and holding processes is necessary. Small-batch or continuous preparation during the service period is suggested. A grill, griddle, tilting braising pan, or large skillet can be used to fry the eggs, depending on the number of servings needed and equipment available. Fresh Grade AA or Grade A eggs should be fried in ample fat heated to approximately 275° F. (135°C.). The fried egg should have a firm white that is free from browning or crispiness; the yolk should be set but not hard or dry, unless so requested by the consumer.

Scrambled

One of the easiest ways to prepare eggs is by scrambling. Large quantities can be cooked in a short time using a griddle, tilting braising pan, oven, steamer, or large skillet. Eggs that are lower than Grade A quality can still be used to produce a high-quality product. Cooking temperature and time are as critical with this method as others. High cooking temperature and long cooking and holding time in a heated serving unit will cause syneresis. An undesirable flavor and greenish color may also occur.

If scrambled eggs must be held at serving temperature for an extended period, a buffer such as powdered citric acid should be added at the rate of 0.1 percent (3 g. per gallon of egg). Cream of tartar can also be used at .5 percent (5 g. or 1/2 teaspoon per gallon of eggs). Many food service operations are now purchasing frozen blended egg products to use in scrambling. The buffers in these enable the product to hold well for extended periods. Frozen egg mixtures require less labor time in pre-preparation and provide a consistent product. If mixtures are prepared on the premises, milk, cream, or medium white sauce can be used to make the egg mixture; the ratio is 1/2 cup (4 ounces) liquid to 1 pound of whole eggs.

For best appearance, eggs should be beaten just enough to blend the yolk, white, and liquid. They should then be cooked over low heat or in the oven, stirring occasionally, to form tender, moist particles.

Baked

Another way to prepare eggs is by baking. Eggs are broken into individual greased baking dishes or greased muffin tins. An attractive way to serve baked eggs is to remove the crusts from a bread slice, butter it, press it into a greased muffin tin, and drop a cracked egg in the center. It should then be baked in a slow oven (325° F. [163° C.]) for 12 to 20 minutes according to the firmness desired.

Omelets

Omelets require greater skill and time in preparation than many other egg products. For this reason, it is not feasible to serve them to large numbers of patients or residents. However, frozen prepared omelets are currently available from several food processors. If resources of time, personnel, and equipment are limited, yet variety in menu items is desired, use of these products should be considered.

Soufflés

Soufflés add interest and consumer appeal to menus. They are similar to fluffy omelets but have a thickening agent (such as thick white sauce or tapioca) added to the beaten egg yolks before the whites are folded in. The soufflé mixture is placed in a well-oiled pan, which is set in water and baked at 375° F. (190° C.). A lower temperature (300° F. [149° C.]) can be used if the pan is not set in water, although this requires more cooking time. Soufflés should be light, fluffy, tender, and delicately browned for serving.

MILK

Milk is an important component of many prepared foods. It requires careful preparation procedures to prevent curdling or scorching. High temperatures and prolonged cooking coagulate and toughen milk protein, change milk flavors, and cause caramelization of the lactose in milk. But the curdling or coagulation of the milk protein can be caused by other things as well. Table salt, or curing salts such as those in ham and bacon, can cause curdling. So do tannins, which are found in many vegetables, including potatoes, and in chocolate and brown sugar. Strong food acids can cause almost immediate curdling. Because milk scorches easily, it should be heated over water or in a steam-jacketed kettle with low steam. Prolonged heating at low temperatures also may darken milk, because of caramelization of the lactose, or cause it to become flat and less flavorful.

There are several techniques that can be used in preparing milk-containing recipes to decrease the risk of curdling. The milk can be thickened with flour or cornstarch, as in white sauce and puddings, to stabilize the milk protein during the cooking process. Salt should not be added early in the cooking process. Acid ingredients should be at the same temperature as the milk, and should be added in small amounts toward the end of the cooking time.

Evaporated milk is whole milk with 50 percent of the water removed. Diluted with an equal quantity of water, it can be substituted for fresh whole milk in most recipes with very good results because it is more heat-stable and resistant to curdling. It produces smooth, even-textured puddings and white sauces.

For reasons of economy and convenience, nonfat dry milk can be used for many cooking purposes. Fourteen ounces of nonfat dry milk and 1 gallon of water produce the equivalent of 1 gallon of fresh skim milk. Adding 5 oz. of butter, margarine, or other fat to this recipe makes the equivalent of 1 gallon of fresh, whole milk in fat and calorie content. For additional protein and other nutritive values, 1/2 to 3/4 cup of nonfat dry milk may be added for each cup of liquid in recipes for many products.

Several methods of combining dry milk into products are possible. In cakes, cookies, quick breads, and instant mashed potatoes, milk solids can be added to other dry ingredients and the water needed is added with other liquid ingredients. For custards, puddings, and similar dishes, the correct proportion of dry milk solids should be combined with the sugar. The water required for reconstitution is added separately. If the milk is to be reconstituted and used in a liquid form, the amount of dry milk specified by the manufacturer's instructions should be weighed and the water needed carefully measured. Once reconstituted, fluid milk should be refrigerated and protected from contamination.

Dried cultured buttermilk is also available and convenient to use in many recipes. It is combined with recipe ingredients in the same manner as nonfat dry milk. Dried cultured buttermilk should be refrigerated after the container is opened.

Many desserts use dairy product foams. When air is beaten into cream or evaporated milk, a semistable foam is produced. Cream of less than 30 percent milk fat will not whip without the use of special methods or ingredients. Whipping cream foams to about twice the original volume, evaporated milk to about three times the original volume. The cream or milk must be lower than 40° F. (4° C.), and bowl and beaters thoroughly chilled. One tablespoon of lemon juice per cup of evaporated milk will help stabilize the foam produced. The lemon juice should be added after whipping.

When substituting nondairy whipped toppings for whipping cream in recipes, it is important to remember that the nondairy products whip to larger volumes. Therefore, substitutions should be made according to the quantity of whipped material required by the recipe, rather than by equal volumes of unwhipped liquid.

CHEESE

Flavorful and rich in nutrients, cheese is a good source of complete protein that can substitute for meat and add variety to menu selection. Like other protein-rich foods, cheese must be cooked at low temperatures. High temperature or prolonged heating causes stringiness and fat separation, which give a curdled appearance to the product. Cheese blends into most recipes more smoothly if it is grated or ground first.

Some recipes use several different varieties of cheese, each with its own distinctive flavor and characteristics. Processed cheese and processed cheese foods often blend into recipes more smoothly, because they have already been heated during processing. However, some of the processed cheeses may lack the distinctive flavor of natural aged cheese. If a strong cheese flavor is desired, a combination of the two can be used. Dried cheeses also are used to heighten the cheese flavor in some products.

VEGETABLES

With the abundant variety of vegetables available in every season and every region, good vegetables that are well prepared should have an almost universal appeal. Well prepared means that the texture, flavor, and appearance are up to standard, serving temperature is right, and the vegetable selected harmonizes with the rest of the meal.

The nutritive value and quality of vegetables depend on the nutrient content of the fresh vegetable, storage, preparation method, and time-lapse between preparation and service. Raw vegetables may vary widely in their vitamin content because of genetic variations, climatic conditions, and maturity at harvest. Some vitamins in fresh vegetables, particularly ascorbic acid and B-vitamins, can degrade severely when vegetables are stored for several days at temperatures well above their freezing points. Carotene, which the body converts to vitamin A, can be destroyed by exposure to oxygen and light. These losses are greatly accelerated when the products lose moisture. With proper refrigeration and storage in containers or packages that reduce exposure to air, these nutrient losses can be retarded. However, it is important to recognize that fresh vegetables, usually regarded by most as representing perfection in vitamin content, can be inferior to carefully processed vegetables unless they are properly handled after harvest and during storage. Mineral content is largely unaffected by storage conditions unless the vegetable is peeled, cut, or soaked.

Other changes can occur during storage of fresh vegetables. Green leafy vegetables lose water and wilt, thus losing appeal and palatability. The sugar in green peas and sweet corn changes to starch, which affects flavor. Extended storage of potatoes at refrigerator temperatures causes a change of starch to sugar, which adversely affects cooking characteristics. Most vegetables require storage at 80 percent relative humidity or above to maintain fresh quality.

PRE-PREPARATION

Because many nutrients are concentrated under the skin of raw vegetables, care must be taken in pre-preparation to minimize their loss. Ideally, vegetables should be pre-prepared just before cooking and/or service. However, this is not always possible, because of limited personnel and time. Vegetables that are cleaned, peeled, chopped, or sliced in advance must be refrigerated in covered containers or plastic bags until needed. Some vegetables darken when peeled and exposed to air, and must be treated with an antioxidant before storage. The commercial antioxidants contain several ingredients, such as sodium bisulfite, sodium erythrobate, and citric acid. In order to avoid severe losses of vitamins and minerals, peeled or cut vegetables should not be stored in water.

Vegetables should be washed thoroughly in cool water before further processing. Leafy green vegetables should be rinsed several times. Long soaking periods in salted water are no longer necessary to remove insects from broccoli, cabbage, brussels sprouts, or cauliflower, because commercial vegetable growers now wash produce before it is shipped. However, these vegetables still need a thorough washing.

Many kinds of equipment can be used to reduce the labor required to prepare raw vegetables. Shredders and mixers with grater and slicer attachments are frequently used. More sophisticated food cutters, choppers, slicers, and vertical cutter-mixers have been designed to uniformly process large quantities of product in a short time. If machine peeling is used for vegetables, the time should be carefully controlled to reduce loss and control cost.

PREPARATION

The overall purpose of preparing vegetables is to make them more digestible and to give them a more desirable flavor. Cooking may be needed to soften cellulose or make the starch more digestible. Cooking methods for various vegetables differ in certain respects, but some general principles apply. A cooking method that best preserves nutrients by a short cooking time and use of a limited amount of water should be chosen. It is not always possible to achieve optimum nutrient retention. For example, steaming under pressure reduces nutrient losses that occur when vegetables are cooked in water, but the higher cooking temperature may increase loss of heat-sensitive vitamins. However, shorter cooking times in low- or high-pressure steam equipment reduce this kind of loss. Flavor enhancement also should be a guide in selecting a cooking method. In most instances, the best method for nutrient retention also produces the most desirable flavor. To preserve nutrients as much as possible and make them esthetically pleasing, vegetables should be cooked only until fork-tender or slightly crisp.

COLOR APPEAL

The vibrant colors of properly cooked vegetables can attract consumers as effectively as any other merchandising device. Conversely, unattractive colors can cause a rejection even before the vegetable is tasted. For that reason, color preservation and enhancement are primary objectives in vegetable cooking. The pigments that create vegetable colors are affected in different ways during cooking—by heat, acid, alkali, and cooking time.

Green vegetables. Chlorophyll, the pigment in green vegetables, is slightly soluble in water and is changed to olive green by acids and heat when the vegetables are cooked in a covered pan or are overcooked. Although alkalis, such as baking soda, intensify the bright green color, they also destroy some vitamins and the texture of the vegetable. Therefore, adding baking soda is not recommended. Steam cooking is ideal for green vegetables because the continuous flow of steam around the vegetable carries off the mild acids that cause undesirable color changes, and vitamin losses into water are eliminated. When steam equipment is not available, green vegetables should be cooked uncovered in a small amount of rapidly boiling water for as short a time as possible.

Yellow and orange vegetables. Yellow and orange vegetables, tomatoes, and red peppers contain carotenoid pigment. This pigment is insoluble in water and unaffected by acid or alkali. Overcooking can dull the color and affects the texture. Corn and carrots contain relatively high amounts of sugars. Because of this, overcooking or extended holding can cause the sugars to caramelize and vegetables to develop a brownish color. Yellow vegetables can be cooked in a steamer or small amount of boiling water, covered or uncovered.

Red vegetables. Anthrocyanin pigments color beets, red cabbage, and eggplant. Anthrocyanins are extremely soluble in water, turn blue in alkaline solution, but become brighter in acid solutions. Adding a small amount of mild acid is an acceptable way to maintain color in red cabbage. However, it is usually not necessary to add acid to beets while cooking, because fresh beets should be cooked with stem, root, and skin on and canned beets merely reheated for a short time. Cooking times for these red vegetables should be short. With long cooking, anthrocyanin pigments turn greenish and eventually lose most of their color.

White vegetables. Light-colored vegetables contain pigments that are colorless, slightly colored, pale yellow, or brown. The group of flavonoid pigments is adversely affected by heat and alkali. In mild acid solutions, they remain white. In the presence of alkali, as in hard water, they become yellow or gray. Although the color change to yellow may not detract from the appearance of cooked onions, the grayish color change that can occur in cauliflower or turnips is unattractive. The addition of a small amount of cream of tartar to cooking water or cooking in the steamer can prevent this color change.

STRONG-FLAVORED VEGETABLES

Onions, cabbage, cauliflower, broccoli, brussels sprouts, rutabagas, and turnips all have strong flavors. Members of the onion family contain singrin, which is driven off when onions are cooked, leaving a sweet flavor. The cabbage family develops sulfide compounds during cooking and becomes strong flavored if cooked too long. Cooking methods for these vegetables differ. Onions can be sauteed in fat or cooked in relatively large amounts of water for the best flavor. Members of the cabbage family can be cooked ideally in the steamer for short periods. However, when steamers are not available, they can be cooked in a small amount of water on top of the range, in shallow pans, uncovered or loosely covered. Rutabagas and turnips should be cooked in a moderate amount of water, uncovered, and only until tender, to keep the flavor as sweet as possible.

POTATOES

Potatoes can be cooked in a variety of ways. Cooked in water, in sauce, steamed, fried, or baked, potatoes are one of the most versatile and well-liked vegetables. Sugar, starch, and moisture content of potatoes vary with the method of preparation. New potatoes and red-skinned potatoes often have a higher moisture content and are not suitable for baking. Russet and other long white potatoes produce a more desirable baked product with a fluffy, mealy texture. Baked potatoes should not be wrapped in foil because foil slows down the cooking process, adds to the cost, and produces a steamed product. The skin of the potato should be oiled or perforated with a fork before baking to allow steam to escape. Specially designed racks for baking potatoes are used in many food service operations. The metal pins on the racks allow potatoes to be placed vertically in the oven and provide faster cooking.

CANNED VEGETABLES

Canned vegetables offer several real advantages to food service operations: moderate cost, year-round availability, consistent quality, reduced energy use, and good variety. However, poor handling can yield cooked products that have lost much of their appeal and nutrients. Canned vegetables are fully cooked and should be reheated only enough for the immediate need, with batch heating throughout the serving period. They can be reheated in the steamer, steam-jacketed kettle, or kettle on the range top. The liquid from the can should first be drained into the kettle and brought to a boil before the vegetable is added. The vegetable should be cooked only long enough to heat through, with very little stirring. A No. 10 can will reheat to 150°F. (65°C.) in about 5 minutes. However, it should not be reheated on a steam table, because it will take too long and will spoil the quality. If cooked vegetables will not be used for extended lengths of time, they should be refrigerated and reheated before use to keep the product in good condition. Imaginative seasoning can greatly enhance the appeal of canned vegetables. Herbs, small amounts of meat, nuts, mushrooms, lemon juice, sauces, or cheese can be used for delicious variety.

FROZEN VEGETABLES

In many instances, frozen vegetables are fresher than fresh vegetables, having been harvested, blanched, and flash frozen within an hour or two. High-quality frozen vegetables provide freshness, beautiful color, portion control, and save labor time and waste. Small-batch cooking is essential for top-quality cooked products.

Many products are available in individually quick frozen (IQF) forms that make it very convenient to cook only the amount needed in a short time. Most frozen vegetables should be cooked from the frozen state. Only a few, like spinach or mashed squash, need tempering in the refrigerator before cooking to allow more uniform heat transfer. Frozen vegetables should be cooked in shallow layers in half- or full-size steam-table pans to eliminate handling time and damage in transferring from cooking to serving container. A full-size (12-by-20-by-2½-inch) pan will hold three 2- to 4-lb. packages of vegetables. As with any other form of vegetable, if frozen vegetables are to be held hot for more than 15 or 20 minutes, they should be undercooked.

Steam is the best method for cooking frozen vegetables. The manufacturer's directions for the type of steamer to be used should be followed. Range-top cooking time should be carefully watched to avoid overcooking, and serving pans should be used rather than large kettles.

Frozen vegetable combinations add excitement to vegetable offerings. In these combinations, blanching times are adjusted to produce a uniform cooking time for the mixture. Package directions indicate cooking time.

EQUIPMENT AND TIME

Although general charts listing cooking times for various types of equipment are available, each facility should use the information provided by its equipment manufacturers. The times given should be tested and posted on a chart beside pieces of equipment used for vegetable preparation. Cooking times will vary according to steam pressure and design of equipment. A timer should be used for accuracy no matter what equipment is used. It is very difficult to obtain the desired quality of vegetables in large-batch cooking either in a steam-jacketed kettle or on the range. Personnel may need to be retrained to use the recommended small-batch methods and in timing batches to match demands of the serving period.

SALADS

Well-prepared salads can add appeal and flavor variety to a menu. They are an excellent means of serving many nutrient-rich vegetables and fruits and provide good sources of fiber. Careful handling and imagination in combining flavors and colors make the difference between appealing and mediocre salads. Using well-designed recipes and careful methods, anyone trained in food preparation can achieve attractive results.

Colors, flavors, and textures in salads should be balanced. Salad underliners of lettuce, endive, or other greens can complement and enhance the appearance of almost any salad. Garnishes and dressings accent salad flavors, color, and eye appeal. There are several basic types of salads, such as mixed green and combination salads, main-course salads, and molded salads, but almost endless variations are possible.

COMBINATION SALADS

The simplest salad is lettuce torn or broken into bite-sized pieces with a savory dressing. But a combination of greens can be used for variety in color, texture, and flavor. Salad recipes that specify weights of ingredients are useful when substituting one green for another as availability or cost changes. The wide variety of salad greens allows plenty of latitude for varying basic combination salads: iceberg, leaf, bibb, Boston, endive (chicory), escarole, romaine, spinach, watercress, and Chinese cabbage. Various other ingredients, such as radishes, tomatoes, cauliflower, red cabbage, fresh mushrooms, green onions, red onion rings, sprouts, cucumber, broccoli, croutons, and hard-cooked eggs, can be added, with exciting results.

All ingredients should be clean, crisp, and lightly mixed to avoid breaking or crushing the ingredients. To prevent wilting of the lettuce, dressings should be added just before service or added by the customer. Whenever possible, a choice of dressings, either prepared on-premise or selected from the wide variety of commercial dressings, should be offered.

MAIN-COURSE SALADS

A salad served as the main course of a meal should contain some protein-rich food, such as chicken, seafood, eggs, cheese, ham, turkey, or other meat. These foods usually are combined with raw or cooked vegetables. For added flavor, meat and vegetable pieces can be marinated in a tart French dressing, drained, and combined with mayonnaise or a cooked dressing before serving. Such mixtures can be used to stuff tomatoes or be served with tomato wedges as a garnish. Care in handling the meat or other protein food is essential to maintain safety. Marinating in the acid salad dressing provides some protection from bacterial growth, but clean utensils and refrigeration also are required.

Julienne strips of poultry, meat, and cheese can be used to top combination green salads for main dish entrees. Salad plates offering a salad mixture accompanied by cold cuts, cheese slices, or fresh fruits are attractive and appealing year-round. In cold seasons, a cup of hot soup or consomme provides a good accompaniment.

In arranging main-course salads, different shapes should be used to make an interesting perspective. The food shapes can be varied for contrast and accented with contrasting and complementary colors. Eye appeal is just as essential as substantial character and a pleasing blend of flavors and textures. Salads should be kept thoroughly chilled at all times.

MOLDED-GELATIN SALADS

Molded salads are usually sweetened mixtures made with flavored gelatin mixes or with plain gelatin. Water or fruit or vegetable juices are used as the liquid. For fast congealing, only enough hot water to dissolve the gelatin should be used before adding cold water or other liquid for the remaining quantity. In very hot weather, or when periods of unrefrigerated holding is necessary, the amount of liquid used can be reduced slightly. Before adding other ingredients, such as chopped vegetables, fruit pieces, or cottage cheese, the mixture should be cooled until it has the consistency of unbeaten egg white. This will keep the added ingredients from sinking to the bottom of the pan. A plain gelatin mixture can be panned or poured into molds without prechilling.

For quantity service, standard 12-by-20-by-2-inch pans should be used so the gelatin can be cut for serving. Individual molds are attractive and can sometimes be used, but they are more time-consuming. All molded salads should be made the day before service.

PREPARATION

Efficient salad preparation and assembly calls for good tools, equipment, and work procedures. Some basic rules should be followed in preparing all salad ingredients. All ingredients should be top quality. They should be kept in the refrigerator except during actual preparation. Salad greens should be thoroughly washed, dried, and stored in vaporproof containers until use. Trays of finished salads should be refrigerated until they are served. All salads can be attractively arranged and garnished by using the natural color and shape of each ingredient to advantage. Maximum sanitation control in work methods and equipment should be observed. Equipment should be used whenever possible to reduce labor time and to produce uniform results.

ASSEMBLY

Most individual salads can be assembled in advance of service, put on trays, and refrigerated until needed. To save time and steps in assembly, all equipment and ingredients should be arranged within easy reach of the employee. Mobile carts can be used to extend work space and to store salad trays. Trays should be stacked on the work counter, and on each tray should be placed all the plates or bowls it will hold. Both hands should be used during assembly, using appropriate portion utensils or disposable plastic gloves for items that must be placed by hand. Salads can be simply and attractively arranged on each plate or bowl, and should be refrigerated until service.

SANDWICHES

Sandwiches are popular in any season and with nearly everyone. They can add variety and interest to menus and provide required nutrients alone or in combination with other foods. Sandwiches can be composed of few or many ingredients, open-faced or closed-faced, cold or hot, and served in a variety of shapes and forms. The essential things to remember are that they should have good flavor, texture, and appearance, and be served fresh at the correct temperature.

INGREDIENTS

Breads. The kind of breads or rolls selected should be harmonious with and enhance the filling used in the sandwich. So many varieties of specialty breads, rolls, and buns are available from commercial sources today that the problem is in which to choose. Bread with close-grained firm texture is desirable to prevent sogginess caused by moist fillings. A coarse, porous bread has a tendency to become stale faster and is more difficult to handle by both the sandwich maker and the consumer. Sandwich or pullman loaves sliced to various thicknesses are often used for making sandwiches because of the uniformity of shape and ease of handling. However, other kinds of whole grain and enriched breads should not be overlooked. Varying the kind of bread or bun used can change the appeal of even the most standard of sandwiches.

Spreads. Butter or margarine is used to enhance the flavor of sandwiches and prevent the bread from becoming soggy when moist fillings are used. Softened or whipped spreads are easier to handle; melted butter should never be used because it soaks into the bread. To whip butter, about ½ cup milk per pound of butter should be added gradually and whipped until fluffy. Whipped butter goes somewhat farther: 1 lb. of whipped butter will spread approximately 96 slices of bread, using 1 teaspoon per slice.

Spreads such as salad dressing, mayonnaise, or combinations of these with other indredients, either homemade or prepared commercially, can be used for flavor. However, the bread should be buttered first to prevent soaking.

Fillings. Sandwich fillings should contain a combination of ingredients with some contrast in flavor, color, and texture. Bland fillings can be sharpened by adding salad dressings or mustard. Fillings that lack color can be enlivened with minced parsley, pickle, pimiento, olives, or green pepper. Crispness and crunchiness can be added with crumbled bacon, chopped celery, nuts, sprouts, or shredded carrot. If desired, a lettuce leaf, shredded lettuce, sliced tomato, or a pickle can be placed on top of the filling.

In many cases, salad dressings are used to moisten the filling, hold the ingredients together, and produce a spreading consistency. Mixed fillings, especially those that contain meat, fish, poultry, or eggs, must be handled in accord with safe food preparation practices. Salad dressing that contains acid helps to retard bacterial growth, but exceptionally clean equipment and refrigeration are needed to reduce the risk of bacterial contamination. Assembled sandwiches should be individually wrapped or bagged, or stored in covered pans in the refrigerator until they are served. However, they should not be covered with dampened towels, because it is questionable from a sanitation point of view and can make the sandwiches soggy.

Cheese and meats for sandwiches can be purchased presliced for uniformity. Some meats—ham, roast beef, corned beef, turkey—can be machine-sliced paper thin and stacked high for appeal and easy eating..

There is almost no limit to sandwich fillings. Food service magazines are helpful for new ideas that could appeal to patients and staff. Attractive sandwiches can be convenient and profitable items in employee and visitor cafeterias, and can add excitement to traditional menu patterns.

ASSEMBLY

Assembly lines should be used to streamline sandwich making. After the steps for sandwich assembly have been determined, the ingredients should be arranged in the proper order. To save steps, time, and motions and have sufficient speed to meet production schedules during sandwich assembly, employees should:

1. Wear disposable gloves, use both hands, and arrange slices of bread in two or four rows on a cutting board
2. Spread butter on bread with spatula covering each slice with a circular motion
3. Use both hands to place slices of meat, cheese, poultry, or tomato on the bread slices in alternate rows
4. Scoop mixture portions onto the center of bread slices and spread with a spatula using one stroke moving in and one stroke moving out
5. Use both hands to place lettuce on top of filling
6. Close sandwiches by turning a slice of buttered bread over the filling-covered slices
7. Stack sandwiches two or three high and cut through the entire stack
8. Transfer unwrapped sandwiches to trays or pans; cover with foil, plastic film, or the pan lid; and store in the refrigerator
9. Individually wrap sandwiches in plastic bags or film before storing

If a great number of sandwiches are to be made, these steps can be divided among two or more employees.

BREADS, CEREALS, AND CEREAL PRODUCTS

Whole-grain and enriched breads, cereals, and cereal products form a significant portion of the daily diet because they supply carbohydrates, protein, B-vitamins, and iron. The wide range of bread and cereal foods offer a great opportunity for menu variety.

YEAST BREADS

To save employee time and labor, most institutions purchase commercially baked bread and rolls, and supplement them with many high-quality mixes for quick breads or frozen dough products for yeast breads. Mixes for quick breads also can be prepared in the institution's kitchen and kept on hand for many purposes.

When facilities have the equipment and labor time necessary, yeast bread products can be prepared. The use of standardized recipes and procedures makes it possible for any experienced person to produce high-quality yeast breads. However, it is essential to understand the functional properties of the various ingredients.

Flour is the basic ingredient in all bread products. It forms the structure and influences the texture, taste, and nutritional value of the product. Flours are tailored for use in specific products. Bread flours produce dough that can take a lot of machine handling. All-purpose flour also will give good results in yeast breads as well as quick breads. Enriched white or unbleached flour should be purchased and used in institutions. Whole wheat and rye flours are usually used in combination with all-purpose or bread flour to produce breads with better volume and texture. Wheat flour is composed of protein, starch, enzymes, fat (in whole grain flour), sugar, minerals, and moisture. Two of the proteins, when mixed with water, form gluten. The amount of gluten formed depends on the kind and amount of protein available in a particular flour. During the bread-making process, the gluten stretched by carbon dioxide formed during fermentation, is developed. After baking, it forms the bread structure..

Starch in the flour is changed to sugar by enzymes and is used by yeast during the fermentation process. Additional sugar is added to yeast doughs to speed up growth of the yeast plants, making the dough rise more rapidly. Sugar also gives a smoother texture, contributes to browning, and helps to tenderize the baked product.

In a bread dough, *yeast* generates carbon dioxide, which causes the dough to expand. Yeast is available in two forms: compressed or active dry. Compressed yeast is a cake of pressed living yeast cells with a small amount of starch as a binder. It is perishable and will remain fresh only for a few days under refrigeration. However, it can be frozen and kept for 3 to 6 months. Granular dry yeast keeps well for several months. In recipes, dry or compressed yeasts are interchangeable. Half as much dry yeast by weight should be used as compressed yeast.

Moisture contributes to the formation of gluten in flour, dissolves the dry ingredients, and permits enzyme actions to take place between yeast and flour. It is usually provided in yeast-leavened doughs by water or milk, and in some by eggs as well. Water dissolves the yeast and starts the fermentation process. Water temperature is critical; 110 to 115° F. (43 to 46° C.) for dry yeast and 95 to 100° F. (35 to 38° C.) for compressed yeast. Higher temperatures will destroy the yeast cells.

Milk improves flavor and nutritive value of yeast breads, but if fresh milk is used, it must be scalded first to denature serum proteins, which tend to soften gluten. It is easier to use nonfat dry milk combined with dry ingredients and add liquid in the form of water. Excess amounts of liquid will make dough sticky; too little liquid results in heavy, nonelastic dough.

Salt flavors the product and toughens the gluten, allowing it to hold more air. Too much salt will reduce the action of yeast or stop fermentation entirely. Omitting salt results in an extremely fast fermentation and a product with a harsh crumb and flat flavor.

Fat is used in small amounts in bread dough. Its function is to lubricate the gluten structure of the dough and help it retain the leavening gas. The result is improved volume and crumb grain and better flavor. Sweet doughs may have higher proportions of shortening, as well as eggs and sugar, producing lighter, more tender finished products.

Two basic methods are used for mixing yeast breads: the sponge method and the straight-dough method. The sponge method includes two mixing processes and two fermentation processes in alternating sequence. Part of the flour, water, yeast, sugar, and shortening is mixed and allowed to ferment. Then this mixture is combined with remaining ingredients, mixed again, and allowed to ferment a second time. In the straight-dough method, all ingredients are mixed at one time preceding any fermentation. This method is the most practical and timesaving.

Bread structure depends on developing the gluten by mixing and kneading. If bread flour is used, more kneading will have to be done to develop the gluten than when all-purpose flour is used. Overkneading is preferable to underkneading.

During fermentation (proofing), a humid atmosphere prevents dehydration or crusting of the dough surface. Temperature control around 85°F. (29°C.) is ideal to ensure adequate yeast growth. After the first fermentation, the dough should be punched down, scaled, shaped, and panned. The second proofing will be more rapid, because more yeast cells are present in the dough. Bread is ready for baking when the dough has doubled in size. A relatively high baking temperature is used to allow the gas in the dough to expand further, firm the structure, and develop a golden brown color.

After baking, the loaves should be removed from the pans and placed on racks to allow steam and alcohol to escape. Bread can be held for long periods if frozen in moistureproof and vaporproof material. For freezing it is recommended that baked bread be wrapped while it is still warm to cut down on moisture losses in the freezer. Dough also can be refrigerated overnight or for at least 12 hours. The first fermentation will occur during refrigeration. By refrigerating dough in this manner, the traditional early morning baking schedule can be avoided. Dough will be ready to shape and bake when employees arrive at more standard starting times, yet products will be ready for main meals of the day. Although dough can be frozen immediately after mixing and before fermentation, formulas must contain more yeast to perform effectively after thawing.

QUICK BREADS

Quick breads, leavened with baking powder, baking soda, or steam, can add appeal to any meal, with a minimum of labor. Prepared mixes for muffins, biscuits, pancakes, popovers, and other items require only the addition of liquid and/or egg to produce high-quality products. Mixes, purchased or made on-premise, minimize personnel skill and time needed.

Two basic methods are used in mixing quick breads: the muffin method and the biscuit method. In the muffin method, all dry ingredients are mixed together. Then all liquids, including oil or melted shortening, are added. The ingredients are mixed only enough to be thoroughly combined. Extended mixing will overdevelop the gluten and cause toughness, tunnels, and holes in the finished product. The muffin mixture should be portioned with a scoop for uniformity.

The biscuit method, used for soft doughs, also involves a minimum of mixing. Solid fat is cut into dry ingredients that have been combined. Liquid is then added and mixed just enough to moisten ingredients. Then the dough is rolled out on a floured board and cut, or rolled directly on the baking pan. The laborsaving method of rolling directly on the baking pan may make it possible to serve freshly made biscuits more often. The dough can be cut into squares or triangles before or after baking. All of the dough can be used without the reworking involved in traditional methods of cutting.

PASTA

Macaroni, noodles, and spaghetti form the basis of many combination entrees. Pastas that have been enriched with B-vitamins and iron should be used. Those made from durum wheat remain firmer and do not stick together as much after cooking. Pastas are cooked in a large volume of rapidly boiling salted water in a kettle or steam-jacketed kettle until the pieces are tender, yet firm. A compartment steamer also may be used. Adding oil to the cooking water keeps the pasta from sticking together and helps prevent boiling over. If the pasta is to be combined with other ingredients for further cooking, it should be slightly undercooked. Durum wheat pastas do not usually need rinsing after cooking. However, any pasta can be rinsed under either hot or cold water, in a colander, to remove excess starch. If pasta is to be served hot, it should be rinsed with hot water; cold water should be used if it will be included in a combination salad.

RICE

Rice is available in brown, milled, parboiled, or precooked forms. Rice combinations with seasonings are also available but are more expensive. The amount of water and cooking time varies according to the type of rice, so it is necessary to check recommended preparation methods for the specific form used. Rice can be cooked in a tightly covered pan on the range, in the oven, in a compartment steamer, or in a steam-jacketed kettle. Rice that is held for later service should be kept in shallow pans to prevent packing. To avoid losing the B-vitamin content, enriched rice should not be rinsed either before or after cooking. Long-grain rice should be used when the rice is to be served plain or combined with entrees.

When cooked, the grains remain firm, fluffy, and not sticky. Leftover rice can be refrigerated or frozen. A half cup of water is then added for each quart of rice when it is reheated for service.

CEREALS

When dry cereal is added to water, the starch granules absorb moisture, become greatly enlarged, and thicken after heating. Instant and quick-cooking cereals have been further processed by various methods that allow them to cook within a few minutes. This additional processing includes grinding or cutting, steam cooking, or the addition of disodium phosphate. Disodium phosphate makes the cooking water slightly alkaline, so the starch granules will gelatinize more rapidly. However, cereals with this chemical added should not be used in low-sodium diets.

The manufacturer's directions should be followed in preparing cooked cereals. The amount of liquid needed and cooking times will vary according to the type of cereal being prepared.

DESSERTS

Imaginative dessert planning and thoughtful preparation can complement the rest of the menu, balance cost, and add nutritional value to the entire meal. Dessert choices balance the satiety level of a menu, such as a heavier dessert with a lighter, less-filling entree; a fruit or light dessert with a hearty meal; and a cool, delicately flavored dessert after a spicy main dish or salad.

Food service operations with limited resources can increase the variety of desserts that can be offered by using mixes and other convenience dessert products. Cake mixes, in particular, yield consistent, uniform results when directions are followed accurately. Manufacturers provide recipes for variations on the basic cakes, which can be substituted for many cakes requiring on-site skilled labor for preparation. Frozen dessert products such as cakes, cheese cakes, pies, and other pastries also have been widely accepted. When deciding whether or not to use a convenience dessert, the cost of the convenience item should be evaluated in comparison to the cost of ingredients and labor to prepare on-premise. In addition, quality should be evaluated objectively to determine which approach is going to yield the most flavorful, attractive product.

Few institutions use convenience desserts exclusively. For high-quality preparation in the facility, standardized recipes, appropriate tools, scales, and standard-sized pans are needed. Employees should be trained in the correct use of recipes and equipment. Cooks and bakers need to understand the preparation principles for the different kinds of desserts and the functional properties of the various ingredients.

CAKES

Cakes are flour mixture desserts that contain a leavening agent to incorporate air into their structure. In butter cakes, the shortening, sugar, and eggs are creamed to incorporate air. Pound cakes are leavened almost completely by creaming. Angel food and sponge cakes are leavened by the foam of egg whites. Air also is incorporated by sifting ingredients and beating or manipulating the batter.

Butter cakes. Cake flour produces better volume and finer texture in cakes than all-purpose flour. For precision, the flour should be weighed instead of measured. Fat is important in the formation of air cells in cake batter. The more completely it is distributed throughout the batter, the lighter or airier the cake. Fat also tenderizes the product. Hydrogenated vegetable shortenings, with emulsifiers added, have better creaming properties than other kinds of shortening. The amount of sugar in the recipe influences the moistness, flavor, and tenderness of the cake. Tenderness is produced by the sugar's interference with both the gluten formation in the flour and the coagulation of the egg protein. When the amount of sugar is increased, more fat is needed for air cell formation and improved volume. Liquid is needed to dissolve the sugar. Recipes with higher fat and sugar proportions need and can tolerate more mixing. Eggs provide structure in the finished product. The amount of egg needs to be carefully balanced in relation to the amounts of sugar and fat. Too much sugar and shortening for the quantity of eggs prevents sufficient gluten formation and protein coagulation.

There are four common mixing methods used in cake recipes. One of these is the *conventional* method in which thorough creaming of the fat and sugar is the first step. Eggs or egg yolks, weighed, are added next. All dry ingredients are sifted together and added alternately with the liquid. If only egg yolks are used, beaten whites may be folded in last. This method, although more time-consuming and complicated than the others, is widely used because it produces very good cakes, with a light, fine, velvety texture.

The *muffin* method is quick and easy. In this method, dry ingredients are weighed, sifted, and mixed together. All the wet ingredients—liquid, eggs, and melted shortening—are stirred into the dry ingredients. These cakes usually have a higher ratio of sugar and fat to flour to prevent formation of gluten strands and toughness because they have to be more thoroughly stirred to blend well. Although the muffin method is easy and fast, it tends to produce a coarse-textured cake that stales quickly.

The *quick,* or *one-bowl,* method is sometimes called the *high-ratio* method because it has increased proportions of both sugar and fat. The dry ingredients, shortening, and part of the milk are combined and beaten at medium speed for two minutes. The remainder of the milk and the eggs are blended into this mixture for an added two minutes. High-ratio cakes have good volume, tenderness, and a moist, flavorful texture.

Many commercial bakers use a fourth method, called the *pastry-blend* method. In this method, fat and flour are blended before other ingredients are added in two stages. First, half of the milk and all of the sugar and baking powder are combined and blended into the fat-flour mixture. Then the eggs and remaining milk are added.

Any one or all of these methods can be used in quantity recipes. As new recipes are tried and evaluated, it is helpful to see which method is used. That will indicate what characteristics can be expected in the end product.

Panning is an important aspect of making cakes. Uniformity in the amount of batter per pan and an appropriate amount per pan are essential to produce uniform portions. If possible, the batter that goes into each pan should be weighed. If there is no scale available for this purpose, the same amount of batter should be measured into each pan. Butter cakes are baked in greased and floured pans, either in the standard 12-by-20-by-2-inch pan or in an 18-by-26-by-2-inch pan for sheet cakes. More variety is possible when the shape of the baking pan is varied from time to time. Layer cakes are easy to make by stacking two 12-by-20-inch cakes or by stacking quarters of a sheet cake baked in an 18-by-26-inch pan.

The correct oven temperature, as specified in the cake recipe, should be used. Baking temperatures for conventional ovens should be lowered by 25° F. (14° C.) for convection ovens. Too high a temperature will cause cakes to peak and crack on top; too low a temperature will cause them to fall. Cakes should be cooled before frosting. Staleness will occur more rapidly if the cake is refrigerated, but some frostings make this a necessity. Freezing retains quality in cakes for a long time and can allow advance production of cakes for service on days when production loads are heavy. Cakes should be frozen unfrosted.

Foam cakes. Feathery light angel food cakes are leavened by egg white foam and contain no shortening. Excellent ready-made mixes have almost eliminated traditional methods of producing angel food cake. However, if they are to be produced from a recipe, the use of the frozen or dry egg white products that have added ingredients to produce better foaming properties should be considered. Batch size should not be too large so that uniform mixing is possible. Combining dry ingredients with egg white foam may be done by hand using a wire whip; machine blending can be done at low speed just until all ingredients are combined.

Sponge cakes are similar to angel food cakes but whole egg foam is used with added lemon juice to stabilize the foam. In either type of foam cake, the extent of beating must be controlled to avoid overbeating. Superfine granulated sugar will produce a cake with finer grain. Accurate time and temperatures are needed to produce a light brown crust. Cakes should be cooled thoroughly in pans before removing for icing and por-tioning.

COOKIES

Methods of cookie preparation are similar to those for butter cakes: sugar, shortening, and egg are creamed; any other liquids are added; and dry ingredients are blended in last. All-purpose flour is suitable for most cookie recipes and butter, margarine, and vegetable shortening also are used. Labor time for portioning cookies is greater than for cakes, but can be decreased by using scoops to portion, avoiding cookies that have to be rolled and cut, and by making larger cookies. Bar cookies frequently are used to eliminate labor time.

Cookies should be baked on bright aluminum baking sheets or pans with low sides. Unless the cookies are very rich in fat and the recipe specifies no pan greasing, pans should be oiled with unsalted fat. Baking sheets should be cooled between each use in the baking sequence. Most cookies freeze well after they are cooled, so when time permits, it is possible to schedule the baking of several varieties at once to handle the needs of several weeks or months.

PIES AND PASTRIES

Pie crust pastry has very few ingredients, but these ingredients must be in just the right proportion to produce a tender, flaky, and flavorful crust. The solid shortening in pastry lubricates the mixture and gives it tenderness and flakiness by blending with the flour and salt in such a way that the flour particles surround small pieces of fat. During baking, the fat melts, resulting in a flaky texture. Salt adds flavor and contributes to firmness of the dough. The liquid produces a gluten structure. Fat should be blended in at room temperature, but cold water is used to prevent fat from melting during mixing. Very soft or melted fat coats the flour completely and prevents it from forming any gluten. The resulting crust will be oily, mealy, and crumbly. Overmixing pastry after water is added should be avoided.

Pies can be made in round pans or, for greater simplicity, in 12-by-20-inch or 18-by-26-inch pans. If large pans are used, a single top crust on the filling results in easier handling during service. These giant pies save assembly time and baking space. If individual round pans are used, pie making can be handled in an assembly-line process.

Pastry dough should be weighed before rolling to achieve uniform crusts with a minimum of waste. Various kinds of pastry rolling or forming machines can eliminate hand labor in forming crusts. If hand rolling is necessary, a lightly floured board should be used and the dough should roll evenly. Pie crust dough should not be stretched to fit the pan; some slack should be provided to avoid shrinking during baking. Shells baked unfilled should be pricked with a fork and chilled before baking to cut down on shrinkage. Double crust pies should have cuts in the top crust to allow steam to escape during baking. Brushing the top crust with milk or beaten egg produces a more golden brown color.

Prepared pie fillings or those made from recipes allow a wide variety in pies. If broken or irregular pieces of fruits are of good quality and flavor, they can be used to advantage in prepared pie fillings.

Pastry and pies can be frozen. The quality of most pies will be better if the pie is frozen unbaked. Most custard or pudding-filled pies should not be frozen unless special starches for thickening are used.

FRUITS AND FRUIT DESSERTS

Fresh, canned, dried, and frozen fruits, either plain or in combinations, are often served for dessert. Fresh fruits in season, carefully selected for quality, can be a regular and popular menu item. When selective menus are used, a fresh fruit should be offered as one of the dessert alternatives. Bowls of whole fresh fruit can be used on cafeteria lines as an attractive merchandising tool and as a simple serving method.

Whole fresh fruits should be thoroughly washed. Precutting clusters of grapes makes them easier to serve, but many fresh fruits need almost no preparation before service. Fresh fruits that are cut can be combined in almost endless variations to produce fresh fruit desserts, or can be combined with canned fruits. Varied shapes and sizes of fruits and complementary flavors and colors should be used. Fresh-fruit desserts should be garnished attractively and the fruits should be kept chilled until service.

When canned fruits are served as a dessert, they should be chilled thoroughly. Sugar should be added if needed. Adding a garnish can dispel the right-out-of-the-can look. Frozen fruits should be thawed in the refrigerator before serving. Canned or frozen fruits can be used in crisps or served warm with whipped topping or a hard sauce.

Crisps are simply some fruit or fruit mixture topped with a mixture of flour, sugar, and fat and then baked. A fruit cobbler is made by spreading a sweetened biscuit dough over layers of fruit and baking until the top is browned. Shortcakes are another simple yet attractive fruit dessert, made in the same way as baking powder biscuits, but using a richer and sweeter dough. Preparation can be streamlined by rolling the dough on 18-by-26-inch pans, baking, and then cutting in squares. Two squares, with fruit in between and on top are stacked to build the shortcake.

OTHER DESSERTS

Readily digested, light, and nutritious desserts are made from various egg and milk combinations: puddings; baked or stirred custards; bread, rice, and other baked puddings; dessert soufflés; and cornstarch puddings. They are easily prepared in quantity and are relatively inexpensive compared with many other desserts. Mixes and frozen egg products also simplify production of these items. Preparation principles and techniques for these foods are described in the section on eggs and milk in this chapter. All desserts in this category should be stored in the refrigerator until service.

Fruit-flavored gelatins are the basis for many easy and attractive desserts. For appealing appearance, plain gelatin may be congealed in shallow layers and cut into cubes. Cubes of various colors can be combined for service, with or without the addition of whipped topping. Partially congealed gelatins can be whipped and poured over a layer of clear gelatin for other simple yet attractive desserts.

Operating
Design
and
Equipment

DESIGN

Economic predictions indicate that the cost of providing services to consumers in health care facilities will probably continue to rise. Because the design of the food service department has a significant impact on operating costs, particularly labor and energy, the physical layout, equipment, and work methods used can be planned to minimize these costs.

The unique nature of each health care facility presents a challenge when designing a food service department that is both functional and efficient. Several common problems plague existing departments: wasted or underutilized space, inadequate or improper storage, inflexible equipment arrangements, energy-wasting equipment, inappropriate equipment capacity or type, excessive cross traffic, labor-intensive layout, and inadequate ventilation or lighting. Application of physical and human engineering principles can improve the operation of existing facilities and guide the design of a new food service department.

PLANNING PROCESS

Although food service directors are not expected to be experts in design and construction, they should be able to communicate to the other members of the planning team the amount of space needed, layout plans, and equipment required to maintain the standards set for the department. The planning process is time-consuming, but careful study of each aspect of the operation can prevent future problems.

The services of a food facilities design consultant should be considered for changes in food service production or tray service, major renovations in the kitchen or cafeteria, or construction of a new food service department. The Joint Committee of the American Hospital Association and the American Dietetic Association recognized the importance of optimizing the capital expenditures while controlling daily operating costs of a food service department and developed guidelines for *Selection of a Consultant in Hospital Food Service Systems, Design and Equipment* (see Bibliography). They include information about the planning process, functions of a consultant, criteria for selection of a qualified consultant, and methods for determining consultant fees.

Before any layout plans can be formulated on paper, the necessary information must be accumulated. The type and amount depends on the extent of remodeling or new construction. Some of the background information the architect and food service design consultant would be concerned about includes the following:

- Goals and objectives of the organization
- Long-range hospital plans
- Number of beds and spatial configuration of the institution
- Number of patient meals served
- Extent of nonpatient services provided by the food service department
- Labor situation

These data are important because they will affect the type of production, assembly, delivery, and service systems used. The optimum system should be compatible with the goals and objectives of the institution. The final decision will be based on projected capital costs, operating costs, ease of administration, and subjective comparison.

Other operational aspects of what has taken place in the past and what is proposed in the future must be considered. The food service manager can provide information about menus served; purchasing policies and practices; production procedures, quantities, and times; and style and hours of service.

Because the menu is the key to the equipment needed and the space required in the production area, further analysis should include:

- Menu pattern and number of selections within the pattern for each group served
- Complexity of menu items
- Type and number of modified diet foods
- Type and number of nourishments

Purchasing policies and practices are important to determine equipment and space needs for low-temperature and dry-storage areas plus production and service. Considerations include:

- Form in which foods are purchased—amount of processing that has taken place prior to purchase
- State of foods at time of delivery—canned, frozen, chilled, dehydrated, or freeze-dried
- Frequency of delivery for all categories of food
- Volume purchased and inventory carry-over from one purchase period to the next
- Issuing and inventory control procedures

The type of production system planned must be studied carefully because this affects equipment, space, and personnel required in the central kitchen. These systems are described in detail in chapter 3. Preplanning analysis includes:

- Total quantity of each menu item needed to yield desired number of portions
- Batch size preferred
- Time required and time available for production

Certainly this list is not all-inclusive; similar data must be gathered for other subsystems in the operation. Then, an operational plan that states organizational constraints and projected needs can be developed and used as a basis for establishing functional work areas.

Work Areas

The location of each work area and the amount of space allocated to this area within the department must be determined for each individual food service facility. The relationship of one work area to another is equally important to minimize distances in employee travel and in the transport of raw materials. A good layout should provide a smooth, orderly flow of both throughout all parts of the operation in as straight, short, and direct a route as possible. Backtracking and cross traffic increase labor time and decrease employee efficiency.

The same principle applies to the amount of space that should be planned for each area. The trend has been to minimize overall dimensions, particularly in the production area, but also in others because of the rising cost per square foot of new construction. This has been possible in many facilities because of the change in types and forms of food purchased and the availability of slimline, modular, and mobile equipment. Easy movement of food, supplies, and people requires consideration of the essential tasks to be performed in each stage of production, assembly, delivery, and service; the number of employees involved; and the equipment required for the activities. In an existing facility, improvements in space utilization often can be made by identifying points of congestion and rearranging equipment or jobs to alleviate them.

To ensure that the best arrangement for placement of work areas has been planned, a chart illustrating the flow of work can be developed on paper. At this point, the actual amounts of space and equipment are not needed. The chart is merely a diagram showing what happens when food and people travel from the receiving area to the point of service and cleanup area. Once the ideal, or at least the best possible, space relationship has been decided, a scale drawing showing the approximate size of each work area and its location relative to other departments within the allocated building space and configuration can be drawn. This task would be performed by the architect in conjunction with the food service design consultant.

The next step in the process is to draw a schematic plan, based on all the important data discussed earlier in this chapter, showing work areas, traffic aisles, and, finally, the location of specific pieces of equipment. This is when it is important for the food service manager to evaluate the proposed layout. Charting the work flow for typical menu items on the scale diagram is an excellent way to assess the feasibility of the plan. It is possible to pinpoint traffic problems that can be the result of misplaced or inadequate equipment, too little or too much space, and poor work flow in general. Suggestions for improvements should be made at this time before actual construction takes place; changes made after the fact are costly and sometimes impossible.

The food service manager should also be familiar with other aspects of building and renovation. These include construction features such as location of the department, floors, walls, ceilings, lights, utilities, ventilation, and, above all, equipment features, design, and space needs.

Location

The food service department should be located with ready access to receiving, storage, dining areas, and elevators. The distance from the food service department to patient floors is a factor in determining a method of food delivery, but new technology in tray distribution has helped to reduce temperature control problems. An area away from the major traffic patterns of other departments is recommended.

Floors, Walls, Ceilings

The floors should be durable, easy to clean, nonslippery, nonabsorbent, and resilient. It is difficult to satisfy all these specifications with one material, and the use of the same material throughout all areas is not esthetically pleasing. For example, a quarry tile floor in the dining area is not conducive to a relaxing atmosphere even though it meets most of the previous criteria. A hard-surface floor answers most of the above demands, particularly for preparation areas. However, it has two main drawbacks: it may be slippery when wet, and because of lack of resiliency, it tends to hasten employee fatigue. Quarry or ceramic tile is usually used in kitchens, and asphalt or vinyl tile or carpeting is used in the dining areas. Careful review of what is available on the market should be made before selection, because new materials with nonskid surface treatment are being developed and improved.

Regardless of the floor material, adequate drains near steam equipment, food cutters, warewashing facilities, and other areas of the kitchen will help to reduce safety hazards and aid in housekeeping tasks. All floors should have a coved base, flush with the wall, for sanitation purposes.

The walls should be hard, smooth, washable, and impervious to moisture. Glazed tile to the ceiling, or at least to a 5- to 8-foot height (with plaster and washable paint above), is preferred for kitchen and service areas. All pipes, radiators, and wiring conduits should be concealed in the walls. In the dining area, it may be desirable to have tile wainscoting on the walls and around columns, and corrosion-resistant metal corner guards to protect the walls. The use of pleasing color combinations enhances appearance and can even help employee morale.

All possibilities of soundproofing should be investigated thoroughly when contemplating construction and before selecting equipment. Kitchens can be very noisy, and this may result in employee fatigue and lower productivity. The use of acoustical materials in ceilings appreciably reduces the noise level. However, selection of the material should be based on ease of cleaning as well as noise reduction.

Lighting

The proper amount and kind of lighting in all work areas are important for cleanliness, safety, and efficiency. A person with expertise in light requirements and types of equipment available should be consulted for proper illumination as well as for meeting the recommended or required lighting codes in production and service areas. For dining facilities, a type of lighting that will create a pleasant atmosphere should be used.

Utilities and Ventilation

Selection and installation of the proper kind of utilities and ventilation equipment are the responsibility of experts in these fields. Food service managers should know what utilities are required for various pieces of equipment and make sure that the right number of connections are located in the right places.

Proper ventilation is also important for food quality preservation, employee comfort, and building maintenance. Excessive moisture or heat can ruin walls and ceilings as well as employee dispositions. Both utilities and ventilation affect energy consumption.

RECEIVING AND STORAGE

Receiving

The location and space needed for receiving depends on the operational policy of the institution. For example, if a materials management department is responsible for the procurement of all goods used throughout the institution, one area will be designated as the receiving point for all deliveries. Because materials used in the food service account for a large proportion of total deliveries, a location close to this department is convenient. If the food service department is responsible only for receipt of its own goods, the loading dock and receiving area should be close to the storage and production areas. In designing a new facility, the traffic flow that surrounds the institution, the space needed for parking delivery trucks, and the building constraints should be taken into account.

The size of the receiving area depends on delivery schedules, volume of goods in a shipment, and the time lapse between receipt and storage. Ideally, all food and supplies should be stored immediately for quality assurance and security, but this is not always possible. Heavy-duty two- and four-wheel hand trucks or semilive skids are essential. Skids are a good investment if large quantity deliveries are received and storage space is available. Cases can be loaded on skids, wheeled to the storage area, and dropped in place, thus eliminating excessive handling.

Accurate scales are needed for weighing all foods purchased by weight. For most operations, platform scales with a maximum capacity of 250 pounds are adequate. A desk or table, clipboards, and file cabinets are additional pieces of equipment that help receiving personnel with their jobs.

Dry Storage

Space for nonperishable foods and supplies may be shared with other departments in the institution or the food service department can have its own storeroom. In either case, a location reasonably close to the kitchen and service areas reduces transportation time. Usually, a short-term dry-storage area is provided near or within the kitchen or as part of an ingredient control center. Determination of the space needs for the system used is based on procurement policies related to product volume, purchase frequency, inventory level, and delivery schedule.

The general construction features to consider when evaluating present facilities or planning new ones include materials used for floors, walls, and ceilings; ventilation and temperature control; lighting; and safety and security.

To prevent access by rodents and insects, floors, walls, and ceilings should be smooth, moistureproof, and free from cracks. Light colors are preferable. Floors should be level with surrounding areas to facilitate use of mobile equipment in moving supplies.

Good ventilation is essential to retard growth of various bacteria and molds, prevent mildew and rusting of metal containers, and minimize caking of ground or powdered foods. Ventilation and air circulation help maintain proper temperature and humidity. Temperatures should be kept between 50 and 70°F. (10 and 21°C.). Several methods can be used to accomplish this. Installation of doors with louvers at floor level allow fresh air to enter the storeroom, and louvers at ceiling level enable warm air to escape. However, this is not adequate in many locales, so mechanical means are used such as intake and exhaust fans or air conditioning.

Water heaters, compressors, motors, or other heat-producing equipment should not be located in the storeroom. All steam or hot water pipes should be insulated; condensation from cold water pipes or cold walls must also be controlled. One or more wall thermometers should be placed strategically in the storeroom and checked at regularly scheduled times to ensure compliance with state and local codes. If humidity seems to be a problem, a hygrometer can be installed to record moisture levels.

Adequate lighting is needed for good housekeeping and inventory control. A level of 15 footcandles is recommended, with fixtures centered over each aisle for best light distribution. Any windows should have frosted glass to protect foods from direct sunlight.

A security sash, screen, or bar should be installed on windows in storerooms located at ground level. Other security measures include provisions for locking doors from the outside but allowing them to open from the inside without a key for safety purposes.

Good organization and the right equipment contribute to maximum use of available space in storage areas. The right equipment may include shelving, mobile platforms, and metal or plastic containers on wheels or dollies. Adjustable metal louvered or wire shelving is recommended to permit air circulation and allow shelf spacing to meet exact heights needed. For safety and convenience, the top shelf should be accessible without the use of a stool or step ladder. Local ordinances usually specify a minimum of 6 inches or more from the floor to the lowest shelf. One- or two-inch clearance between the wall and shelf is needed for air circulation and cleaning.

Shelving may be mobile or stationary and should be adjustable for variations in type and quantities purchased. Selecting the right width and length of shelves is important. Widths range from 12 to 27 inches and, if space allows, shelves can be placed back to back for easy access from both sides. Single-unit widths of 20 to 24 inches can easily accommodate two rows of number 10 cans on a single shelf. Clearance between shelves should be at least 15 inches to allow stacking of two number 10 cans on top of each other. Length of shelves varies from 3 to 3-1/2 feet or more. Calculation of the dimensions for packaging each item, weight per unit, and inventory quantities should be used as a guide to determine total linear feet needed.

If large amounts of dry-food items are stored, mobile platforms and dollies are useful for moving and storing these goods until opened. Metal or plastic containers with tight-fitting covers are useful for storing broken lots of flour, cornmeal, sugar, and other cereals and grains. Food from packages that have been opened should be stored in food grade containers and the contents clearly marked on the outside.

A separate storage area should be provided for cleaning supplies, chemicals, paper goods, and other nonfood materials. Space needs, equipment requirements, and sanitary construction features are just as important for these goods as for food. For safety purposes, approved types of fire extinguishers should be located in or nearby all storage areas, and employees should be trained to use them.

Refrigerated Storage

To meet quality and sanitation demands, several kinds of refrigerated units should be placed for convenient use throughout the food service department. Standard refrigeration, which operates between 32 and 40°F. (0 and 4°C.) and low-temperature units with a range of 10 to 0°F. (-12 to -18°C.) are needed. Rapid refrigeration systems that can quickly chill, freeze, and thaw foods are needed if cook/chill or cook/freeze production systems are used. Standard refrigerated and low-temperature units are built for storage of food to prevent deterioration, not for quick chilling or freezing foods. All types of refrigerated and low-temperature systems are available in walk-in and self-contained units. Selection should be based on need, flexibility, and convenience.

Walk-in coolers and freezers

Important features to consider when assessing cooler and freezer demands include the refrigeration system used, construction materials and design, optional features, and the amount of usable space inside.

The basic components of any refrigeration unit are the evaporator, refrigerant, compressor, and condenser. In walk-ins, the condenser and motor are usually located in a remote area. They should be built to provide even temperature, balanced humidity, and good air circulation. Because of continuing changes in design and operating efficiency of refrigeration systems, professional help should be obtained before selecting a unit.

All floors, ceilings, walls, and doors should be constructed of durable, vaporproof, and easily cleanable materials. The type and amount of insulation used on all these parts are important. Foamed in-place or froth-type insulation is used by many cooler manufacturers, but the thickness may vary. All doors should be provided with a good seal to prevent condensation and loss of energy. Clear, heavy vinyl, overlapping door strips hung inside door openings also reduce energy consumption by keeping cold air in when the door is opened. Locking hardware on the outside is needed for security; an inside safety release prevents entrapment when the door is locked from the outside.

Ideally, floors of walk-in units should be level with adjacent flooring. However, models are available with built-in interior or exterior ramps. Nonskid strips on an incline are needed for added safety. Automatic audio and visual alarm systems outside the unit or in a remote location are essential. Built-in thermometers on the outside of the unit should also be checked at regularly scheduled intervals.

Optional features on some walk-ins include reach-in doors in addition to the regular door plus view-through windows. If the walk-in is located in the production area, the reach-in feature could be convenient for in-process holding or obtaining frequently used ingredients. View-through windows should not frost or fog. Units constructed with modular panels assembled on premise are recommended over permanently installed models to allow for future relocation and/or expansion.

Space requirements for standard and low-temperature walk-in units vary considerably among food service operations. Specific needs depend on the types of foods offered on the menu, the amount of preparation built in before purchase, and the volume of perishables and frozen goods purchased and delivered at specified times. Analysis of these factors and usable space provided by stationary or mobile shelving can be used as a guide. The cubic feet of storage space needed can be calculated using the following formula:

$$\frac{\text{Interior cubic feet}}{\text{of space required}} = \frac{\text{Total pounds of food stored}}{\substack{\text{15 pounds of food per} \\ \text{cubic foot of storage}}}$$

One cubic foot of refrigeration space will store approximately 30 pounds of food. However, because a considerable amount of space is taken up by aisles and unused space between shelves, 15 pounds per cubic foot is used in this formula.

Requirements for walk-in freezers are similar to those for coolers except a greater amount of insulation is needed. Freezer units installed with the door opening into a walk-in cooler can be very inconvenient and eliminate storage space on one wall.

Self-contained refrigerators and freezers

Standard and low-temperature self-contained refrigerator units provide convenient storage at point of use. Where space is at a premium or in small institutions, these should be considered in place of walk-ins. Many options are available, so construction features, size, and where and how the unit will be used should be considered before purchasing.

Self-contained units are built with the refrigeration system mounted at the top or bottom. Bottom-mounted models reduce the amount of convenient space. A properly sized compressor, condenser, and evaporator are needed for uniform temperature control regardless of the load. Foamed in-place or froth-type urethane insulation of 2-1/2 inches or more is recommended for walls, ceilings, and doors. A one-piece, durable, seamless lining in the interior cabinet is needed for easy cleaning. Exterior finishes vary among manufacturers; vinyl in a choice of colors, stainless steel, or other durable metals are used.

Refrigerators and storage freezers are designed as reach-in or pass-through and roll-in or roll-through units, which are convenient in areas between production and service. Solid or glass doors may be hinged on the right or left. One-piece molded door gaskets that provide a positive seal are recommended to conserve energy. Full- and half-door models with self-closing and safety stop features are available. A system for locking all doors is needed for security. An exterior dial thermometer and audiovisual temperature alarm should be installed in all units. Adjustable legs facilitate leveling of reach-in and pass-through cabinets; single units may be equipped with casters for mobility. Other design options include provisions for interchangeable interiors that accommodate adjustable, rustproof wire shelving; tray or pan slides; roll-out shelves and drawers; and flush-with-floor models for mobile carts and food service racks.

Quick-chill and freezing systems

Refrigeration systems capable of chilling precooked foods to 45°F. (7°C.) in less than 4 hours are available in one- or two-section roll-in units. Rapid chilling is accomplished with circulating fans installed within the cabinet. High-velocity air, forced horizontally over the surfaces of the food product, eliminates formation of layers of warm air that can slow heat transfer.

Self-contained or remote quick-chill models can be purchased. Cabinet finishes, insulation materials and thickness, door gaskets, hinges, locks, and other features are similar to those found in conventional storage refrigerators. One model automatically reverts to a 38°F. (3°C.) storage refrigerator at the end of the quick-chilling process. Standard equipment includes a chill timer and several temperature probes. An external probe selector switch temperature indicator and audiovisual alarms are optional.

Foods can be frozen by blast or cryogenic freezing systems. Self-contained roll-in models or large chambers with a conveyor belt are available. Product temperature is lowered to 0°F. (-18°C.) or lower by high-velocity circulating air and a mechanical refrigeration system in blast freezing. In a cryogenic freezer, liquid nitrogen or carbon dioxide in a liquid or gaseous state and convected air circulation quickly remove heat from the product. Design and construction features of the cabinet are similar to those of other refrigeration systems. Comparison of the capabilities of the mechanical parts used to lower temperatures and time required in various models should be made before selecting a freezer.

Tempering refrigerators

Food service departments that primarily use frozen foods should consider specialized equipment for tempering (thawing) foods rapidly. Conventional refrigeration systems require a great deal of time for this process. Individual units have been designed to thaw foods rapidly by using high-velocity airflow and a system of heating and refrigeration. Products are safe throughout the process because cabinet air cannot exceed 45°F. (7°C.) at any time. Upon completion of the tempering process, the cabinet can operate as a conventional refrigerator. Conventional refrigerator models also are available with accessories designed to convert them to tempering equipment through the use of special controls. This type may be more suitable to food service departments that use a limited amount of prepared frozen foods.

FOOD PRODUCTION CENTER

The food production center is the heart of any food service department. Modern facilities are designed to combine all pre-preparation and preparation activities in the same area to save labor time, reduce space needs, and eliminate possible duplication of some types of equipment. The location of the production area should be in close proximity to raw ingredient storage areas and on a direct route to assembly and service areas. Adequate space and equipment are needed for the production and holding of foods prior to distribution and service.

The area and shape of the floor space allocated to production will influence equipment arrangement and work flow patterns. The shortest possible route from one area to the next with a minimum of backtracking or cross traffic by personnel is preferred. In large rectangular kitchens, work and materials can flow in parallel lines by using an island arrangement of cooking equipment. In square or small kitchens, a U-shaped, L-shaped, or E-shaped arrangement may be better for efficient space utilization.

The main cooking equipment, such as ranges, ovens, braising pans, fryers, and so forth, is usually grouped together. Steam-jacketed kettles and compartment steamers are placed close by for convenience. Compact central arrangements of such equipment facilitates construction of effective exhaust hoods over all cooking surfaces and steam equipment. Aisles between equipment should be wide enough to park carts, turn them around, and permit employees to use them without blocking traffic.

Space for vegetable and salad preparation, baking, and preparation of food should be allocated within the main production area. Dividing the open space into operational areas by equipment arrangement rather than by partitions is an effective way to create a sense of spaciousness, improve air circulation, simplify cleaning, permit better supervision, and allow greater flexibility for equipment additions and use of mobile equipment.

PREPARATION EQUIPMENT

The types, styles, capacities, and construction features of needed equipment will vary, depending on food service policies and standards. The major pieces of production equipment commonly used in health care institutions are described below.

Ovens

Equipment that is essential for production of high-quality foods includes one, two, or more ovens using either similar or unlike principles of heat transfer. Oven cooking requires little attention from food service employees, can be energy efficient for large quantities of food, and, simply, is the only method usable to achieve the quality desired for some products. The most common method of cooking foods in ovens is by radiation or convection; microwave energy is used primarily for reheating individual portions of ready-prepared foods in institutions. Several types of ovens are available.

Convection ovens are versatile, efficient, and space-saving equipment with high-volume output. Convection ovens have replaced many of the more traditional ovens in many food service departments. Basically, this oven consists of a closed cooking chamber, gas or electric heat source, and a motor-driven fan, usually on the rear wall, to circulate heated air within the oven cavity. Because the rapidly moving air prevents the formation of an insulating layer of spent heat from developing above the food items being cooked, it speeds cooking time and allows for a heavier load than conventional ovens. In addition, the convection oven can operate at lower temperatures because the circulating heat is more efficiently used. Fuel use is lower than with other kinds of ovens for production of an equivalent volume of food.

Variations among brands include different systems of air circulation, heat supply, and control; chamber size; and temperature and moisture control. Some convection ovens have two-speed fans that permit changing the rate of air flow or that can be turned off completely, thus converting the oven to a conventional one. Others have a heat source control that regulates the rate at which air is reheated when the oven is partially or fully loaded. This feature affects the amount of fuel used. All ovens have thermostatic and timer controls.

Interior capacities are designed for volume production, with five or six shelves standard and more available. Two convection ovens can be conveniently stacked to reduce space requirements. Door style can be selected to suit available space. Single doors, with either right or left hinges, double French doors that are side hinged with one or two handles, or

Dutch doors can be obtained from various manufacturers. Solid metal doors or those with tempered glass to permit visual inspection of foods may be purchased.

The total capacity of the oven depends on the dimensions of the oven cavity, the number of racks, space between racks, and the heat input to the oven. Capacity will also depend on the depth of the pan being used. Ovens built to hold nine racks with 18-by-26-by-1-inch pans could only accommodate ten 12-by-20-by-2-1/2-inch pans, side by side on five shelves. Optional features of some large and compact models include provisions for roll-in mobile racks or baskets to minimize food handling.

Other criteria for selection include materials used for interior and exterior surfaces to facilitate cleaning; type and amount of insulation; ignition system for gas models; sturdiness of hinges and door handles; accessibility to components for inspection, adjustment, repair, or replacement; and temperature distribution throughout the oven cavity.

Deck ovens require more space than other ovens but can be stacked in double or triple units. However, convenient and safe working heights should be maintained. Therefore, the top and bottom units should be easily accessible without extensive reaching or stooping. Various oven widths and cavity heights are available to accommodate sheet pans, standard size pans, and roast pans. Individual thermostatic controls for each compartment are recommended. Heat balance within the oven will be improved if there are top and bottom heating units for each deck. Thermostats should be sensitive enough to provide quick recovery to the preset temperature. Interior and exterior finishes must be durable, well constructed, and easily cleaned. On gas ovens of all types, ignition systems that eliminate fuel waste through a constantly burning pilot light should be present.

Range ovens, located beneath surface cooking units, are not recommended for use in institutions because of wasted space within the oven cavity, poor accessibility for placing and removing products, and inconvenience in cleaning.

Rotary and **reel ovens** may be suitable for institutions producing large volumes of baked goods. Flat shelves are rotated horizontally in a rotary oven, whereas in reel ovens, shelves rotate on a vertical axis. The conventional system of radiant heat transfer is used. Door openings are located at a convenient height for product removal. Various sizes and capacities are available to fit the needs of users. Before selection of this type of equipment is made, careful analysis of energy requirements, space, projected utilization, and cost versus other types of ovens is necessary.

The deck, range, and rotary and reel ovens, whether gas or electric, are operated under the principle of heat first being passed directly through the oven chamber (radiated) to cook the food and then being vented to the outside. Some convection of heat does take place naturally to help in the cooking process. However, the heated air velocity is much less than in a convection oven.

Ranges

Traditionally, designers of food service facilities planned the layout of the food preparation center to include several utility ranges. With the choices of cooking equipment on the market today, a limited number of surface cooking units are used in renovated or new facilities. However, if space is needed for preparation of small batches of food for modified diets or ingredients used in some recipes, modular units, either gas or electric, should be considered. Modular ranges in 12- to 36-inch widths mounted on casters can be placed side by side or individually at the point where they are needed at the present time or moved easily when changes in the operation take place.

Electric utility ranges are available in two styles: solid tops that apply heat uniformly over the entire top, or round heating elements that are set into the tops with individual thermostatic controls. Combinations of solid tops or round units with griddles or broilers are also available. On a solid-top range, it should be possible to heat only a portion of the top at a time. High-speed heating capacity is important for all types of utility ranges. Tubular units should be removable for complete cleaning as well as the drip pan under the elements. Units may have roast ovens or pan storage beneath the cooking top. All units should be constructed of durable metals that can be easily cleaned.

Construction of gas ranges is similar to their electric counterparts; solid tops, open burners, or a combination of both are available. The solid top should be capable of heating the entire surface uniformly, whereas the open burner directs the flame to the bottom of utensils. When selecting gas ranges, construction materials, ignition systems, thermostatic controls, safety features, and ease of cleaning should be considered.

Tilting Braising Pan or Skillet

The tilting braising pan is one of the most versatile pieces of cooking equipment introduced in food service departments in recent years. Braising pans have replaced or reduced the need for ovens, range tops, grills, and other surface cooking equipment in many facilities because they are designed to grill, fry, sauté, stew, simmer, bake, boil, and even warm an endless variety of foods. The rectangular, shallow, flat-bottomed vessel is constructed with heavy-duty stainless steel with welded seam construction and may be heated by electricity or gas. Pans are designed with a contoured pouring lip and most models have a self-locking tilt mechanism to facilitate removal of cooked products and cleaning. Units range in capacity from 10 to 40 gallons. Small units may be table mounted; larger sizes can be wall mounted or freestanding on tubular legs with or without casters. Braising pans are energy efficient and reduce cooking time by as much as 25 percent on many combination food items. Human energy also can be conserved because a significant volume of pot and pan washing is eliminated.

Steam Equipment

Energy-conscious managers have found that steam equipment, properly used, results in significant fuel savings as compared with surface or oven cooking. Equipment operated by steam includes low-pressure, high-pressure, or no-pressure (convection) compartment steamers, and steam-jacketed kettles. Any one of the compartment steamers may be purchased as individual units, combination units, or with steam-jacketed kettles. Each classification is discussed separately.

Low-pressure compartment steamers

In most models, steam is injected into the compartment at approximately 5 to 7 pounds pressure per square inch (psi). This means that food is cooked at a temperature of 227 to 230° F. (108 to 110°C.). There is a wide range of models to choose from in relation to size, capacity, and special features such as controls, shelving, heat source, and so forth. One-, two-, or three-compartment steamers are available as self-contained units or directly connected to a remote steam source. Self-contained units generate their own steam through the use of a boiler powered by gas or electricity. Selection would be based on the sources of energy supply available in the institution. Self-contained units do have the advantage of greater mobility if rearrangement of the layout is desired at a future date. However, a self-generating unit should be limited to two compartments for ease of handling cooked products; the height of a three-compartment steamer is inconvenient and unsafe for most personnel.

Steamers are equipped with either metal grate shelves or multipan supports to hold standard full-size, half-size, or smaller pans in each compartment. Manual or automatic timers for each compartment are needed. An automatic timer cuts off the steam supply at the end of the preset cooking period and the steam and condensate are exhausted. If a manual timer is selected, the bell or buzzer should sound off loud and long enough to be easily heard in a busy kitchen. Doors should be equipped with one-piece, easily replaceable gaskets; self-engaging latches are necessary for ease of opening and closing doors. Steamer interiors should be of stainless steel and exterior finishes of baked enamel or other durable materials for sanitation purposes.

High-pressure steamers

This type of equipment is highly suitable for small-batch cooking of fresh or frozen foods. Energy is conserved because cooking time is reduced by forcing steam directly into foods at a high velocity. High-pressure steamers operate at 15 psi and at a 250°F. (121°C.) temperature. Size and capacities range from compact countertop or freestanding single units to multiunit combinations of large, medium, and/or small compartments for large-volume operations. Like low-pressure steamers, they may be purchased as self-generating units or may require a direct steam source. All models come equipped with automatic timers and shut-off valves and safety features that prevent personnel from opening the door before pressure is reduced to zero. Other features to consider before purchasing a high-pressure steamer include doors that can be opened easily, replaceable gaskets, removable or easily cleaned pan holders, and finishes that are durable and easily sanitized.

Convection steamer

A fairly recent advancement in technology to assist management in improving food quality and efficiency is the pressureless forced convection steamer. The principle of cooking fresh or frozen food items separately or at the same time in this piece of equipment is based on unpressurized steam being forced around the food, vented out, and then replaced continuously with freshly heated steam. A layer of cold air is not allowed to form above the food product, thus rapid and uniform cooking takes place. General design features are similar to those for compartment steamers; the steam supply may be generated in self-contained units by gas or electricity or come from a central steam source. Single- or two-compartment units, countertop or freestanding models are available. Some manufacturers offer units that can be switched from pressureless to low-pressure cooking units. Overall dimensions, capacity, pan racks, slides, timers, and construction materials are other features to consider before purchasing.

Steam-jacketed kettles

For years, kettles heated by steam enclosed between the inner and outer walls of the kettles have been used as laborsaving equipment to produce good-quality food using a minimum amount of time and energy. Steam-jacketed kettles are suitable to all types and sizes of food service operations because they can be used for browning, simmering, braising, boiling—just about any type of cooking method except frying and baking. Food placed in a steam-jacketed kettle is cooked by heat conducted through the walls of the kettle, rather than by direct contact with steam. Kettles are constructed with stainless steel double walls, through which steam flows, and may extend the full height (fully jacketed) or partial height (partially jacketed) of the kettle.

There are two types of steam-jacketed kettles: stationary kettles, from which food must be ladled or drawn off through a valve at the base of the kettle, and titling kettles, from which food can be poured. Tilting or trunnion kettles can be manually operated or may have a power tilting mechanism, especially useful for large capacity models. Capacities range from 2-1/2 gallons to 120 gallons; depths of kettles also vary. In the larger sizes such as 40 and 60 gallons, broader, shallow depths may be easier for employees to use and clean. The smaller sizes, such as 2-1/2 to 10 gallons, are very convenient for use in vegetable and bakery preparation units and in small operations. In general, the capacity that best suits the batch sizes needed in the operation should be selected.

Manufacturers offer many optional features, such as removable or counter-balanced lids, automatic stirrers and mixers for 20- to 80-gallon sizes, basket inserts for cooking several different products at the same time, and pan holders for ease of removing products for service. Steam-jacketed kettles may be purchased as self-contained or direct-connect steam models, individually or in combination with other steam equipment. Some kettles are built to allow cooling of foods after cooking and before removal. A cold-water line is connected to the kettle and when the steam is turned off, water circulates in the jacket. Food service operations using a cook/chill system may be wise to consider such a piece of equipment to reduce microbiological hazards.

Deep-Fat Fryers

Properly prepared deep-fat fried foods provide menu variety and can increase volume in nonpatient cafeterias and snack bars. Several kinds of gas-fired or electric fryers are available with a wide range of capacities and features. Freestanding counter models or built-in single or multiple units are available. Capacities range from 15 to 130 pounds; the type of fat—solid or liquid—that may be used in each varies by manufacturer.

Accurate thermostats and fast heat recovery features are essential for product quality and prevention of fat deterioration. Some models provide a cool zone at the bottom of the kettle where crumbs and other sediment can collect, thus prolonging the life of the fat. An easily accessible drain for removal and filtering of fat and cleaning the fryer is also important. Other features to consider are automatic timers, basket lifts, and, for safety purposes, the location of the on/off switch.

Other specialty types of fryers are available for more rapid cooking of foods. This is accomplished by frying under pressure. Pressure fryers are equipped with tightly sealed lids; moisture given off by the food or steam under pressure is retained during the cooking process to yield a tender yet crispy product in less time than in conventional fryers.

Mixers

The time and laborsaving attributes of mixers make them essential pieces of equipment for bakery, dessert, and some entree production. Mixers come in sizes ranging from 5- to 20-quart bowls in bench models to 140-quart bowls in floor model machines. Capacity selection should be based on volume needs, handling convenience, and product quality desired. Bowls are raised or lowered by hand lifts on small-capacity mixers or by power lifts on larger ones. Timed mixing controls with automatic shut-off are available. Some models are built with transmissions that allow speed changes while the mixer is in operation. Speed controls range from three to four or more changes in large models.

Standard equipment with most mixers includes one bowl, either heavily tinned or stainless steel, one flat beater, and one wire whip. Optional accessories may include bowl adapters to accommodate smaller bowl sizes, splash covers, bowl extenders, bowl dollies, and mixer agitators such as dough hooks, pastry knives, and other specialty whips and beaters. To make this equipment even more versatile, mixers are constructed with a hub on the front of the machine. Attachments such as a slicer, dicer, grinder, chopper, strainer, and shredder can be purchased to increase productivity and reduce human energy. When purchasing more than one mixer or another kitchen machine, the same hub size should be selected so that attachments can be used interchangeably.

Food Cutters

Various types of specialized food cutters or choppers can supplement mixer attachments or perform functions not otherwise possible. High-speed vertical cutter-mixers perform cutting, blending, whipping, mixing, and kneading functions. Capacities of these floor machines range from 25 to 130 quarts. The unit can be mounted on locking casters or be permanently installed. Various cutting and mixing blades are available. One model is equipped with an easily removable plastic bowl inserted into the outer metal bowl to facilitate removal of food. The metal bowl also tilts for easy emptying. Bowl covers can be of solid metal construction or transparent plastic. Counterbalanced bowl covers interlock with the motor for safety. Because of the extremely high speed of the knife blades, large amounts of food can be prepared in seconds by merely switching the start and stop controls. Vertical cutter-mixers should be located near a hot and cold water supply and convenient floor drain for cleaning.

Several other types and brands of food cutters are available to make production jobs more efficient. Careful study of the construction features and the functions that can be performed by each must be undertaken before making a selection. The basic mechanical operations of these machines are based on revolving knives and bowls or rotating plates with horizontal or bias feed entries, or a combination of both. Capacities range considerably, thus food processing requirements must be analyzed carefully. Food cutters may be obtained in table or pedestal models. Attachments for grating, dicing, slicing, or shredding are also available for some brands. Good safety features are built into every reputable manufacturer's models. However, this does not eliminate the need for continuous training and supervision of personnel safety.

Food Slicers

These power machines are designed to slice meats and other foods uniformly. Manual or automatic controlled models are available with gravity or pressure feeds. In gravity feed machines, the food carriage is slanted and the weight of the food pushes it against the blade. On pressure feed slicers, the operator must force the food against the blade. Most automatic machines have more than one carriage speed and can also be operated manually. A dial for adjusting cut thickness is standard on slicers. Optional features include chutes for foods like celery or carrots that are to be cut crossways or fences for the carriage that allow placement of two or three rows of similar items for simultaneous slicing.

Safety features and ease of operating and cleaning should be checked before a slicer is purchased. Safety features should ensure maximum protection against contact with the knife when the slicer is in use and when sharpening the blade. Any food slicer should be easy to disassemble and reassemble for cleaning.

Worktables

The type and size of worktables needed in the food production center are based on the specific tasks to be performed, number of employees using the space available, best work heights, and storage need of small equipment or food supplies. Well-planned and properly located tables can save labor time and reduce employee fatigue. A 12- to 14-gauge stainless steel work surface is preferred; lighter weights are not as durable. In centers where a great deal of chopping or slicing is done manually, cutting boards or table surfaces of hard rubber or durable plastic cause less damage to both knives and tabletops. Such surfaces can be easily cleaned and sanitized, and should be used instead of laminated hard maple tops that are more difficult to clean.

Tables equipped with locking heavy-duty casters provide greater flexibility for rearranging the work center and facilitate cleaning. In determining the length and width of tables, the employees' normal reach and need for space in which to arrange supplies and/or pans should be considered. Tables 6 feet long or less are recommended if they are to be on wheels. Standard 30-inch widths accommodate most preparation tasks. Tables with straight 90-degree turned-down edges can be placed together without gaps for food particles to collect and will fit tightly into corners. For wall arrangements, tables with a 2-inch turn-up on the back are available. Adjustable feet, undershelves, tray slides, roller-bearing self-closing drawers, sink bowls, and overhead shelves or pot racks can be selected as optional features. Undershelves and drawers may be constructed of galvanized metal, painted or anodized metal, or stainless steel. The high cost of specially designed and fabricated tables strongly suggests the advisability of thorough investigation of the many options possible in the purchase of standard manufacturer models.

Portable stainless steel or less-expensive but durable plastic or fiberglass bins are convenient for bulk storage in food production centers. Worktable designs should be planned so that bins can be rolled beneath the work surfaces where needed. Portable drawer units are also available and offer convenient storage for small utensils and tools as well as easy movement from one part of the work center to another.

Baking Equipment

A separate baking unit may not be necessary in a small institution or in large operations where most bread and pastry items are purchased ready to serve. However, if any on-premise production of baked goods takes place, some equipment is necessary. This would include a baker's table, portable bins, scales, mixers, and other appropriate small equipment, as well as cooling racks and equipment storage space. Any specialized bakery equipment that is needed will depend on the type and volume of goods produced. In operations where a great deal of baking is done, consideration should be given to the purchase of laborsaving devices such as a dough divider-rounder, electric dough rollers, and sheeters that are capable of handling many types of doughs and proofing equipment. Proofing cabinets are available in various sizes. Units may be manually or automatically controlled to maintain proper temperature, humidity, and air movement around the dough.

Mobile Equipment

Equipment on wheels can increase kitchen efficiency, save labor time and effort, and lend a great deal of flexibility to work center arrangements. Manufacturers offer a wide variety of mobile equipment with general or specialized functions. The exact quantity, type, and size of each piece must be selected with the specific needs, layout, and budget of the particular operation in mind. The following list suggests some of the types of mobile equipment that can be used to increase efficiency in an operation:

- Bowl stands for hand-mixing bowls that come with or without a pan rack below
- Heavy-duty utility carts with two or three shelves that are available in a wide range of sizes
- Open or enclosed pan and tray racks with angle or channel supports for 12-by-20-inch or 18-by-26-inch pans
- Food holding cabinets, insulated or uninsulated, with optional cooling plate insert or heater-humidity unit
- Equipment stands with optional attachment storage below or on accessory poles or racks

- Pot storage racks with slatted or solid metal shelves
- Tray and flatware carts, separate or in combination, with varying number of openings for silverware cylinders, in stainless steel or stainless with vinyl laminates
- Dollies for dish racks, cup racks, garbage cans, mixer bowls, case lots of food
- Dish carts, open or enclosed, unheated or heated, with or without self-leveling features
- Hand trucks or platform carts for moving heavy, bulky items to and from storage areas
- Tray carts for patient meals

The following construction features should be considered before selecting mobile equipment: durability of construction, load-carrying capacity, size relative to aisle width and space within the work centers, quality of wheels and casters, bumpers, and ease of cleaning. Construction materials may be aluminum or stainless steel depending on the type of mobile equipment needed.

Sinks

The exact number of compartment and hand sinks needed will depend on the extent and complexity of the kitchen layout and the requirements of local public health codes. Several recommended construction features include:

- Stainless steel sinks (14 gauge) with coved corners in each compartment and integral drainboards on each side
- Ten-inch splash back over drainboards and sinks
- Hot and cold faucets for each compartment unless a swing faucet serves more than one compartment
- Separate drain system for each compartment with an exterior activated lever drain control and a recessed basket strainer for the drain
- Compartment size variable but pot and pan sinks should be at least 11 to 14 inches deep and capable of accommodating 18-by-26-inch pans
- Approximate sink height of 34 to 36 inches to the top of the rolled rim for convenience of employees
- Rear or side overflow for each compartment
- Garbage disposal in one compartment of adjacent drainboard for sinks used in preparation or warewashing area (drainboard location is more desirable for pot and pan sinks to avoid loss of one compartment for waste disposal)
- Tubular legs with adjustable bullet feet
- Rack or undershelf, if space permits

The number and location of hand sinks will depend on the size and shape of the kitchen as well as the number of employees. They should be conveniently located near entrances to production and service areas and within work centers to help prevent employees from using sinks in the preparation and warewashing areas. The sink size should be small enough to discourage use for cleaning small food service equipment. Foot- or knee-operated controls are recommended and may be required by local codes.

WASTE-HANDLING EQUIPMENT

An efficient method of disposing waste materials is needed for economic and sanitary purposes in any food service operation. Equipment available to simplify cleanup tasks include mechanical waste disposers, pulper-extractor units, and trash compactors. The type or types selected depend on not only the volume of waste materials generated, but also the local codes and ordinances. For example, mechanical disposers that grind and flush solid waste through drain lines into the sewage system are prohibited in some communities. The number of disposer units needed and the placement of each one in the facility should be considered carefully before purchase. Food service operations that produce large quantities of foods in an extensive amount of space may need one placed in several of the functional work areas such as pre-preparation, salad, cooking, and warewashing; small facilities can get by with one located in warewashing and another in some other area.

Heavy-duty **mechanical disposers** range in size from one-half to 5 horsepower or more; the size selected should be based on the intended use. A 1-1/2- to 3-horsepower unit is recommended for the dishwashing center; smaller units may be acceptable in other areas where the load is smaller. However, horsepower is not the only factor to consider when purchasing a new unit. Because disposers can jam, one that has a reversible rotor turntable that can be operated by a manual switch is recommended to increase the life and efficiency of the grinding elements. Easy access to and replacement of the cutter blocks are also helpful.

Disposers can be table mounted with cones or installed in sinks or trough arrangements as in dishwashing areas. Sink installation is least desirable, particularly when sinks are at a minimum. Resilient mountings between the disposer and the cone are needed to prevent vibration and reduce noise. In all disposers, an adequate water supply is necessary to flush waste. Some models feature a dual directional water inlet for this purpose. Accessory components that may be desirable include a silver saver splash guard and overhead prerinse spray.

A **pulper-extractor** is designed to reduce the volume of solid waste and trim handling costs. Food scraps and disposable materials, excluding glass and metal, are pulped by rotating discs and shearing blades in a wet processing unit. The pulp slurry is picked up by a mechanical steel screw that extracts the water. Waste material is forced into a discharge chute and dropped into waste containers. The water used to wash waste is recycled through the pulping unit and an automatic water level control allows replacement of the small amount lost in the operation. This type of waste system may be used, in combination or instead of other disposers, where sewage and refuse disposer systems are inadequate.

Models are available as freestanding, separate units or can be installed under the counter. Capacities—rated as pounds per hour that can be handled—vary by manufacturer and should be studied before selection is made.

Another type of waste disposer used in some facilities is the **compactor**. Solid waste, including paper, glass, and metal containers, can be reduced in size by crushing under pressure with a mechanical compactor plate. Compression ratios vary from 4 to 1 to 20 to 1. However, the type and density of waste materials affect the actual amount of reduction. The volume of trash generated in a facility should be determined before capacity is selected because several sizes are available in either portable or stationary units. Whatever types of units are used, written instructions and trained employees are necessary for safe operation of all units.

VENTILATION EQUIPMENT

A good ventilation system is essential for maintaining a clean, comfortable, and safe environment. Any equipment that produces heat, odor, smoke, steam, or grease-laden vapor should be vented through an overhead hood with a blower (fan) to move air through exhaust ducts that lead to an area outside of the food service facility. Fire protection equipment is also essential.

Hoods come in canopy or back shelf styles. Canopy hoods are either wall mounted or centrally hung over a battery of equipment. The back shelf hood, or ventilator, is placed at the back of equipment and extends only part of the way over the surface rather than over the entire piece. Design and placement of each type are important for employee convenience and safety as well as operating efficiency.

The size of a canopy hood is based on the overall dimensions of the equipment to be covered and requirements of local codes. A minimum of 6-inches overhang is adequate. A practical rule of thumb is 2 inches for each foot of hood clearance. The clearance between the surface of the equipment and lower edge of the hood must be sufficient for employee safety yet provide an effective exhaust system. A minimum of 6 feet 3 inches and a maximum of 7 feet is recommended for the distance between the floor and lower edge of the hood.

The back shelf hood does not require an overhang. It extends the width of the equipment and is approximately 18 to 22 inches in depth from the back of each piece. Clearance above the work surface varies according to the type of equipment needing ventilation, hood design, and exhaust air volume. Because this type of hood is smaller in size and closer to the cooking equipment, fire hazards may be reduced and maintenance is easier.

Both hoods are built with a filtering or extracting system to prevent grease deposits and other suspended particles from accumulating and creating a fire and health hazard. In the filtering system, corrosion-resistant metal mesh screens or baffle filters are installed at angles of 45 degrees or more inside the fabricated hood. Hot vapors passing through these filters condense and the grease runs down into drip pans rather than being exhausted into the ducts and creating a fire hazard. Two types of filters available are low velocity and high velocity; selection is based on the expected volume of airflow per minute. The size and number of filters needed depend on the style and dimensions of the hood. Hoods built to accommodate standard-size filters are more economical. Filters should fit tightly together within the holding frame and be placed in a position for easy removal. Structural integrity of the filter should be considered. Those that can hold up under extreme temperatures and can be easily cleaned are recommended.

Grease removal by the extraction method is achieved by high-velocity air forced through specially designed baffles in the hood. A centrifugal force is created by the air making rapid turns within the unit. Water spray or cool air, controlled manually or automaticaly, helps saturate and solidify grease vapor. These units are usually self-cleaning and thus reduce labor time needed for maintenance.

The design and construction of exhaust fans and ducts have become extremely important for energy conservation. To maintain a balanced ventilation system, proper air movement is necessary. A continuous supply of make-up air must replace any that is expelled through the system for comfort, cleanliness, preservation of equipment, and for the building itself. However, if this make-up air is withdrawn too rapidly, drafts can occur and energy usage increases.

Technological advances in system design for reduction of energy consumption continue to be made. The basic premise behind these energy savers is to reduce the amount of air drawn from the kitchen. Separate air supply ducts and exhaust ducts are in the hood; untempered air flows down the ducts, draws off heat and fumes under the hood, and is expelled. Some air from the kitchen is used but it is much less than by conventional methods. Anyone responsible for planning the renovation of an existing facility or building a new one should seek professional help in selecting the most economical, efficient, and safe ventilating and heat recovery system.

SMALL EQUIPMENT

Adequate and appropriate equipment and utensils are required for follow-through on control in preparation and service. These are usually referred to as expendable equipment because they have a short life (although some last for years) and no depreciation account is kept for replacement. Some of this equipment includes measures, pans, cutlery, cutting boards, scales, thermometers, and portioning utensils.

Measures

Liquid and dry measuring equipment come in sizes ranging from one cup to one gallon. Liquid measures should have a pouring lip and dry measures should have a level top. Measures should be made of durable, well-constructed materials. Because lightweight metal dents and bends, it destroys accuracy in measuring. Both measures and measuring spoons are available in either stainless steel or heavy-duty aluminum. Although aluminum may be satisfactory, the extra cost of stainless steel may be balanced by the longer life of that metal. Glass measures should not be used in institutional food service departments for safety reasons.

Pans

Preparation equipment should be standardized as much as possible. Perhaps the most important application of that principle is to the selection of pans. Most standardized recipes are based on the standard pan that measures approximately 12 by 20 inches—the size that fits the openings in the hot food serving table or cart. Standard pans are used for many purposes such as cooking, holding, and storing foods under refrigeration. These pans are available in 2-1/2-, 4-, 6-, and 8-inch depths. The most shallow pan is used for many entree, vegetable, and dessert items. Shallow pans are also better for foods that may be held on the serving line for longer periods. Deep pans hold such large quantities of food that over-cooking of vegetables or some main dishes can occur during the serving period. Deep pans are better for stews, soups, chili, and so forth that can be scooped or ladled on plates in the serving line.

There are also smaller pans of several sizes that are based on the 12-by-20-inch serving table opening: half-sizes measuring 12 by 10 inches (two would fill an opening); one-third size measuring 12 by 6-2/3 inches (three to fill an opening); and other smaller sizes.

Considerations other than size that apply to pan selection are type and weight of the metal and design. Stainless steel and aluminum pans are available. For stainless steel pans, usually 18- to 22-gauge metal is used. Eighteen-gauge is the heaviest and is most desirable for oven cooking because it is less likely to warp. Stainless steel pans of this gauge are heavier to handle but much more durable.

Standard pans come with solid or perforated bottoms. Perforated pans should be used for cooking almost any frozen vegetable in a compartment steamer. For service, the perforated pan is placed inside a regular pan to prevent the cooked vegetable from becoming liquid soaked or overcooked. This prevents decreased quality and possible nutrient loss. If solid bottom pans are the only ones available in a kitchen, perforated inserts can be purchased to serve the same purpose.

Design is important for storing. Pans that taper slightly from top to bottom nest well and can be stacked without danger of wedging together. Covers come in several designs: flat, hinged, and domed. Usually only one cover is needed for each well in the hot serving table.

Besides the serving table pans, sheet pans (bun pans) are also needed. Sheet pans are 18 by 26 inches or 20 by 24 inches with a depth of 3/4 inch to approximately 2 inches. Shallow pans are ideal for baking cookies, buns, rolls, and biscuits as well as for refrigerated storage use; depths over an inch accommodate sheet cakes, meats, and poultry. Sheet pans are usually 16-gauge aluminum, which is strong enough for baking, for storing portion foods in the refrigerator, and also for serving as trays on carts.

If pots, kettles, saucepans, and stock pots are needed for food preparation, heavy-gauge metal pans are more durable and will help reduce the possibility of scorching and sticking. Saucepans and stock pots are available in various thicknesses of aluminum and stainless steel as well as other metals. Although the bright appearance and durability of stainless steel is desirable, it does not conduct heat as evenly as heavyweight aluminum when used in surface cooking. Also, handles should be sturdy. Large saucepans should have an additional bracket handle on the side opposite the long handle to make lifting easier and safer.

Pan sizes that are appropriate to the kind of cooking that will be done and that match burner sizes on ranges that have circular heating units should be selected. Four-quart saucepans are a useful size for many purposes. However, the small pan capacity selected should be based on portion sizes and total quantity needed of any product. Lids should also be purchased for pans that are used in surface cooking because they help to reduce cooking time of some products, which results in fuel conservation. There are many other kinds of pots and pans available, but if much of the cooking is done in the oven or in steam equipment, the ones discussed above are probably sufficient.

Cutlery

The quality of a knife is determined by the material of the blade and handle and their shape and construction. Most knife blades are made of steel and carbon. A high-carbon steel blade has the finest cutting edge *if* it is properly cared for and sharpened. When chrome is added to the alloy, the result is stainless steel; when vanadium is added, the blade is stronger and tends to hold its cutting edge longer.

Handles may be of wood, plastic, wood and plastic combinations, or even bone. Possibly more important than material in knife handles is the construction of the knife, that is, how the handle is attached to the blade.

High-quality knives have a continuous piece of metal extending from knife tip through the handle. This is called full-tang. In such knives, the handle is usually two pieces that are attached to the blade with heavy rivets. The blade must be well fastened into the handle or it will loosen with use.

Even though a food cutter or chopper may be available, several types of knives are needed for small jobs or jobs that cannot be done by more sophisticated equipment. Such knives usually include French cooks' knives that have a 10-inch blade for chopping, paring knives, utility or boning knives with slim 5- or 6-inch blades for trimming, and carving knives for slicing. Employees should be trained to use the correct knife for cutting, chopping, or slicing jobs.

Slicing machines are most efficient for slicing large quantities of cooked meats and poultry; electric carving knives, made for heavy-duty use, might be a possible second choice for a small operation. However, hand carving and slicing is the least efficient. Whatever knives are chosen, they will need sharpening at frequent intervals, either by hand or a convenient and inexpensive electric knife sharpener. Good knives need proper care and must be washed, dried, and stored properly in knife racks after each use.

Cutting Boards

Wherever knives are used, boards should be available for preserving tables and preventing dulling of knife blades. Boards must provide sanitary cutting surfaces that are thoroughly cleanable and that will not absorb juices from foods or provide places for food particles to lodge. Hard composition rubber or plastic cutting boards are superior to the wooden variety and are the only kind recommended. The small 10-by-12-inch boards are convenient for employees to use in cutting small amounts of food. In the cooking or salad preparation areas, where large quantities of food may be sliced or chopped, 18-by-24-inch boards are adequate. There are other sizes available, so individual needs must be assessed before selection.

Scales

Scales are needed for checking deliveries, weighing ingredients in food preparation, and controlling serving portions. Scales become even more important after considering the losses that can result from overportioning and the damage to product quality from inaccurate weighing of ingredients. Use of scales helps managers control costs.

Scales must be accurate, easy to use and read, durable, and easy to clean. Types used in food service facilities include floor scales, suspended platforms, overhead tracks (in large facilities), built-ins, and portion, counter, or table scales. Most scales are expensive but well worth the money.

Receiving area scales were discussed earlier in this chapter. Baker's scales, which weigh from 5 to 20 pounds, are most useful for operations that do a great deal of baking. For all-purpose use in preparation areas, a 25- to 50-pound capacity scale that will weigh in fractions of an ounce is ideal. For checking portion sizes, a scale that weighs up to 2 pounds and that has 1/4 ounce gradations will help control the accuracy and uniformity of serving sizes.

Thermometers

For the control of food quality, thermometers must be used. Oven thermometers, with a 200 to 600° F. (93 to 315° C.) range, check accuracy of oven thermostats. Meat thermometers that are inserted into large pieces of meat and poultry tell when the right degree of doneness has been achieved. A thermometer that has a tubular metal stem filled with a nontoxic liquid and that is equipped with a dial temperature indicator for easy reading should be selected.

Thermometers for refrigerators, freezers, and dry storage areas are also needed. Newer models of cold storage equipment include them built in, if specified. Periodic checks using a freestanding, shelf thermometer will validate accuracy.

There are also quick-reading pocket thermometers for checking temperatures from 0 to over 200° F. (18 to 93° C.). Quick-reading pocket thermometers are particularly useful for quality control and microbiological safety of food held on the serving line as well as during the cooling phase of foods that should be quickly chilled to 45° F. (7° C.) or lower. This is because the temperature of the food being checked will read out quickly on the dial. After each use, the thermometer should be sanitized to prevent cross-contamination. An inexpensive chlorine solution or some other sanitizing agent can be employed. Deep-fat thermometers are essential for frying equipment that is not thermostatically controlled. However, purchase of this type of equipment is not recommended.

Portioning Utensils

Kitchens need scoops, ladles, and spoons for quality and quantity control and labor efficiency. Scoops are particularly necessary for standardizing portions of foods such as cupcake and muffin batter, puddings and fruit cups, sandwich fillings, meatball mixtures, mashed potatoes, and some vegetables and salads. Scoops are numbered from 6 to 60; the number on the scoop refers to the number of scoops to equal one quart. Equivalent measures of scoops in cups, tablespoons, and teaspoons are available in most quantity food cookbooks and manufacturers' catalogs.

Portioning ladles, usually made of 18-gauge stainless steel, are available in sizes of 1, 2, 4, 6, 8 ounces and larger; most are engraved with the number of ounces on the ladle. Large ladles, holding 1 to 4 quarts, may be needed to transfer foods from the steam-jacketed kettle that does not have an adequate draw-off valve, or stock pot to serving pans.

Besides scoops and ladles, stainless steel spoons are necessary. They come with varied handle lengths and with solid, slotted, or perforated bowls. The perforated or slotted spoons are essential for serving drip-free vegetables onto a plate or compartment tray. Because these spoons are not identified by a number, the portion size of each food to be served should be measured or weighed. Employees should be instructed in the correct portion size before service.

Many other types of expendable equipment are needed to make the job of production and service easier on personnel. Detailed information on such equipment is available through catalogs and equipment suppliers. Careful consideration of needs and personal contact with manufacturer or supplier representatives are advisable to obtain the best quality merchandise for the money.

FOOD ASSEMBLY

The work space, equipment, and layout needed for the assembly of food for patients and residents requiring tray service depend on the type of service and delivery systems selected. Centralized tray assembly is used extensively in health care facilities because assembly lines can be designed to accommodate virtually all sizes of institutions. The more labor-intensive decentralized system may still be used when physical limitations within the food service department prevent the installation of a tray makeup line. (See chapter 3 for further discussion of service systems.)

All assembly areas require careful planning to achieve maximum efficiency and to ensure delivery of high-quality meals at a reasonable cost to consumers. In a centralized service system, the assembly area should be positioned in close proximity to kitchen production, storage, dishwashing facilities, and the tray cart storage. Easy access to food and materials and minimization of transportation time greatly affect quality and costs. Analysis of the basic functions to be performed and equipment necessary to simplify tasks will help determine space requirements. Factors to consider during the planning stage are:

- Number of patients or residents to be served at each meal
- Composition of the menu (number of food components offered and selected for general and modified diets)
- Type of tray service used
- Time limitations for tray assembly
- Amount and shape of space available or planned for tray makeup and support equipment

To ensure that each tray is properly prepared, the components of a centralized assembly line should include a conveyor or tray makeup table, hot and/or cold food serving carts or tables, and auxiliary equipment for holding and dispensing trays, dishes, utensils, covers, condiments, and so forth. In some cases, limited preparation equipment for hot beverages and toast are needed. Individual equipment needs will vary, of course, from one installation to another. Mobile units are recommended for easy rearrangement and cleaning purposes.

Tray makeup lines may be long or short, but ample space should be provided to accommodate peripheral equipment and service personnel. The key elements of the line are the conveyor (if one is used) and placement of the peripheral equipment. Traditionally, straight-line conveyors have been used because they are more economical. When space is critical or configuration of the available area is unusual, units with one or more turns or carousel conveyor systems can be purchased.

Conveyors may be automated or may operate by gravity feed. Small hospitals and extended care facilities may find the latter adequate. Automated conveyors are made with a continuous solid or slatted belt made of sturdy material that is resistant to animal fats, oils, and acids. An adjustable speed control and an automatic shut-off are necessary at the checker end to prevent tray pile-up. Gravity-feed conveyors are available with skate wheels or rollers in a variety of lengths.

Easy maintenance of conveyors is necessary. Heavy-duty noncorrosive removable scrap pans aid in cleaning. Some conveyors are equipped with a wash system contained within the unit.

Single or double stationary or movable overhead shelves can be added to some tray makeup lines to reduce floor space requirements of peripheral equipment. Side work shelves of various lengths also can be added. Individual tray carriers attached to a continuous-drive chain mechanism revolve around a rectangular table. The number of tray holders varies according to the tray size and length of the assembly system. Flat or sloped shelves placed above the revolving trays hold the food to be assembled within easy reach of personnel and reduce the needed floor space.

Planning for the right type and arrangement of support equipment is essential. It can make or break the operation regardless of how sophisticated the beltline may be. The key position on the line is the tray starter station. Equipment for holding trays, paper supplies, eating utensils, menus, condiments, and so forth should be within easy reach if a continuous supply of trays are to advance. A variety of starter units are available and may be made up of several component parts. Self-leveling tray dispensers and mobile carts or stand-type stations for holding cutlery and condiments are helpful. The configurations of these stations can be adapted to a variety of requirements. Correct height of these units is needed for visual control of the line.

Hot-food serving tables or carts with heated pan wells are needed to provide optimum performance. These may be placed at right angles or parallel to the conveyor. Electric receptacles on the conveyor should be conveniently placed and wired to accept the voltage, cycle, and phase of support equipment. Slimline units that are easy to reach over are better for the parallel arrangement. All wells should be sized to hold standard 12-by-20-by-2-inch or deeper pans and have the capability of holding inserts for smaller pans needed for the variety of modified diet foods. Mobile units with two, three, or more wells are available. Each well should have its own temperature control to keep each type of food at the proper serving temperature and to eliminate energy waste if all units are not needed at each meal. Wells should be of the dry-heat type for better control. The size and number of units purchased should be based on menu requirements, such as the meal at which the greatest number of hot food items will be held, easy reach for placement of food by personnel, and balanced work load by servers.

Backup equipment for holding foods hot also is needed in most facilities because batch cooking of all foods is not possible or practical. Some units are enclosed with heated compartments underneath. If space permits, hot-holding cabinets placed directly behind the service line are more convenient. All hot-holding equipment must be well insulated and have good temperature controls. Employees responsible for turning on units should know the preheat time and follow good practices to reduce energy waste. Too often, hot food wells are preheated far in advance and left uncovered, resulting in heat loss in the unit and higher temperatures in the kitchen environment.

Cold-holding equipment is just as necessary as hot-holding equipment. In fact, chill systems require only this type to keep foods microbiologically safe. Although the same principles of construction and arrangement previously mentioned apply to chill systems, the type and style may vary according to menu requirements. Some food service departments may use carts with refrigerated wells, chest coolers for beverages and frozen desserts, or portable tables for holding cold preplated salads and other foods placed on 18-by-26-inch trays. Reach-in or roll-in refrigerators located close to the serving line help keep cold foods cold and save employee energy.

Other support equipment for perfect food assembly includes units for holding cups, saucers, glasses, dishes, and covers if these are necessary for the delivery system. Open and enclosed carts or self-leveling enclosed dispensers are available in various sizes and capacities. Heated units are recommended for dinnerware used for hot foods; unheated carts are suitable for room temperature dish storage. Heated units equipped with a separate thermostatic control for each section are more energy efficient. If all dishes in a unit are not needed in a meal, they do not have to be heated. The control mechanism should be capable of warming dinnerware to 165° F. (74° C.) or higher according to the type of material used. Access to the thermostat and temperature controls should be convenient for regulating and repairing the equipment. Electrical cords on mobile dispensers should be retractable for safety. Polyurethane tires are best for equipment carrying heavy loads.

Self-leveling plate units should be equipped with springs that can be adjusted to suit the weight of the dinnerware. A manually actuated control located at the top of the units makes adjustment easier. Some models are difficult to adjust. Strong guideposts at the top help prevent dish breakage when dispensers are wheeled from the dishwashing to assembly area.

Unheated open carts are practical and less expensive for dishes used in the salad and dessert portioning area. Single or double carts, with or without plastic-coated dividers, accommodate various sizes and shapes of tableware. If open carts are used, plastic covers should be provided to keep dishes sanitary when not in use. Cups and glasses can be stored on mobile carts or dollies that hold the racks in which they were washed. Self-leveling units are more convenient for employees but also more expensive.

Hot beverage-making equipment and toasters may be located near the end of the assembly line or in the cafeteria, dining room, or floor galleys. The prime requisite for serving both is temperature control. To minimize heat loss, beverages should be served last in insulated servers or cups. Ideally, toast should be made at the point of service.

A wide variety of makes, models, and sizes of coffee makers are available. An important consideration for selection is the amount of coffee needed within a certain period. If all coffee is made in a central location, one or more urns with a capacity of several gallons may be needed. When a small quantity of fresh coffee is called for in continuous or intermittent service, half-gallon batch brewers are ideal. Other key factors in balancing equipment and demand are the personnel available to make coffee, physical dimensions in existing facilities, and capital allowed for initial investment.

Coffee urns come in three basic types: manual, semiautomatic, and fully automatic. The more sophisticated models help ensure quality control by eliminating human error and reducing personnel time. However, trained personnel can produce good coffee with less-expensive equipment. Precision controls that regulate brewing time as well as brewing and holding temperatures are important features.

In semiautomatic models, the water that is siphoned and sprayed through a nozzle over the coffee grounds and the replacement water for the urn jacket are automatically controlled. Timing of the brewing cycle and the drawing off and repouring of a portion of the brewed coffee for proper blending requires manual operation.

Fully automatic urns control the entire process: water spray, water refill, brew time, temperature, and agitation are accomplished through a simple push-button action.

Urn capacities range from 3 to 10 gallons in single or twin units with a hot water draw-off faucet for making tea. Faucets may be placed on one side or both sides of urns or even on the ends to accommodate any serving arrangements. Urns can be permanently installed either above or below the counter, or mobile units may be selected. The source of heat supply can be gas, electricity, or steam, depending on the make and model of the urn.

Batch brewers are capable of making superb coffee in a short time through automatic controls that accurately measure both time and temperature of the brewing cycles. Some models require both water and electrical connections; others are the simple pour-over type that require manual addition of water above the coffee grounds. These drip-coffee brewers come in single units that are capable of holding one decanter on the base, or with modular add-on warmer units beside, above, and/or as part of the base. Whatever type of coffee maker is chosen, high-quality construction is necessary for cleaning and maintenance.

The preferred serving temperature and texture of toast is difficult to achieve in food service departments where the time lapse between preparation and service is considerable. If toast must be made in the production or central assembly area, a rotary toaster, capable of producing a large quantity in a short time, is preferable. Gas and electric models are available for toasting both bread and buns. An automatic sensing and compensating device is helpful for maintaining desired color during consecutive cycles and voltage fluctuations. Employees must be made aware of preheat and production times to avoid serving cold, dry, or soggy toast.

A better method is to perform this operation at the point of service, using a heavy-duty conventional toaster. Two-slice, four-slice, or a combination of these units can provide more flexibility and certainly a better product with a little extra labor time. Models are available to accommodate bread and buns of varying thicknesses. All types of toasters should be constructed of materials that are durable, easy to clean, and have good controls.

The principles for equipment selection and maximum utilization of space in a centralized tray assembly area apply just as much to a decentralized system. Variations in the type and capacity of equipment will vary with the service system selected and the number of patients or residents served from a floor galley. Space for storage of food trucks, tray carts, dinnerware, trays, and all other equipment needed for limited preparation or service must be planned for efficient use of personnel and quality assurance.

Dining Areas

Patient and resident

Some hospitals and most extended care facilities allocate dining space for ambulatory patients and residents either within the patient care area or near the central kitchen. The service and dining room furnishings are affected by type of service, such as table or cafeteria; number of people served at each meal; menu variety; location of the dining room; health concerns, such as disabilities of clients; and functions, other than serving food, that take place in the area.

Regardless of the type of service system used, mobile hot and cold holding carts or tables are more versatile and flexible than stationary equipment. Adequate space is needed for holding trays, dishes, utensils, and beverage containers. Some on-site preparation equipment, toasters, beverage makers, egg cookers, and so forth may be desirable for quality control of food. If cafeteria service is used, height and width of the counter and tray slides are important for convenience and safety of the client. Nursing home residents confined to wheelchairs will need a low tray slide if a self-service system is used.

Attractive, colorful furnishings help patient and resident morale. Tables suitable for seating two, four, or more persons are suggested. Space between tables should allow easy movement of people and cleanup equipment. Height of tables should be comfortable yet be able to accommodate wheelchairs for nursing home residents. Chairs should be comfortable and sturdy but not too heavy for clients to move.

Personnel and guests

Cafeteria service is the most economical way of serving a large number of people with limited resources of personnel and time. Speed of service and presentation of high-quality food are two major concerns of consumers. Management must share this concern as well as be aware of costs related to service. Location of the service area, layout of the line, equipment, and employee work methods affect consumer satisfaction and efficiency and economy of the food service system.

Locating the cafeteria close to the central kitchen reduces transportation time and can help control food quality. Batch cooking of vegetables and some other foods is recommended for quality reasons but is difficult to do if the service area is far away from the cooking center. Close access to dishwashing facilities is recommended also.

Service lines can be of various sizes and configurations, depending on the number of people served, service time allotted per meal, complexity of the menu, and the dimensions of the available physical space. Conventional service lines are straight or L-shaped. Variations in new and large facilities include circular, scatter, or open square design. Flow of traffic is important in whatever configuration is chosen.

The length of the service counter depends on the menu pattern and the amount of food displayed. Adequate space should be provided for attractive display and preservation of food quality. Mobile hot- and cold-food holding units lend themselves to rearrangement when greater efficiency and speed are needed. Whether stationary or mobile, the hot-food holding section should contain an adequate number of wells for accommodating 12-by-20-inch standard pans to a depth of 6 inches.

Dry-heat wells provide better control. Individual, accurate temperature control dials for each unit help in energy conservation. The cold-food section should provide appropriate storage or dispensers for salads, desserts, bread, butter, condiments, and beverages. Mechanical refrigeration may or may not be needed in this section. For example, if the facility is small and few persons are served in a short time, a service refrigerator nearby could provide adequate sanitary conditions for holding foods at the proper temperature up to serving time. Hot- and cold-food sections should have a sneeze guard to meet the local sanitation code.

Additional space is needed on or near the line for trays, eating utensils, napkins, beverage containers, and so forth. These should be located for easy accessibility by the customer, but not where traffic flow will be interrupted or slowed down. The same principle applies to location of cash registers. A line can easily form if there are not enough cashiers. In the meantime, the customers' food gets cold.

Behind the service line, adequate space and equipment must be provided for dishes, food storage, and food set up. Mobile self-leveling dispenser units for dishes help reduce labor, handling, and breakage. Some should have the capability of being heated; others are merely dish storage units. Hot-food holding cabinets or drawers within easy reach of servers save time and help maintain quality of foods that must be held for short periods. Pass-through units from the kitchen are convenient. Likewise, pass-through, reach-in, or roll-in refrigerators are needed for cold foods. In some facilities, where fast-food items are served, grills or griddles are available for short-order cooking. These do require more labor, but the trade-off is food quality and customer satisfaction. If this type of service causes delay, a separate station may be set up, away from the general traffic flow, or work methods used by commercial fast-food operations can be instituted.

Overall space requirements must be carefully analyzed for easy movement of customers and employees working in the serving area. Space behind the line should be wide enough for transportation equipment and for efficient use by employees. Customer space must also be wide enough for bypassing the line, if this is allowed, and for easy access to the dining area. A periodic check of waiting times at various stations and customer counts per minute will indicate bottlenecks that can be eliminated by equipment rearrangement or menu changes.

Once customers are served, adequate space in a pleasant, attractive dining room should be available. Health care personnel usually have a very limited amount of time to relax at meal breaks. Therefore, waiting for a table or overcrowding is not conducive to good morale. The size of the dining area depends on the number of people expected to be seated during a given time and the rate of turnover. Generally, a minimum of 10 to 14 square feet per person is advised.

Also, the type of furnishings used or to be used should be considered. The usual table styles are those capable of accommodating two, four, or more persons. Attractive booth arrangements similar to those used in commercial establishments can add to the decor and good space utilization. Rather than one large room, dividers in the form of partial partitions, sliding or accordian doors, or large healthy plants or dwarf trees can give the feeling of seclusion and relaxation that people may prefer. Wall color and flooring materials are also important. Employees who use the facility can help with ideas as to whether bright, cheery colors or more subdued tones are preferable; professional decorators and talented food service employees are other good sources for ideas.

SERVICE SUPPLIES

Selection of appropriate service supplies (trays, dinnerware, tableware, hollowware, glassware, and disposables) is important for presentation of attractive meals. Initial investment and replacement costs because of use, breakage, or loss are vital factors to consider.

The kind and size of trays required for patient and resident service will depend on the delivery system used (see chapter 3). The type of tray used can be one of the following:

- A single, uninsulated tray that holds the entire meal
- A single, uninsulated tray that is divided into two compartments: one for cold and room-temperature foods and the other for hot foods
- A single, insulated or uninsulated tray divided into compartments
- Two individual uninsulated trays: a large one for cold and room-temperature foods and a smaller one for hot foods that are combined at the point of service

Regardless of the system used, preserving food quality is of prime importance. Trays should be constructed of durable materials that will not bend, dent, warp, or lose shape through continuous use. Hard rubber, plastic, and molded fiberglass trays in a variety of shapes and sizes are manufactured to withstand repeated warewashing. Attractive colors that are plain or have designs permanently molded under a protective surface layer eliminate the need and associated cost of placemats at all meals.

The type of dinnerware chosen may be permanent, single-service disposable, or a combination of these. Permanent ware should be durable, easy to clean, stain resistant, and attractive. Colors and designs should be compatible with trays and food items served. If conventional dinnerware is purchased, vitrified china is recommended. Three weights are available: thick, hotel, and medium. However, weight does not necessarily indicate strength; quality of materials and manufacturing methods determine durability.

Managers who prefer the appearance of china but also want to minimize breakage costs have found that dinnerware made of the components of glass and modified to resist breakage, crazing, chipping, and staining is very satisfactory. A variety of sizes and shapes, plain white or with a design, are available. Food service departments using microwave ovens for heating foods just prior to service find these very compatible.

Another type of dinnerware, which is light in weight and easy to handle, is made of melamine plastic. This type saves energy because initial costs are lower than that of conventional dinnerware and it is break resistant, even with rough handling. It also reduces the noise level in handling. Plastic dishes, however, lose their finish with use. This makes them susceptible to stains and scratches and difficult to sanitize.

The tableware (flatware and hollowware) chosen for institutional use should be designed for durability and attractiveness. Eating utensils made of stainless steel meet both of these criteria as well as the added advantage of cleanability. They are easy to care for because they do not tarnish like silverware. The size of flatware selected for tray service should be based on ease of handling and size of tray. A uniform size used for both patient and personnel service reduces sorting and washing time.

The types and sizes of beverage containers needed vary among food service departments. Good-quality plastic juice and water tumblers can be appropriate for part of or all meals in some facilities, whereas glass is preferred in others. Whichever is chosen, beverage containers should be durable, easy to clean, and suitable to the portion size served in them.

Single-service disposable dinnerware and tableware are used in part or exclusively by some food service departments. Acceptability by clientele and supply, labor, and storage costs should be analyzed before a decision is made as to the extent of use. Disposables are available in a variety of materials, colors, and designs. Attractive geometric, floral, or modern patterns can enhance tray or cafeteria service; plain white can detract from the appearance of the finest quality of food. Based on service needs, these items should be selected for strength and rigidity. Plates used for entrees should resist cut-through, sagging, and soaking of gravies or broth. Beverage containers should be suitable for holding cold foods cold and hot foods hot. Eating utensils must be sturdy enough to see a customer through the meal without breaking. Adequate storage space and sanitary conditions must be provided for disposable dinnerware as well as permanent dinnerware.

WAREWASHING

The costs inherent in the labor, equipment, and supplies required for sanitizing pots, pans, and serviceware make the warewashing facility one of the most important areas of the food service department. Centralized washing, located in close proximity to the tray assembly area, cafeteria, dining room, and production areas, eliminates duplication of equipment and personnel. More effective supervision and control of sanitation also are permitted.

Cooking Utensils

Some space should be provided for washing, or at least scraping and presoaking, pots, pans, and other preparation equipment even though a dishwasher is used for the final wash and sanitizing cycle. An area close to the main production equipment is most convenient. The basic equipment includes a three-compartment sink with drainboards on each side, a waste disposer, and portable carts and/or racks for soiled and clean ware. Adequate space arrangement will promote good work flow.

As discussed earlier in this chapter, all sink compartments must be large enough for washing, rinsing, and sanitizing utensils and equipment. However, some equipment is just too large to fit into any sink. In this case, provisions should be made for cleaning through pressure spray methods. All equipment washed manually must be allowed to air dry. Stainless steel wire racks with adjustable shelves are ideal. Mobile racks or carts are advisable for transporting clean ware to point of use if storage space is not available or if it is more convenient to store them elsewhere.

Large facilities serving many meals per day may find that a mechanical unit capable of washing and sanitizing production equipment is helpful. These are available as single-tank, stationary, or moving rack models. The necessity of purchasing such a machine should be carefully scrutinized because of space requirements and cost.

Serviceware

The dishroom layout should be planned to provide good work flow, minimize labor time, and ensure employee convenience and safety. Arrangement of equipment can take any form: straight line, L-shaped, oval, square, rectangular, or triangular. The shape depends on the equipment used, space available, and methods of soiled dish return and clean dish removal and storage. Before the type and arrangement of equipment are planned, a self-analysis of policies, practices, and food service needs should be made. Factors influencing selection of dishroom equipment and space arrangements are:

- Type of service—Is it tray, cafeteria, table, buffet, or a combination of these services? Each style requires different types and amounts of serviceware.
- Number of persons served—Are there fluctuations from meal to meal and day to day? Service demand will affect the type and amount of serviceware used and will in turn affect dishwasher capacity requirements.

- Type and number of menu items served—Are there variations among the types of service at one meal as well as from meal to meal? The style and quantity of dishes, trays, and so forth affect needed dishwasher capacity. Storage space for carts and dollies also will vary based on these requirements.
- Length of meal service and time—Is serviceware used more than once during each meal or is it stockpiled and washed later? Serviceware inventory, dishwasher capacity, and space requirements will vary based on these practices. Many facilities use a combination system whereby cafeteria dishes are washed continuously throughout the two major meals, but patient serviceware is processed at one time after each meal.

Adequate space is needed for scraping, sorting, and racking soiled dishes. Tables that are 2 to 2-1/2 feet wide, the same height as the dishwasher (34 inches is convenient), and long enough to hold the prewash and waste disposal unit should be provided. Some dishroom arrangements include slanted, overhead shelves for holding glass and cup racks while they are being loaded. Convenient placement of these can help to reduce employee fatigue and utilize space efficiently.

Table space for air drying clean dishes held in racks, carts, and dollies is needed. Table heights and widths should be the same as those mentioned above; length will vary according to the type of dishwasher used and washing load. Flight-type machines require less table space because dishes are removed from the conveyor and placed in storage units almost immediately. Specialized equipment also may be used, such as portable soak sinks, a glasswasher, and a pulper-extractor waste disposer. All these require space and should be carefully planned in the overall design.

All floors and walls should be constructed of materials that are easy to sanitize. Distance between walls and stationary equipment must be wide enough for easy cleaning and for mobile equipment. The floor is particularly important because it can be a safety hazard with water and other debris. Nonskid flooring or mats that are acceptable according to local codes will help alleviate the problem. Adequate floor drains should be strategically placed to avoid accidents.

Employee comfort and sanitation are essential. Hand-washing facilities should be conveniently placed to prevent contamination of clean tableware and safeguard employee health. One of the most important considerations in planning this area is the ventilation system. Dishwashing is not the most pleasant job but excessive heat and steam make it worse. Dishwashers with exhaust hoods attached at each end allow steam and hot air to escape through the ducts rather than in the dishroom area. Installation of an air conditioning system is advisable for renovated or new facilities.

Dishwashing Machines

Many makes and models of dishwashing machines are manufactured to meet volume, labor, and space demands. According to the Food and Drug Administration's Model Food Service Sanitation Ordinance, 1976, mechanical cleaning and sanitizing of utensils and equipment may be done by spray or immersion dishwashing machines. Institutional food service departments use spray machines; some commercial operations use the immersion machines. Most machines use hot water for sanitizing; models built to reduce energy consumption use chemical sanitizers. Spray dishwashers are classified as single-tank stationary rack or conveyor or multitank conveyor units.

The **single-tank stationary rack** machines have revolving wash arms above and below the wash racks to distribute water thoroughly over, under, and around each dish. Separate rinse sprayers above and revolving rinse arms below are available in some models. Others use the same nozzles for the wash and rinse cycle. These are called single-temperature washers; both wash water and rinse water are dumped after each cycle. Single-tank models that use approved chemicals in the rinse water, rather than 180°F. (82°C.) hot water, are called chemical sanitizing machines. Wash and rinse cycles for single-tank machines may be automatically or manually controlled. Standard equipment includes dial thermometers, for wash and rinse, that are conveniently located for monitoring by employees. Doors may be located on both sides for straight-through operation or on the front and one side for corner installations. Many other standard and optional features are available. Because the capacity of single-tank models is limited, they are suitable only to very small operations.

The **single-tank conveyor** machine is similar to the stationary one except that a drive mechanism carries the tray rack over the sprays and through the machine at a timed rate. Left-to-right or right-to-left operation can be specified. An integral prewash unit also can be built in.

Multitank conveyor units have two or more tanks for prewash, wash, and rinse. These models are built to accommodate dish racks, or a continuous conveyor with pegs or rods that holds dishes upright as they travel through the machine. Racks also may be used for cups, bowls, and tableware to reduce labor time. Each tank increases the length of the unit. Flight-type dishwashers are the longest because of the space needed at the loading end of the machine for soiled dishes and at the drying end for the clean ones. Larger units also include a final rinse as well as a power rinse; some models have drying mechanisms at the exit. As with single-tank machines, many additional features are included as standard or optional equipment. Most multitank conveyor dish machines are large enough to handle the majority of cooking utensils and other equipment. In fact, utilizing dish machines in this manner can reduce labor time and costs and ensure sanitary conditions.

To generate the required final rinse water temperature of 180°F. (82°C.) for both single-tank and multitank machines, a booster heater is usually necessary. The energy supply may be gas, water, or steam. Placing the booster heater as close to the machine as possible and insulating water lines help to eliminate line temperature loss. All machines have an attached data plate indicating required temperatures for wash and rinse plus water pressure at the manifold of the final rinse. Frequent checks of temperature and pressure gauges are necessary if dishwashers are to be kept in good operating condition. Minimum temperature requirements for clean wash water and pumped rinse water in spray machines, as stated in the Model Food Service Sanitation Ordinance, are discussed in chapter 4.

All dishwashing machines should be approved by the National Sanitation Foundation. Once they are installed and in operation, preventive maintenance is necessary to continue to meet federal, state, and local codes and regulations.

A great deal more information than is presented here is needed before making a decision about the type and size of dishwasher needed. Equipment experts can help food service managers with the technical aspects and preferred features of dishwashing machines. However, managers must be aware of the department's needs and space requirements in order to make the best selection.

Cart Washing

The trend toward the use of more mobile equipment has created the need for space and cleaning equipment for compliance with sanitation standards. An area close to the dishroom is usually convenient. Space allowance is needed for easy access to all sides of carts, food trucks, and so forth. Hot and cold water connections and a steam supply for sanitizing are needed. The area should be constructed with adequate drains and with walls and floors that will not be damaged by cleaning compounds or water. Employees assigned to this job require training and supervision to prevent damage to electrical equipment and especially for their own safety.

Housekeeping

Sanitation never stops. Trash collection and removal, floor sweeping, mopping, waxing, sealing, and numerous other housekeeping jobs keep the food service department in perfect condition. Adequate space for cleaning supplies and equipment, close to or within the immediate kitchen vicinity, makes the job easier. A sink for washing mops and a separate area for air drying should be provided. The same area can be used for cleaning trash containers, or a separate room may be better, particularly if cans are used for garbage. Mechanical can washers are available and advisable for ease of sanitizing.

EQUIPMENT SELECTION AND PURCHASE

Many kinds of equipment were discussed in this chapter in order to provide some basic information concerning the types of equipment and arrangements available that aid the food service manager in achieving the standards of high-quality food. Equipment represents a large monetary investment. Therefore, it should be studied carefully before a purchase is made. Well-chosen equipment, used and maintained properly, will provide many years of service.

Because of the many variables associated with food service departments, the person responsible for planning and selecting equipment should have a great deal of knowledge of the needs of the department and what will best fulfill these needs. Overequipping or selecting the wrong kind of equipment is poor management practice and contributes to unnecessary and excessive costs. The amount and type of equipment needed will depend on several factors, such as type and size of institution, menu pattern, style of service, financial resources, and plans for future expansion.

The menu influences choice of equipment in numerous ways. One of the basic questions that should be answered is why a specific piece is necessary. If it will save time, money, and improve quality and personnel performance, then further study to justify size, capacity, and space needs can proceed. Analysis of menu items listed in the cycle menu, number of servings needed, batch size, and production time requirements will aid in this decision.

Another important aspect is cost, not just the purchase cost but also those costs that will be incurred in installation, operation, maintenance, and repair.

Equipment requiring electricity or gas must be compatible with the institution's supply unless utilities are so outdated or inadequate that renovation is planned. For example, the institution's wiring and circuits must be able to supply the voltage required for operation of electrical equipment. A piece designed for a 230-volt circuit will lose about 20 percent efficiency if it is connected to a 208-volt circuit. A motor designed for 208 volts may burn out at higher voltages. Consequently, voltage, whether alternating or direct current, and phase—the source of alternating current in the circuit—available in the kitchen must be known before ordering equipment. Some equipment requires a single phase of alternating voltage; others require three phases, that is, three separate sources of alternating current that are arranged to handle larger power and heating loads. If gas equipment is preferred, an adequate gas supply must be available for peak operating periods and connections available in a convenient place.

The importance of design and construction to ensure proper performance without costly repairs cannot be overlooked. Equipment should be functional and durable as well as being attractive and compatible with other equipment in the facility. Careful study of information supplied by manufacturers in catalogs, bulletins, brochures, and specification sheets is necessary. Contact with other food service managers and equipment specialists is also helpful. If standard stock items do not meet the institution's needs, custom-built equipment can be considered, but it is generally more expensive.

Safety and sanitation features of equipment are extremely critical in selection. All equipment should be constructed and installed in a manner that complies with the requirements of the Occupational Safety and Health Act (OSHA) of 1970 and other federal, state, and local regulations and codes. Several national not-for-profit organizations have been in existence for a number of years: their main thrust is to establish standards and controls to ensure sanitation and safety of equipment and the operating environment. Among these are: the National Sanitation Foundation (NSF), Underwriter's Laboratory (UL), American Gas Association (AGA), National Board of Fire Underwriters (NBFU), and American Society of Mechanical Engineers (ASME). Equipment bearing the seal of approval of any one or more of these organizations is recommended.

SPECIFICATIONS

When the decision to purchase equipment has been made, all information related to the type, size, capacity desired, installation, and conditions of purchase must be communicated to the vendor. This should be in a written form to eliminate any possible misunderstanding of what should be delivered. Specifications can be brief or extensively written documents depending on organizational policies. The important point is to write them simply and concisely, giving only those details that are necessary to ensure delivery of the equipment desired.

Some procurement policies prohibit the use of trade names; this procedure is usually followed in organizations using a formal bid system. If this method is used, a great deal of care must be taken to ensure that equipment does meet food service requirements. If brand names can be stated, but the clause "or equal" must be included so that competition will not be eliminated in competitive bidding, other manufacturers with reputations for quality, dependability, and service should be listed. Another solution is to require bidders to submit complete, detailed specifications of what they propose to furnish and then compare these statements with the original specifications to be sure that they are really equal. The burden of proof should be placed on the seller. Too often items are purchased based on price alone. Equipment should be purchased for quality and performance.

As mentioned previously, specifications stating responsibilities for installation and testing of equipment in the operation are essential. Demonstration of the use and care of equipment is also very important. All work desired must be in the written contract. Follow-up in the performance of each piece and utilization by personnel is the responsibility of the manager. Full knowledge of what is stipulated in the warranty, particularly the time, replacement of parts, and service included, will save money in the future.

MAINTENANCE AND RECORDS

Each piece of major equipment needs preventive maintenance from the time it arrives in the facility. It is the responsibility of the manufacturer, food service manager, and operator to keep equipment operating at top efficiency. When new equipment is purchased, the manufacturer must provide an operator's manual. The information contained in this manual should include principles of operation, instructions for cleaning and care for daily maintenance, long-term preventive maintenance procedures and schedules, problems that may occur with a description of what to check to alleviate the problem, and a parts list with the location of service centers where replacements can be obtained. The second responsibility of the manufacturer is to see that a qualified representative explains and demonstrates proper operation and care to the manager, maintenance personnel, and employees when the equipment is installed. The buyer should specify these obligations in the purchase contract.

The responsibilities of management are more extensive. These include keeping equipment records, establishing preventive maintenance procedures and schedules, assigning and training personnel to perform activities according to directions, and supervising inspection and follow-up procedures. Steps in setting up a preventive maintenance program include:

1. Recording all pertinent information related to the equipment purchased on a permanent record card or sheet as shown in figure 43, next page. If this record is complete, accurate, and up to date, it will serve as an invaluable aid in ordering new parts, having repairs made, checking warranties, making the decision to replace equipment, and performing equipment inventories.
2. Reading the instruction manual and thoroughly understanding the operation and care of the equipment.
3. Writing out operating instructions for personnel who will be using the equipment. These should be simply written and easy to understand. Instructions for cleaning equipment and supplies to be used should also be included. After personnel are trained, these instructions should be posted near the equipment for easy reference.
4. Developing a maintenance and inspection schedule. Instructions should be explicit and complete and should include diagrams indicating the location of key points or parts. It should also indicate what, when, and how activities are to be performed.
5. Training personnel responsible for performing maintenance tasks. It is important that employees understand the instructions and time schedules.

```
┌──────────────────────────────────────────────────────────────┐
│  Item of equipment_____ │
│                                                                 │
│  Trade name_____Manufacturer_____  │
│                                                                 │
│  Model No._____Serial No._____Motor No._____  │
│                                                                 │
│  Capacity_____Attachments_____  │
│                                                                 │
│      Operation:  ☐ electric    ☐ gas    ☐ steam    ☐ hand      │
│                                                                 │
│  Purchased from _____☐ new  ☐ used  Cost $_____   │
│                                                                 │
│  Purchase date_____Guaranteed for_____Free serv. period___│
│  ─────────────────────────────────────────────────────────────│
│     Date            Description of repairs           Cost       │
│  ─────────────────────────────────────────────────────────────│
│   _____     _____    _____    │
│   _____     _____    _____    │
│                                                                 │
└──────────────────────────────────────────────────────────────┘
```

FIGURE 43. Equipment Record Card.

6. Developing a follow-up method of inspection. A master check-off sheet that lists the equipment, activities to be performed, and employees is helpful. However, other types of systems also work well. The key is to develop a system that works best for the institution involved.

7. Reviewing records periodically and taking action before a complete breakdown takes place. No food service equipment can function forever without service. If service is required too frequently for any piece of equipment, the records should be checked. Repair costs may far exceed replacement costs in the long run. Accurate records provide management with quantitative data that can be presented to administrators for requesting new equipment.

8. Filing all manuals and other information received from the manufacturer in a location convenient to the food service manager and maintenance department personnel. These should be part of the permanent equipment file for the life of the equipment. If the maintenance department is in charge of routine inspection and care, an up-to-date file may also be located in that department. Files should be reviewed periodically and old materials discarded.

Preventive maintenance is preventing trouble. Employees properly trained in the operation and care of equipment can be a valuable asset to management in this respect. Breakdown of equipment is not only damaging to product quality in some instances but also frustrating and possibly unsafe for personnel. After instruction, many employees can practice preventive maintenance on the equipment they use. All employees should learn to report suspected malfunctions, unusual noises, or other problems with equipment.

When repairs are needed, the maintenance department personnel in many health care facilities are trained for routine inspection, care, and repair of minor problems. Large institutions may have a staff member who is specially trained to perform these duties. Having skilled personnel within the organization certainly helps to reduce the time needed to repair the equipment. However, money and storage space may be tied up in inventory of spare parts and personnel. Alternative methods for equipment maintenance and repair are contract service agreements with the equipment manufacturer or vendor or informal agreements with a local repair service. The important fact is that factory-trained workmen and spare parts are available within a reasonable distance of the food service operation to eliminate lengthy delays in equipment repair. The cost, convenience, and delay time for each type of service should be evaluated before a maintenance decision is made.

ENERGY MANAGEMENT

Throughout this chapter and in many of the others, energy conservation has been mentioned because it is one of the most important concerns that the food service industry faces. Energy conservation does not just happen: it takes careful planning from purchase of new equipment through training and supervising employees in the use, care, and maintenance of the equipment. The example the manager sets about energy saving will be reflected in employees' actions. A careless or inefficient employee can waste a lot of costly energy.

The beginning of a conservation program is knowing how much energy is being used. Unfortunately, most food service departments are part of a larger system, located in one building or several, and metering devices are not available to each department. In fact, many food service managers never see a breakdown of gas, electricity, or water costs. Rather, a percentage of the total cost for all utilities is allocated to each department. Perhaps this will change in the future but in the meantime an estimate can be made, at least for major pieces of food service equipment, by completing an energy survey. To do this, a list of the types of equipment, rated input of energy, hours operated per day, and the fuel charge rates must be collected. Some of this information is easy to obtain: the most difficult or time-consuming may be the actual operational time for some pieces of equipment. Calculations obtained in this manner are only estimates but can serve as a basis for control.

The next step is to observe current practices and work methods of employees in each area of the department. Numerous guidelines are available in current literature and from equipment manufacturers that can be useful for developing a checklist for a particular facility. By using common sense and good management practices, employees can be trained to be aware of energy-wasting methods. Regular care and maintenance of equipment pay dividends in performance and length of service. All of them save energy and operating costs.

Bibliography

CHAPTER 1—
ORGANIZATION AND MANAGEMENT

Boyd, B. B. *Management-Minded Supervision.* 2nd ed. New York City: McGraw-Hill Publishing Co., 1976.

Haimann, T., and Hilgert, R. *Supervision: Concepts and Practices of Management.* Cincinnati: South-Western Publishing Co., 1972.

Hospital Administrative Services. *HAS Six-Month National Data Book for the Period Ending December 31, 1979.* Chicago: AHA, 1979. Catalog no. 1797.

————. *Monitrend.* Ongoing monthly comparative data reports for hospitals, extended care facilities, ambulatory-care facilities, rehabilitation hospitals, and psychiatric hospitals.

Joint Commission on Accreditation of Hospitals. *Accreditation Manual for Hospitals.* Chicago: JCAH, 1981.

Lateiner, A. *Modern Techniques of Supervision.* Stamford, CT: Lateiner Publishing Co., 1975.

Position paper on recommended salaries and employment practices for members of the American Dietetic Association. *J. Amer. Diet. Assn.* 74:468, 1979.

CHAPTER 2—PERSONNEL MANAGEMENT

American Hospital Association. *Developing Policies and Procedures for Long-Term Care Institutions.* Chicago: AHA, 1975. Catalog no. 3170.

American Society for Hospital Food Service Administrators. *OSHA Reference for Food Service Administrators.* Chicago: AHA, 1976. Catalog no. 1420.

Bobeng, B. J. Job enrichment in job design. *J. Amer. Diet. Assn.* 70:251, 1977.

Boles, K. Writing a policies and procedures manual for the dietary department. *Hospitals, J.A.H.A.* 42:86, Nov. 1, 1968.

Henderson, P. Labor staffing guidelines for long-term care facilities. *Hospitals, J.A.H.A.* 50:79, Jan. 16, 1976.

Hospital Research and Education Trust. *Training Program.* Chicago: HRET, 1967.

Being a Food Service Worker: Student Manual.

Training the Food Service Worker: Instructor's Guide.

Visual Aid Training Supplement to Training the Food Service Worker.

———. *On-the-Job Training: A Practical Guide for Food Service Supervisors.* Chicago: HRET, 1975.

Joint Commission on Accreditation of Hospitals. *Accreditation Manual for Hospitals.* Chicago: JCAH, 1981.

Welsh, J. N. Four-day workweek implemented. *Hospitals, J.A.H.A.* 49:89, April 16, 1975.

CHAPTER 3— FOOD PRODUCTION AND SERVICE SYSTEMS

American Hospital Association. *Shared Food Services in Health Care Institutions.* Chicago: AHA, 1976. Catalog no. 2636.

Bobeng, B. J., and David, B. D. HACCP models for quality control of entree production in foodservice systems. *J. Food Protection.* 40:632, 1977.

Foodservice Systems: Product Flow and Microbial Quality and Safety of Foods. Columbia: Univ. of Missouri, North Central Regional Research Publication no. 245(RB 1018), 1977.

Herz, M. L., and others. *Analysis of Alternative Patient Tray Delivery Concepts.* Natick, MA: U.S. Army Natick Research and Development Command, 1977.

Joint Commission on Accreditation of Hospitals. *Accreditation Manual for Hospitals.* Chicago: JCAH, 1981.

Koncel, J. A. Surveying the status of hospital vending operations. *Hospitals, J.A.H.A.* 50:90, Aug. 16, 1976.

Koogler, G. M., and Nicholanco, S. Analysis of a decision framework for prepared food systems. *Hospitals, J.A.H.A.* 51:95, Feb. 16, 1977.

Matthews, M. E. Cook/chill food production systems: current research on quality of food, Cassette-A-Month, no. 11. American Dietetic Association, 1979.

_____ . Quality of food in cook/chill foodservice systems: a review. *School Foodserv. Res. Rev.* 1:15, 1976.

Peddersen, R. B., and Doctor, B. Departmental review leads to changes in operational systems. *Hospitals, J.A.H.A.* 50:99, July 1, 1976.

Weisman, C. ASHFSA president predicts. *Food Manage.* 13:50, 1978.

CHAPTER 4—FOOD PROTECTION PRACTICES

Food and Drug Administration. *Food Service Sanitation Manual.* Washington, DC: U.S. Department of Health, Education, and Welfare, Pub. no. 78-2081, 1976.

Joint Commission on Accreditation of Hospitals. *Accreditation Manual for Hospitals.* Chicago: JCAH, 1981.

Longree, K. *Quality Food Sanitation.* 3rd ed. New York City: John Wiley & Sons, Inc., 1980.

National Institute for the Foodservice Industry. *Applied Foodservice Sanitation.* Chicago: NIFI 1978.

National Restaurant Association. *Sanitation Operations Manual.* Chicago: NRA, 1979.

National Sanitation Foundation. *Maintenance and Measurement of Product Temperature in Food Service.* Ann Arbor, MI: NSF, 1979.

_____ . *Thermometers in Food Service: A Pocket Guide.* Ann Arbor, MI: NSF, 1980.

Post, E. J., and Vincent, J. *Sanitation and Personal Hygiene Handbook.* Madison: Wisconsin Department of Public Instruction, bulletin no. 0401, 1980.

CHAPTER 5—FINANCIAL MANAGEMENT

American Society for Hospital Food Service Administrators. *Determination and Allocation of Food Service Costs.* Chicago: AHA, 1976. Catalog no. 1495.

—————. *Hospital Food Service Management Review.* Chicago: AHA, 1980. Catalog no. 1410.

—————. *Preparation of a Hospital Food Service Department Budget.* Chicago: AHA, 1978. Catalog no. 1615.

Drake, R. L. Determination and allocation of food service costs. *Hospitals, J.A.H.A.* 49:75, Sept. 16, 1975.

Kaud, F. Budgets that work. *Food Manage.* 15:38, Feb. 1980.

—————. Operating budgets are valuable in managing finances. *Hospitals, J.A.H.A.* 51:69, Nov. 16, 1977.

Keiser, J. and Kallio, E. *Controlling and Analyzing Costs in Food Service Operations.* New York City : John Wiley & Sons, Inc., 1974.

Ruby, J. B. Financial management planning in a small hospital. *Hospitals, J.A.H.A.* 51:77, Nov. 16, 1977.

CHAPTER 6— MANAGING A NUTRITION SYSTEM

American Dietetic Association. *A Guide for Professionals: The Effective Application of Exchange Lists for Meal Planning.* Chicago: ADA, 1977.

—————. *Guidelines for Consultant Dietitians.* Chicago: ADA, 1977.

—————. *Patient Care Audit: A Quality Assurance Procedure Manual for Dietitians.* Chicago: ADA, 1978.

—————. *Patient Nutritional Care in Long-Term Care Facilities.* Chicago: ADA, 1977.

American Hospital Association. *Recording Nutritional Information in Medical Records.* Chicago: AHA, 1976. Catalog no. T015.

Christakis, G., editor. Nutritional assessment in health programs. *Amer. J. Public Health.* 63:19, Nov. 1973.

Turner, D. *Handbook of Diet Therapy.* 5th ed. Chicago: University of Chicago Press, 1970.

Wisconsin Department of Health and Social Services. *Diet Manual for Small Hospitals and Nursing Homes.* Madison, WI: WDHSS, Public Health Nutrition Program, Bureau of Community Health and Prevention, 1979.

CHAPTER 7—MENU PLANNING

Axler, B. H. *Foodservice: A Managerial Approach.* Lexington, MA: D. C. Heath & Co. and the National Institute for Foodservice Industry, 1979.

Boyd, G. M., and others. *Standardized Quantity Recipe File.* 6th ed. Ames: Iowa State University Press, 1971.

Eckstein, E. F. *Menu Planning.* 2nd ed. Westport, CT: The AVI Publishing Co., Inc., 1978.

Kotschevar, L. H. *Foodservice for the Extended Care Facility.* Boston: Cahners Books, 1973.

_____. *Management by Menu.* Chicago: National Institute of the Foodservice Industry, 1975.

Matthews, M. E., and others. Master standard data quantity food production code. *J. Amer. Diet. Assn.* 72:612, 1978.

West, B. B., and others. *Food for Fifty.* 6th ed. New York City: John Wiley & Sons, Inc., 1979.

West, B. B., and others. *Food Service in Institutions.* 5th ed. New York City: John Wiley & Sons, Inc., 1977.

CHAPTER 8—FOOD PROCUREMENT

Darrah, L. B. *Food Marketing.* New York City: Ronald Press, 1971.

Economic Research Service. *The Bill for Marketing Farm-Food Products,* ERS-20. Washington, DC: U.S. Dept. of Agriculture, 1974.

_____. *The Food and Fiber System—How It Works,* AIB 383. Washington, DC: U.S. Dept. of Agriculture, 1975.

_____. *Marketing America's Food,* ERS-446. Washington, DC: U.S. Dept. of Agriculture, 1972.

Food and Farm Policy—A Fresh Look, NCR 38. Madison: University of Wisconsin-Extension, 1974.

Kohls, R. L. *Marketing of Agricultural Products.* London: The MacMillan Co., 1969.

The Michigan Food Distribution Industry Now and in 1985, Res. rept. 190. East Lansing: Michigan State University Agricultural Experiment Station and Cooperative Extension Service, 1973.

Protecting Perishable Foods during Transport by Motortruck, Agricultural Handbook 105. Washington, DC: U.S. Dept. of Agriculture, 1970.

U.S. Department of Agriculture. *Food for Us All: The Yearbook of Agriculture.* Washington, DC: U.S. Dept. of Agriculture, 1969.

_____. *Handbook of Agricultural Charts,* AH 561. Washington, DC: U.S. Dept. of Agriculture, 1979.

Your Food—A Food Policy Basebook, Pub. no. 5. Columbus, OH: National Public Policy Education Committee, Cooperative Extension Service, 1975.

CHAPTER 9—FOOD SELECTION

American Egg Board. *A Scientist Speaks about Egg Products.* Park Ridge, IL: AEB, 1981.

Esheach, C.E. *Foodservice Management.* 3rd ed. Boston: CBI Inc., 1979.

Food and Nutrition Service. *Food Purchasing Pointers for School Food Service,* PA-1160. Washington, DC: U.S. Dept. of Agriculture, 1977.

———. *Food Storage Guide for Schools and Institutions.* PA-403. Washington, DC: U.S. Dept. of Agriculture, 1975.

Food Purchasing Specifications for Foodservices. Madison: Wisconsin Dept. of Agriculture, Trade, and Consumer Protection, 1978.

Kotschevar, L. H. *Quantity Food Purchasing.* 2nd ed. New York City: John Wiley & Sons, Inc., 1975.

Meat Buyers Guide. Tucson, AZ: National Association of Meat Purveyors, 1976.

Meat in the Food Service Industry. Chicago: National Live Stock and Meat Board, 1975.

Mennes, M., and Vaninger, B. *Purchasing Fruits and Vegetables for Foodservices.* C2813. Madison: University of Wisconsin-Extension, 1977.

Pedderson, R. B. *SPECS: The Comprehensive Foodservice Purchasing and Specifications Manual.* Boston: CBI Publishing Co., Inc., 1977.

The Professional Chef: Foodservice Buying and Specifying Guide and Product Directory. Chicago: Cahners Books, 1979.

Warfel, M. C., and Waskey, F. H. *The Professional Food Buyer: Standards, Principles, and Procedures.* Berkeley,CA: McCutchan Publishing Corp., 1979.

CHAPTER 10— QUALITY ASSURANCE IN FOOD PRODUCTION

American Dietetic Association. *Standardizing Recipes for Institutional Use.* Chicago: ADA, 1967.

American Hospital Association. *Improving Work Methods in Small Hospitals.* Chicago: AHA, 1975. Catalog no. 1910.

Food and Nutrition Service. *Guide for Writing and Evaluating Quantity Recipes for Type A School Lunches.* Washington, DC: U.S. Dept. of Agriculture, 1969.

Longree, K. *Quantity Food Sanitation.* 3rd ed. New York City: John Wiley & Sons, Inc., 1980.

West, B. B., and others. *Food Service in Institutions.* 5th ed. New York City: John Wiley & Sons, Inc., 1977.

CHAPTER 11—
FOOD PRODUCTION PROCESSES

Dunn, Charlotte M. *Fish and Seafood—Dividend Foods.* Pub. Info. Report no. 118. Madison: University of Wisconsin Sea Grant College Program, 1974.

Fennema, O. Loss of vitamins in fresh and frozen foods. *Food Technol.* 31:32, Dec. 1977.

Institute of Food Technologists. *The Effects of Food Processing on Nutritional Values.* Scientific Status Summary. Oct. 1974.

Kotschevar, L. H. *Standards, Principles, and Techniques in Quantity Food Production.* 3rd ed. Boston: Cahners Books, 1974.

McWilliams, M. *Food Fundamentals.* 3rd ed. New York City: John Wiley & Sons, Inc., 1979.

Meat in the Foodservice Industry. Chicago: National Live Stock and Meat Board in association with the National Association of Meat Purveyors, 1975.

National Turkey Federation. *The Turkey Handbook.* Reston, VA: NTF, 1975.

Paul, P. C., and Palmer, H. H. *Food Theory and Applications.* New York City: John Wiley & Sons, Inc., 1972.

Peckham, G. C. *Foundations of Food Preparation.* 3rd ed. New York City: Macmillan Publishing Co., Inc., 1974.

Powers, J. M. *Basics of Quantity Food Production.* New York City: John Wiley & Sons, Inc., 1979.

Sanstadt, H. Let's do it with vegetables. *Cooking for Profit.* 11:14, 1978.

Terrell, M. E. *Professional Food Preparation.* 2nd ed. New York City: John Wiley & Sons, Inc., 1979.

United Fresh Fruit and Vegetable Association. *Conserving Nutrients in Fresh Fruits and Vegetables.* Washington, DC: UFFVA, 1977.

West, B. B., and others. *Food Service in Institutions.* 5th ed. New York City: John Wiley & Sons, Inc., 1977.

CHAPTER 12—
OPERATING DESIGN AND EQUIPMENT

Avery, A. *A Modern Guide to Foodservice Equipment.* Boston: CBI Publishing Co., 1980.

American Hospital Association. *Selection of a Consultant for Hospital Food Service Systems Design and Equipment.* Chicago: AHA, 1977. Catalog no. T011.

———. Workshop on *Planning for Design and Renovation of Health Care Food Service Departments,* conducted by AHA, Jan. 1980, Tampa, FL.

Food and Drug Administration. *Food Service Sanitation Manual,* Pub. no. 78-2081. Washington, DC: U.S. Dept. of Health, Education, and Welfare, 1976.

Food and Nutrition Service. *Equipment Guide for On-Site School Kitchens,* PA-1091. Washington, DC: U.S. Dept of Agriculture, 1974.

———. *Food and Storage Guide for Schools and Institutions,* revised, PA-403. Washington, DC: U.S. Dept. of Agriculture, 1975.

Jernigan. A. K., and Ross, L. N. *Food Service Equipment.* 2nd ed. Ames: Iowa State University Press, 1980.

Kazarian, E. A. *Work Analysis and Design for Hotels, Restaurants, and Institutions.* 2nd ed. Westport, CT: AVI Publishing Co., Inc., 1979.

———. *Food Service Facilities Planning.* Westport, CT: AVI Publishing Co., Inc., 1975.

Kotschevar, L. H. *Foodservice for the Extended Care Facility.* Boston: Cahners Books, 1973.

Kotschevar, L. H., and Terrell, M. E. *Food Service Planning: Layout and Equipment.* 2nd ed. New York City: John Wiley & Sons, Inc., 1977.

Myers, J. R. *Commerical Kitchens.* 6th ed. Arlington, VA: American Gas Association, 1979.

National Restaurant Association. *Sanitation Operations Manual.* Chicago: NRA, 1979.

Stevens, J., and Scriven, C. *Food Equipment Facts.* Valley Falls, NY: Scriven Duplicating Service, 1980.

West, B. B., and others. *Food Service in Institutions.* 5th ed. New York City: John Wiley & Sons, Inc., 1977.

Wilkinson, J. *Complete Book of Cooking Equipment.* Boston: Cahners Books, 1972.

INDEX

DATE DUE

GAYLORD			PRINTED IN U.S.A.